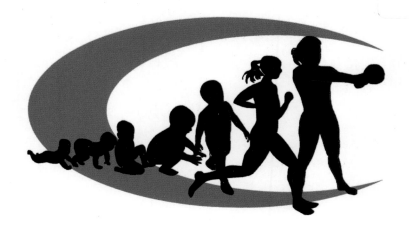

Movement Restoration

Improving Movement Always and in All Ways.

by:

Brandon Hetzler

Karen Rakowski

Jim Raynor

The content of this book has been taught very selectively within very select organizations over the past 4 years. The information within these pages serves as the cornerstone for the Masters of Athletic Training degree at Missouri State University as well as the foundation for the clinical rehabilitation philosophy for the Mercy Sports Medicine department. Even though, the content has not been shared publicly, it has been tried and tested in the most stringent environments for many years.

Published by Movement Restoration, LLC

5364 S. Woodfield Ave

Springfield MO 65804

Hetzler, Brandon. Rakowski, Karen. Raynor, Jim.

ISBN 978-0692274569

DISCLAIMER

The authors and publisher of this book are not responsible in any manner whatsoever for any injury that may occur through following the instructions contained in this material. The activities may be too strenuous or dangerous for some people. The readers should consult a physician before engaging in them. All healthcare professionals should know their State Practice Act and refer to that regarding what can and cannot be done.

At the end of each of the Neurodevelopmental sections there will be a blue box with links to YouTube videos showing what each section highlighted. You can attempt to type that into your browser, or you can go to our YouTube Channel, which is MovementRestoration.

Introduction

This Movement Restoration Project is the result of two things: multiple failures with our patients and being tasked with developing an ACL rehab protocol, which in hindsight was also a failure. While this text is itself a collection of many years worth of discussions, meetings, and random thoughts it has been the process of putting of putting what we do everyday onto paper that has lead to the most profound ideas we have had. Since we started this project 5 years ago, we have taken very rough ideas and polished them, refined them and blended them all into this approach. What we have attempted to do is bridge the gap between what some really smart people before us have done in the worlds of anatomy, human development, assessing movement, and training people.

Many people have tried to complicate things. What we have done is the opposite - we tried to refine and simplify everything back to the most basic components, and then spend time getting really good at that. From assessment, to corrective exercise, to strength - we have taken the road back towards simplicity. Through this process we have had many challenges, which we have attempted to face with integrity and reserve. Since we began on this journey we have seen several individuals come out with products very similar to ours - some even using "Movement Restoration" in the description of their products. While we have spent the past several years presenting our material at various conferences and workshops -all with our name (Movement Restoration Project) and logo in the presentation- as well as in the bio of several different articles I have written, we were still surprised by the mimicry. Often times, we were tempted to do exactly what they did - just throw out a series of exercises and claim how they heal everything from old age to gingivitis. However, we wanted something better with a higher quality. We wanted to highlight the "system", not the exercises.

The beauty of this text is that if you follow the principles, then you can include any exercise, tool, training modality, or piece of exercise equipment into our approach to make what you do better. We were asked "why should I come to your workshop, what exercises will I learn?" The answer, was you should come to our workshop not looking to learn any exercises. Our goal is to teach a philosophy where anyone can plug any piece of exercise equipment (kettlebells, barbells, bodyweight, free weights, suspension trainers, sandbags, etc) in and instantly improve their efficiency. The exercise examples we do list utilize kettlebells and bodyweight - these are our preference. But, like everything else we do, our inclusion of these are more based on the philosophy behind these tools and not the tools themselves. We have also spent the past 2 years teaching this material as part of the Masters of Athletic Training degree at Missouri State University as Graduate faculty members. Having to repeatedly answer questions like "I understand what you are teaching us, but why are you teaching it to us?" has forced us to look very hard at our material.

We have spent years and several thousands of dollars to find and explore information from many text books and workshops. The systems which we are tied the closest to also are the systems in which we have had the most discussion with about this product. Many hours have been spent in discussion with Pavel Tsatsouline and Mark Toomey at StrongFirst ™ Inc. regarding the strength philosophy we have included. Gray Cook, Lee Burton and Brett Jones have spend significant amounts of time as part of Functional Movement Systems listening to our presentations and have had several discussions regarding how we utilize the FMS tool and have blended their tool into our philosophy of corrective movements. As you read the text, there are parts that will refer to other organizations from which we have drawn ideas from or have found follow very similar philosophies that are based on the same principles we follow. We hope you can see the similarities between these organizations as well as how in the end we are all working towards the same outcome - *Better Movement*. Allow yourself to "Be Moved".

PART 1
The Neurodevelopmental Sequence (NDS)

The Neurodevelopmental Sequence (NSD) is the sequential, predictable manner in which movement develops across every continent and race of people on the planet. This is how everyone develops movement skills. Simultaneously, as movement develops the brain is developing. Both movement and brain development rely on each other - as movement develops and increases the amount and type of sensory experiences that the infant is experiencing the brains need for further stimulation is driving the development of new movements. Children do not crawl because mom and dad teach them to crawl, they crawl because they want to get to some item that has gotten their attention. Movement is driven by the need to expand our world and continuously increase stimulus. This increase in stimulus can be through vision, touch, smell, taste, and hearing. Each of the five senses play a vital role in the development of the brain and in the development of movement. From the infant that exhibits a startle reaction when they hear a loud noise, to the child who manages to grab their toes so they can put them in their mouth, to the toddler who likes putting objects in his ear and then rolls on the ground because of the sound it makes. Movement is a sensory experience. The growth of the brain neural tissue and neural networks are sculpted to match the efficient movement solution's that the infant comes up with every time they accomplish a task. The beauty of this is that once a skill is learned, that skill is never forgotten - although the execution of the skill may be impaired due to nervous system or muscular system defects (Cech). Everyone has heard the saying "it's just like riding a bike". This simple saying has a very deep meaning that is rooted in how our brain retains movement skills. This fact is also a key to restoring movement that has been lost due to injury or habitual postures.

During the first 2 years of life there is an astounding amount of development that takes place within the body, both from a developmental standpoint and from a neurological standpoint- but one is dependent upon the other. By the age of two, 80% of the brain is intact (Melillo). By comparison, between the ages of 2 and 6 years old, that number only rises to 90%. Movement and the brain both grow and develop together in conjunction with the other, and dependent upon the other. Researchers have found that children who do not play much, who are rarely touched, and are unable to interact with their environment develop brains that are 20-30% smaller than normal and ultimately have delays in other cognitive functions (Melillo)(Blakeslee). What has also been observed is that when neurons are excited together, they become linked functionally. This leads to the saying "neurons that fire together, wire together." (Melillo)(Doidge). It has been known that during these first 2 years of life, the brain is very open to change and remodeling - a term called plasticity. By age 6, there will be upwards of 1,000 trillion neural synapses which is much more processing power than any computer on the planet. What is being observed recently, is that this plasticity is present for the duration of the life span (Doidge)(Melillo)(Doidge). The brain has the ability to change both physically and chemically when given the proper stimulation. These forms of stimulation are: smell, sound, vibration, light, taste, temperature, touch, pressure, and gravity. In addition to this, repeated muscle activity is the single most important element of brain development (Melillo). All of these are the stimulus that infants seek during those formidable first years, and are the same stimuli that can be manipulated in adults to increase the rate at which neurological changes (movement changes) can take place.

The NDS is a universal and predictable pattern of motor development that occurs from before birth until around the age of 2. At birth, two reflexes are present that significantly affect movement for the duration of life - breathing and gripping. The human infant is one of the only species on the planet that is born unable to do anything purposeful. Infants are 100% dependent upon their care givers for food, transportation, shelter, and everything else needed for survival. An infant enters the world with just enough brainpower to keep their heart beating, the lungs breathing, the bowels moving, and other essential systems functioning. The brain is the only organ that is not fully developed at birth The portion of the brain that is fully functioning, is the lower brain - the region of the brain stem (the "lizard brain'). The entire goal of the infant is based around survival.

Every infant greets the world with the best sound a parent can hear - a scream. This "scream" is actually the second accomplishment that the infant achieves within the first few seconds of life, the first is a giant inhale. After the amniotic fluid is cleared from the mouth, nose, trachea and lungs the first breath of life is taken. Up until this point, the lungs are filled with fluid. That first breath is truly the breath of life. The beauty of this is that all of the muscles of inspiration that are taught in every anatomy class across the planet are unable to function. Except one. The diaphragm.

This diaphragmatic breathing is the only option. At this stage in life, no other muscle can assist the diaphragm. One major reason is that at this point of life, there is no purposeful movement, which means these other accessory muscles of inspiration have not developed the strength, the timing, the activation pattern, or the endurance to assist with breathing. The only reason the diaphragm functions is via a survival reflex. This is seen as "belly breathing" - every baby that breaths, does so by expanding the belly. This diaphragmatic breathing is crucial for deep spinal stabilization later in the NDS.

In infancy, every movement seen in an infant is driven by a survival reflex - touch a babies cheek and they turn their head as they seek nutrition (Rooting reflex), a sudden change in an infants head position will elicit system wide extension and abduction followed by system wide flexion and adduction and they exhibit a flexion response (Moro Reflex), pressure on the palm of the hand results in strong flexion of the fingers (Palmar Grasp Reflex), and a noxious stimulus to the bottom of the foot results in flexion of the entire lower extremity (Flexor Withdrawal Reflex) (Bertoti). All of these examples are reflexes that are present in utero and are seen until up to the 6 month point. All are associated with some aspect of survival. The father that puts his finger in the hand of his son, is not really getting a conscious response from his son when he feels the squeeze to his finger, but is experiencing a reflexive response. However, this reflexive gripping is very important for beginning to develop shoulder stability via irradiation of the gripping forces all the way up to the rotator cuff. These early survival reflexes, gradually begin to be integrated into purposeful movement as the infant gets older and begins to have the capacity to respond to their environment. Every movement that infants make gives them a stimulus input and a perception about their environment. They then use this gained information to learn how to and to make other movements/actions possible. "Movement is the vehicle that drives spatial and temporal correlation and thus learning and skill performance."(Cech).

It has also been shown that movement and cognitive function are closely tied together. If children are not allowed to move their brains to not develop appropriately (Melillo). This largely is related that if movement is limited -or restricted early in life- the quantity of stimulus to the brain is limited. The homunculus is a representation of how the brain is divided in both sensory and motor components. Certain areas of the body are afforded more or less space of neural real estate based on the level of sensory input that each body provides to the brain. The areas of the body with the largest sensory representation in the Homunculus are, in order:

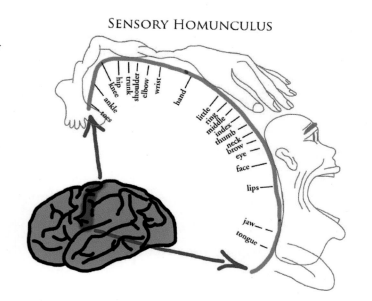

SENSORY HOMUNCULUS

1. Lips/tongue
2. Hands
   - thumb
   - index finger
3. Feet

From a motor standpoint, the areas in order are:

1. Lips, tongue
2. Hands
   - Thumb
   - Index finger

Children learn to explore their environment by interacting with it. As they gain control of their hands, the first thing they do is put things in their mouths. Everything goes to their mouth - their hands, their feet, their toys, books, cloths, rocks, and anything else they find. They do this to get more information about it - it is in closer proximity to their eyes so they get more visual input, they get taste, texture, consistency, and smell of the object. All of this -along with their caregivers response- is filed into their cortical real estate as characteristics of the item they are investigating. If this does not happen, they do not learn about their environment. It has also been shown that intelligence is contingent upon the proper development of the brain's frontal lobe which depends on movement (Melillo). If the frontal lobe is not stimulated by movement during the most critical time period of brain development (the first 5 years of life) then problems can be seen that have far reaching effects. Neural strategies for balance, body sense, and movement can fail to develop normally when babies are not allowed to move freely (Blakeslee).

The sequence of movement that is observed is directed by how each infant is interacting with and responding to their environment and gravity. Every movement involves a shifting of weight from one area to another. These weight shifts stimulate touch receptors, proprioceptors (and via these proprioceptors stimulates the vestibulocochlear system), vision, and our sense of equilibrium (the labyrinths within the ear). Throughout the NDS, these areas are continually stimulated in different postures and patterns. For clarity, postures are the developmental posture that will be discussed in the next few paragraphs. Patterns are repeatable movements that happen in each of the different postures and can be single joint or multi-joint in nature. For example many movement patterns can be seen in the supine posture - arm flexion, lower body extension, segmental rolling, etc.

The sequence of these developmental postures are:
1. supine
2. prone
3. quadruped
4. sitting
5. kneeling
6. vertical stance

FUNDAMENTAL LEVEL   TRANSITIONAL LEVEL   FUNCTIONAL LEVEL

BREATHING, GRIP, MOBILITY   SUPINE   PRONE   QUADRUPED   SITTING   KNEELING   VERTICAL STANCE

THE POSTURES

COPYRIGHT MOVEMENT RESTORATION PROJECT 2012

These postures are connected through different movements that gradually increase the scale and ease of locomotion:

1. Breathing Reaching of the limbs
2. Head movements
3. Rolling - connects Supine and Prone
4. Crawling - Connects quadruped to sitting
5. Pushing Down - connects quadruped/sitting to vertical stance
6. Cruising - connects vertical stance to gait
7. Unsupported Bipedal Gait (Walking) - the beginning of the locomotion patterns seen in a vertical stance.

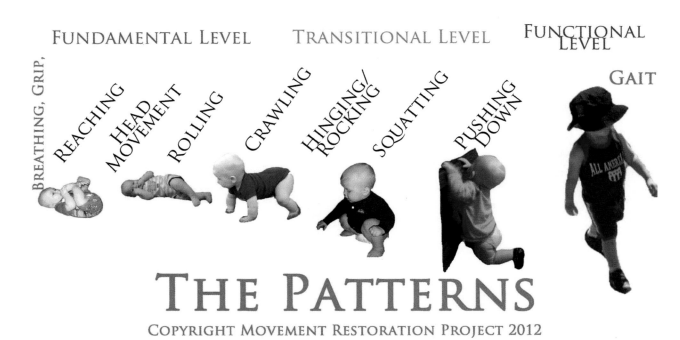

FUNDAMENTAL LEVEL   TRANSITIONAL LEVEL   FUNCTIONAL LEVEL

BREATHING, GRIP,   REACHING   HEAD MOVEMENT   ROLLING   CRAWLING   HINGING/ROCKING   SQUATTING   PUSHING DOWN   GAIT

THE PATTERNS
COPYRIGHT MOVEMENT RESTORATION PROJECT 2012

When the entire NDS is put together what we get is this very predictable sequence of movement development that serves as a roadmap for restoring movement for the duration of a lifespan. The 'postures' rely on and help establish specific mobility and stability; the 'patterns' layer in the motor control to each postural level. The entire NDS is:

1. Breathing/Grip
2. Reaching of the limbs
3. Head Movement (visual development)
4. Supine
5. Prone
6. Segmental Rolling
7. Quadruped
8. Crawling/Creeping
9. Transitional Postures
   A. Sitting
   B. Kneeling
   C. Squatting
10. Vertical Stance
11. Cruising
12. Unsupported Bipedal Gait

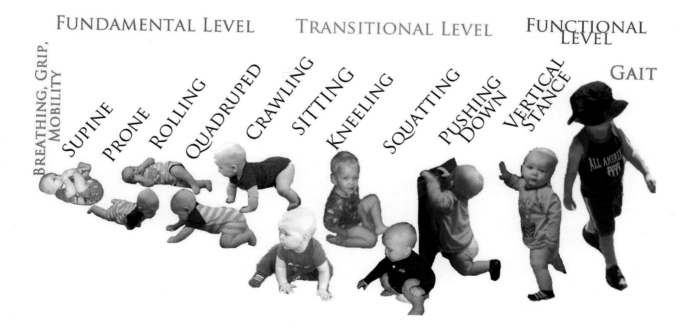

This sequence is a sequence. Meaning that until one skill is developed the higher level skills will not be developed. In certain instances, steps in the sequence are missed. Movement continues to develop but what happens is that the specific developmental needs that are missed at the skipped level are not developed. Often times, these defects are not noticed until later in life when problems occur (developmental, motor, educational, etc).

For example, the stability that is developed during segmental rolling is dependent upon the mobility and stability that is gained during the supine and prone postures. This segmental stability is then a building block as the infant attempts to progress up to the quadruped posture.

The Implication of the NDS

What does this have to do with anything after the age of 2? Traditionally, when a movement skill is lost due to injury, detraining, stroke, or any other reason, the manner in which physical rehabilitation/physical therapy (the verb, not the profession of Physical Therapy) has been done to treat these losses have been based on an isolation approach or more recently a regional approach. Both approaches have seen limited success. The fact that the number 1 predictor of injury is previous injury and the number 2 predictor of injury is asymmetry highlights the defects of these two approaches.

Both the isolation approach and the regional approach each neglect one major contributor to movement - the brain. All movement is an output from the brain in response to some stimulus within the environment. If how the brain processes these stimulants is ignored, the resultant movement will be less than optimal. Other body systems, such as the skeletal, muscular, cardiovascular, and pulmonary systems, develop and interact with the nervous system so that the most efficient movement pattern is chosen for the movement task (Cech). There are no motor programs, and the brain should not be thought of as a computer or as hard-wired (Cech). All movement is based off of the situation at hand and the ability of the brain to process all of the important stimulus at the moment the movement needs to occur. Because of this, the idea that neural plasticity may be a constant feature across a life span opens the doors to new concepts in how restoring movement can be achieved.

Movement is not a pre-programed, scripted activity. Movement occurs in real time - meaning, as the movement is occurring all of the stimulus that is reaching the brain has the potential to alter the movement in light of the task that is taking place and in the environment in which the movement is occurring in (Cech). Because of this every time a movement takes place, there is potential for change. Every movement is either making poor movement patterns worse, or creating new and more efficient motor patterns - movement is either continually getting better or getting worse. As Gray Cook has been known to say: "Poor movement can exist anywhere in the body, but poor movement patterns can only exist in the brain."

The Movement Restoration (MR) approach of incorporating the NDS into clinical applications for addressing movement problems is based off of the above information. Addressing movement as a behavior, acknowledging that more than the musculoskeletal system is involved, and realizing that every repetition of every movement is either taking the patient towards better movement or worse movement are three basic concepts that serve as the tenants for this approach. The rules of the MR approach are:

1. If movement is accidental, pain is inconsequential. (Pain changes everything.)
2. Movement is a behavior.
3. Movement starts and ends with the brain.
4. Every repetition matters - each rep is either re-enforcing a bad pattern or strengthening a good pattern.
5. Movement output occurs in response to a rich sensory environment.
6. Isolation does not exist anywhere in the body - the brain has a tendency to favor patterns.
7. Shoes restrict sensory input, and therefore interferes with the re-acquisition of movement.
8. If improved movement does not "Stick", it has not really been improved.

If Movement is Accidental, Pain is Inconsequential.

Gray Cook has long promoted that pain changes everything. From a neurological standpoint, when pain is present the brain will do whatever is necessary to avoid pain. At the same time, rarely do people walk in the door saying "My Movement is Dysfunctional, fix me". What we get is "I hurt" or "*blank* hurts". Many times, pain is viewed as the priority - fix the pain and everything will get better. After more than a decade of this approach, it is clear that covering up or fixing pain

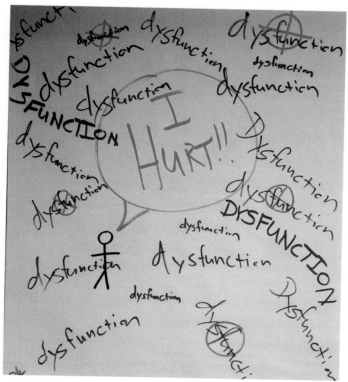

has little bearing on movement quality. The discussion turns into a chicken and egg argument - does the pain cause the poor movement, or does the poor movement cause the pain. Bottom line, it does not matter - both have to be resolved. The MR approach favors addressing movement first. Now, this does not mean move into and through pain. What it means is find and address what is causing the pain, not just the site of pain. Thomas Myers text *Anatomy Trains* has essentially re-written the standard anatomy text book. He did not discover any new structures, but he reformatted how we look at the structures. His fascial lines approach has essentially tied distant parts of the body directly together. For Example, his Superficial Back Line connects the forehead to the bottom of the big toe through a route that stretches over the entire posterior aspect of the body. With the current knowledge of trigger points and the understanding that trigger points can be active (painful) or latent (not painful) combined with the knowledge that everything is truly connected to everything else, there is an understanding that latent trigger points can have very distant far reaching areas of referred pain or active trigger points.

Humans are set up for survival. Pain and movement are intricately tied together. The nerve fibers that transmit pain to the brain are the same fibers that carry sensory information to the brain regarding movement. How many times does an athlete sprain their ankle but are able to continue playing, only to have so much pain the next day that they can barely walk? The level of tissue damage has not changed, but all of a sudden their pain level has increased. Yes there may be more swelling, but in the end the tissues damaged are the same. The biggest difference is that they are no longer moving, and now those nerves that transmit both pain and movement information are not longer carrying movement information - just the pain. Now, the only stimulus reaching the brain is "OUCH, MY ANKLE HURTS!!" From a survival standpoint, movement stimulus overrides pain stimulus - this allowed primitive man to continue to have the ability to run away from T-Rex after spraining his ankle. If pain took the processing priority in the brain, then Mongo would have sprained his ankle and been unable to run away from T-Rex and T-Rex would have had a Mongo snack.

This survival aspect characteristic also gives us predictability when pain is present. In painful situations, breathing patterns change - the breath is held. Muscles around the areas of pain tend to become more active in an attempt to stabilize, brace, or protect the damaged or painful tissues. How humans deal with pain is rooted in one of the primitive survival reflexes mentioned earlier, the Moro reflex (startle reflex). This is the foundation of how the CNS deals with any threat to the body - either from pain, sudden changes to the surrounding environment, or sudden threats (loud noises, impacts, etc). The actual Moro reflex disappears around the 6 month mark, but continues to serve as how humans deal with actual and perceived threats to the body. Imagine sneaking up behind someone when they think they are the only person in the room. You either grab them from behind or loudly and forcefully yell "BOO!" What is their response - physiologic flexion. They will drop into a partial squat, shorten their abs, bring their shoulders and head toward their knees and their hands will rise up - systemic flexion. This serves as a way to protect the vital organs. The eyes begin to blink rapidly (to keep a clear visual field) and the breath is held (to stabilize the body against whatever the threat is). Constant pain, or poor movement, or poor habitual postures can lead to this reflex being more of a constant state of readiness in some individuals. Dr. Vladimir Janda was the first to describe what is now widely known as Upper-Crossed Syndrome and Lower-Crossed Syndrome. These two dysfunctions consist of the body moving into a systemically flexed posture where the anterior structures shorten and the posterior structures are force to elongate and weaken. Several diagnoses of pain result from these dysfunctions, ranging from knee pain, to shoulder pain, to jaw pain, to headaches, to low back pain, and several more. In all of these instances pain is often the by-product of poor patterns of movement. But at the same time, the pain continues to cause poor patterns of movement which results in more pain.

The MR approach favors addressing movement by tailoring soft tissue work to the fascial lines that are affected, and then using this window of opportunity to improve movement pattern quality. It is a very focused approach to movement, that relies on several of the other 'rules' we have established and that will be discussed in detail momentarily. The bottom line is finding the cause of the pain. The best way to do this is through movement screening. If pain is present the Functional Movement Screen (FMS) **_should not be used._** When pain is present the correct assessment tool is the Selective Functional Movement Assessment (SFMA). The intricacies and implications of each will be thoroughly discussed in later chapters. If pain is present, there MUST be a referral to a licensed medical professional. Non-licensed, non-medical professionals are not able to treat pain legally, ethically, or morally.

Movement Patterning

Within the brain, movement does not exist in isolation. Patterns of movement, however, do exist - these are referred to as movement maps (Doidge). The idea that the brain recognizes and controls movement and not individual muscles is not a new concept. The problem has been in this theory and its application. For example, the right index finger has a brain map that controls its movement; there is not a brain map for the flexor indices, nor any of the other muscles that attach on the index finger. In the text The Brain That Changes Itself, the author discusses the implications of a study into brain mapping using a group of monkeys to explain how this works - they took a monkey and inserted electrodes to the surface of the brain where the index finger map was. They then surgically attached the index finger to the second finger. After a period of time, they re-examined the brain map of the monkeys index finger. What they found was that it had moved and was blended into the brain map for the monkeys middle finger. (Doidge)

"We are what we repeatedly do" is a very true quote. This can work for either the good or the bad. From the perspective of restoring movement, it is of the utmost importance that every repetition reinforces a correct movement pattern. Often times, professionals get hung up in the sets and reps of certain exercises or are so focused on their client "feeling" the effects of their workout/training session that they lose sight of what their original goal was - improving movement.

Movement is a Behavior

Movement has always been thought of as a by product of a healthy musculoskeletal system. If the structures within these systems are healthy and normal, then movement will be normal. The medical specialty of orthopedics is the greatest example of this. Tear an ACL? Reconstruct it. Fracture the femur into 52 pieces? Enough rods, pins, and screws will hold it back together. While this specialty is vitally important, if movement were only based on orthopedics then why is previous injury the first predictor of future injury? Insuring that the structural anatomy is as normal and as healthy as possible is the very important first step. If someone has shoulder pain due to a labral tear, there is only so much that any corrective strategy can do to relieve the symptoms. In the end, the labrum is still torn and the only way to address that is with a skilled orthopedic surgeon. To quote orthopedic surgeon Victor Wilson - "We heal with steel." Surgically correcting any structural problem is VITALLY important, but putting things back together is only one step in restoring movement.

In addition to needing structural integrity, movement needs many things in order to function as normal and as efficient as possible. These include:
- adequate tissue quality and mobility
- adequate sensory input
- adequate feedback on the outcome of the movement
- adequate perception of movement

The first, is somewhat orthopedic in nature. However, many people fail to address tissue quality prior to addressing movement. If there is a spasm within a muscle, or there are adhesions that limit tissue mobility within a region the overall movement being performed will be compromised. If the spasm causes pain, this will change the overall movement pattern. Pain changes everything (Cook). Everything humans do is either to avoid pain or is in search of pleasure. If there are tissue adhesions limiting tissue mobility, this too can cause pain, which again will alter the movement pattern because the brain will try to avoid whatever is causing pain. The last three bullet points all include aspects of the CNS: sensory input, feedback, and perception. All of these require an adequate CNS. Multiple systems are involved with these requirements - the proprioceptive system, the vestibulocochlear system, the visual system, the cranial nerves, nociceptors, the cerebral cortex, the frontal lobe, the limbic system, mirror neurons, and several more. All-in-all, movement is much more complicated than the standard orthopedic view many professionals have.

Movement Starts and Ends with the Brain

Movement is a sensory experience. Every movement is initiated by some type of stimulus. For example performing a squat. The specific stimulus to squat might be related to a toddler seeing something on a couch and wanting to stand up, or a teenagers desire to have stronger legs, or it may be hearing a fire alarm while seated in a chair, or it could be from sitting on a plane for 8 hours and all of a sudden there is a pain in your legs, then again, it could be because the trainer you pay $75 an hour to just watched a YouTube video titled *"193 Ways to make your clients pay you $95 an hour"*. In each instance, there is a stimulus to move. That stimulus has to be strong enough for the brain to send the signals out to the entire body that says "hey, its time to squat". While the squat is being performed, the brain is constantly taking in input from every bodily system to adjust each repetition of the squat so that it is appropriate for the situation. After the squat, there is an "after-action" review where the brain asks itself - "did that have the desired outcome, did I accomplish the task at hand?" If the answer is 'yes', then that situation is filed away until the next time a similar stimulus is presented and the movement is repeated, but in a manner that is less variable and more refined. If the answer is 'no', then the situation is filed away until the next time a similar stimulus is presented and the movement is repeated with the same level of variability. Novice movers show a high level of variability with their movements (Cech). They are still working through the development of an efficient movement solution. Those that have spent time performing a movement do so with a level of ease, grace, and precision that gives observers the impression that what they just saw was simple. In any instance the brain initiates, tracks, adjusts, and stores every movement.

Every Repetition Matters.

At various workshops, Brett Jones (ATC, Master StrongFirst Instructor, FMS Instructor, and the most entertaining person that he knowns) has been known to state "I only ask for everything from my clients." Brett has mastered the kettlebell as a training implement, and has performed several thousand kettlebell swings. He is *still* in search of a "better" swing. "I'm still looking for the perfect swing. I came close once in 2009." While he often says this to get a laugh, there is much truth in this. However, the quest is not necessarily for "perfect", but for "better."

As it was alluded to earlier, every movement has the potential for change - either for the better or the worse. One clear indicator of the quality of movement is the breathing patterns of the person moving. At times, breath holding is paramount to the success and safety of certain sports related activities. For example, an olympic weightlifter at a competition is not going to exhibit smooth, relaxed, controlled breathing after they have just cleaned a weight that equals double their body weight. Breath holding is providing them with key spinal stability as they attempt to grind out of the bottom of their catch position. However, a majority of the times this is not the case in individuals outside of their sporting activities. Remember, breath holding under stress is taking the person back towards systemic flexion (the Moro Reflex). Once this is seen in an individual as movement is being corrected, it is an indicator that their stress level has been taken too high. Breathing is the only manner in which humans can directly affect their nervous system. Breathing is an autonomic function, just like heart beat, blood pressure, and all the other homeostatic functions. Breathing is unique in that there is conscious control over this function - by controlling the breathing the autonomic nervous system can in essence be 'dialed down'. Controlling and maximizing the breathing cycles can be used as a valuable manner to manage the level of arousal (or stress) that is being introduced to the body. Several martial arts have taken advantage of this and use breath as a way to control their movement.

Making sure that breathing is regulated and the appropriate levels of stress are present for the given activity is the first step in assuring quality in whatever the desired movement is. The second step is making sure that the individual has the requisite Range of Motion (ROM) and mobility to get into the position that they need to get into. For reference, ROM here refers to joint specific cardinal plane movements. Shoulder flexion, internal rotation, external rotation, extension, ABDuction and ADDuction are all required ROM's for normal shoulder movement patterns to occur. Mobility is full freedom of movement based on unrestricted range of motion. If ROM or mobility in a region (or outside of a region, but along connected fascial lines) then the body is going to find the needed mobility by sacrificing other areas of the body. A great example is shoulder mobility, specifically the ability to get the arm fully overhead. If -as is often the case- thoracic extension is lacking, the body will sacrifice the lumbar spine in an effort to get the arm overhead. Excessive lumbar hyperextension will be seen bringing the thoracic spine backwards, allowing the arm to appear overhead. Lay this person flat on he ground with their lumbar spine pressed into the ground and what was an overhead position quickly becomes a German Salute from World War II.

Once adequate mobility is present, stability is needed. Many definitions of stability exist, many use the term 'stable' to describe stability. A different way of thinking of stability is that stability is how an individual utilizes their given range of motion. Stability is 100% dependent upon mobility. If a person does not have the mobility to get into a position, there is no reason to be able to stabilize there. Once adequate stability is present the final key is motor control. Essentially, this is how mobility and stability play nicely together in order to accomplish smooth, precise, controlled, coordinated movements.

If breathing, mobility, stability and motor control are not emphasized prior to and during every repetition then the resulting movement will demonstrate compensations and dysfunctions based off of whatever component is lacking.

Movement output occurs in response to a rich sensory environment.

Providing adequate and appropriate sensory experiences for individuals is very important to the quality of the movement outcome. Ask too much of them, or provide too much stimulus for their CNS to process and they will go into a sensory overload and movement quality will implode. This is often seen as and described as sensory overload or "overthinking" an activity. Provide too little stimulus and they will not be engaged in the activity. Finding the appropriate balance is pivotal to the success of the movement that is being sought from the individual. Tactile cues, visual cues, proprioceptive cues and verbal cues all are options, however many people fall back on to the verbal cues to correct movement. The problem with verbally trying to correct-or instruct- movement is that there are a lot of assumptions.

- Assumption #1 - the movement was seen at the correct angle at the correct time.
- Assumption #2 - the individual coaching the movement can verbalize exactly what they saw.
- Assumption #3 - the person trying to improve their movement is listening and paying attention.
- Assumption #4 - the person trying to improve their movement understood what the coach was telling them.
- Assumption #5 - The person trying to improve their movement can process and implement what they were told.

And, coaches expect all of this to occur DURING movement. The great strength coach Dan John has been known to say "you can't think your way through an explosive movement." In reality, this can be expanded to almost any highly coordinated movement, regardless of the speed.

The only stimulation that is constant across the life span is gravity-gravity is present 24 hours a day / 7 days a week. The human body is continually adapting to and overcoming gravity. The entire NDS is about the infant developing the ability to overcome gravity. Gravity is present 100% of the time - unless you are a diver or an astronaut you cannot escape it. This overlooked fact is extremely important. Every movement that is made stimulates the brain and provides feedback regarding how the body or a body part feels in relation to gravity. Manipulating gravity can increase or decrease the difficulty of any activity and it can increase or decrease what each individual "feels". Children (or adults) who cannot feel themselves have a poor sense of gravity and, as a result are not very good with what is termed "balance". (Balance is essentially the product of how the brain sorts through visual, proprioceptive, and vestibulocochlear stimulus -in that order of priority). These individuals will be clumsy, and will have poor bodily control.

Individuals can respond better to what they feel. Gray Cook often says that "the language of movement is feel." It is the clinician or the coaches job to provide the right level of 'feel' for the movement so that the individual being corrected can understand their movement flaw. This is often the "AH-HA" moment people have, that moment they feel what they are doing wrong. THIS IS WHAT THIS POINT IS ALL ABOUT.

Visual input has often been used to stimulate movement, but this has often revolved around an individual watching themselves in a mirror. Over roughly the last decade new knowledge has shown that this may not be the best mechanism to capture the visual input the brain is receiving. In the late 1990's research began discussing neurons within the brain that are known as mirror neurons. These are the neurons that allow us to mimic and imitate others. Think of the toddler that wants to be just like his daddy, and does everything (for good and for bad) that he sees his daddy do. The role of these neurons during a child's development is crucial, but these neurons remain present throughout the lifespan. Anytime humans see someone doing something, or experiencing something the neurons in the brain of the observer that their brain would use to perform the same action become active - as if they were watching themselves perform the action. This allows in individual to gain valuable information by "watching" someone perform the desired task. Often times, verbal cueing can be replaced by the simple instruction of "watch me, and be my mirror image."

Isolation does not exist anywhere in the body

Every system of the body is connected. Thomas Myers has shown that muscles that are separated by extreme distances have very important fascial connections that bind the functions of these isolated muscles together. To perform what is even considered an isolated movement - say elbow flexion- several things have to happen at the exact same time and in a very coordinated manner to occur. Certain areas have to stabilize, certain areas have to shorten, certain areas have to lengthen, the sensory input has to be processed, and all of this has to constantly work together for this 'isolated' movement to occur. As we are learning, nothing in the human body is that simple. The brain does not recognize isolation, movement does not occur in isolation, and even in 'isolated' movements there is the exact opposite of isolation occurring. Why then, does it make sense to try and isolate certain movements? The only time this makes sense is in the very specific world of bodybuilding where the the outcome is dependent upon how the body looks - not how the body functions.

Shoes Restrict Sensory Input

In the lower body, the largest amount of sensory input comes from the feet. Therefore, any activity that takes place in any standing posture is affected by the quality of this sensory input. Because of this, a majority of movement patterning exercises should be performed barefoot. While shoes allow for a wide range of activities, they alter the sensory input that the brain receives. (While being barefoot is optimal, certain instances require shoes - public gyms for example). Having a firm, solid connection with the ground is vital in order for the brain to receive quality sensory input. This is seen in many forms of martial arts, where it is referred to as "rooting." The goal is to establish a strong connection with the ground - the more force that can be imparted into the ground results in the ground returning more force into the body.

The feet are very adept at managing and handling the stress of being barefoot during the performance of daily activities. The medial longitudinal, lateral longitudinal, and transverse arches are very capable of absorbing the forces that the body creates. There are those that argue of the need to support and assist the arches with orthotics. This approach raises the question: is this support needed because of an actual anatomical (structural) change in the foot, or rather a weakness that has developed in the muscles that support the arches? Thomas Myers text Anatomy Trains highlights and discusses the latter of these two options. Quoting the text *The Brain That Changes Itself:*

> "According to Merzenich, shoes, worn for decades, limit the sensory feedback from our feet to our brain. If we went barefoot, our brains would receive many different kinds of input as we went over uneven surfaces. Shoes are a relatively flat platform that spread out the stimuli, and the surfaces we walk on are increasingly artificial and perfectly flat. This leads us to dedifferentiate maps for the soles of our feet an limit how touch guides or foot control. Then we may start to use canes, walkers, or crutches or rely on other senses to steady ourselves. By resorting to these compensations instead of exercising our failing brain systems, we hasten their decline.

As we age, we want to look down at our feet while walking down stairs or on slightly challenging terrain, because we're not getting much information from our feet"

As humans age, falling becomes a greater and greater concern. At the same time, the remedy becomes "orthopedic" grandma shoes for support, walkers, and canes. As people age, they are taught to fear the ground. This coupled with a natural decline in strength has potentially fatal consequences. A recent study (Roshanravan, Robinson-Cohen et al.) directly ties mortality rates with a simple sit to stand test - the ability to get down to the ground and back up again.

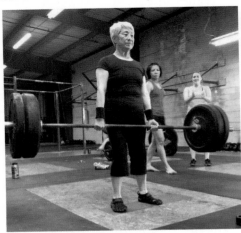 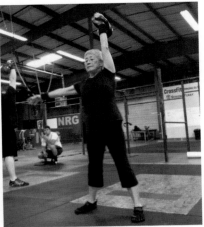

This is Sondra Fair. At the ripe young age of 70+, she attended and passed StrongFirsts Level 2 Instructor Certification course. For perspective, she snatched a kettlebell 50 times in 3 minutes, pressed 1/3 her body weight, and passed skill tests where the emphasis was on strength. All of this after 3 grueling days of intense physical training. She also has attended and passes the SFG Level I Instructor course, and their BodyWeight Course. Sondra does not use a walker, she bends them into pieces of artwork to sell an a local craft fair (that is completely made up, but would not be a surprise.)

Keeping the feet as healthy as possible, and allowing them to provide quality sensory input to the brain is vital for movement and for aging gracefully. In all of his years of training athletes and instructing at various workshop across the planet, Jeff O'Connor claims to have never seen a true "Flat foot". He has seen many feet that are weak, but none that have had structural changes to the arch. His quick test to asses the presence of an arch is outlined in the following to pictures:

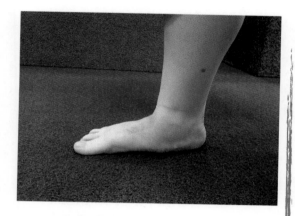
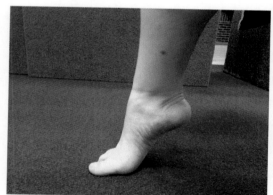

These pictures are of the same individual taken about 30 seconds apart. She has been told by several medical professionals that she has a "Fallen Arch".

Notice the lack of an arch in the first picture, but a prominent arch in the second. Is this truly a structurally flat foot, or is this a condition involving a weakness of the muscles that support the arches?

If improved movement does not "Stick", it has not really been improved

Corrective exercise has become very popular and made many people lots of money. Those that oppose corrective movement make a very valid point that if the corrective exercises are removed, the problems tend to come right back. Why is this? If corrective exercise works, then why when it is removed do the problems it was being used to correct tend to return? Are they then really 'corrective' exercises or are they 'camouflage' exercises used to hide or cover up the problems? The definition for corrective is "designed to correct or counteract something harmful or undesirable." If the improvements that corrective exercises elicit disappear, did the prescribed exercise meet the definition of "corrective"?

Everyone wants the one exercise to fix the one problem. However, movement problems tend to be multi-layered. A simple one exercise to fix all problems is not possible. Appropriately addressing mobility restrictions, stability deficits, and motor-control deficiencies is the protocol to follow. Functional Movement Systems uses the terms **RESET, REINFORCE, RELOAD**. Reset the mobility restrictions, reinforce the new mobility by improving stability, and reload the pattern by improving motor control. The key to seeing long term staybility (our own term for the ability to maintain a correction over a period of time) is following this sequence. Addressing just one area will often result in seeing immediate changes, however, these changes will not stay around. This reset, reinforce, reload is vital. When new mobility is created, there is now a new range of motion that the brain does not have a stabilization strategy for - the brain has developed a movement map that includes a mobility restriction. If mobility is increased, and no stability is provided for the new range of motion, then the brain will default back to the current movement map which does not include this new range of motion and the gained mobility will be lost. When mobility is increased, this opens a window of neural opportunity to create a new movement map. To do this, a stabilization strategy has to be immediately implemented to capture this window of opportunity. Once a new stability strategy has been incorporated it must be "cemented" into the cerebral cortex. This is accomplished by reloading this new movement map - because of Hebb's Law (muscles that fire together, wire together) adding an appropriate load and/or repetition to a new movement pattern will allow the newly gained mobility and stability strategy to become a permanent part of the movement map.

DEVELOPMENT OF FUNDAMENTAL MOVEMENTS

<u>DIAPHRAGMATIC BREATHING AND GRIP</u>

Breathing marks our entrance into and our exit from this world. Breathing and gravity are the only constants across the life span - movements change, knowledge changes, and experience level changes. Everything flows from our ability to breath - and breathing is a reflection of everything we do. When this ability is restricted, or taken away, survival becomes the priority. This affects everything. Breathing is the only autonomic action in which there is a conscious control over. Breathing can be regulated based on the situation, or it can just happen unconsciously. While other autonomic functions can be manipulated, there is no ability to directly control them. Breathing mirrors the status of the person (Key).

Why is this important? Most individuals have occupations (or are in school) that are defined as sedentary, meaning they are not on their feet for eight hours a day. This translates to a majority of the population being in a seated position for roughly 40 hours each week. Systemic flexion is the position that most people spend a majority of their time in - work or school, the commute to work or school, sitting at home, etc. This habitual posture feeds into Janda's Upper Crossed Syndrome - the head sits forward, the shoulders are rounded, and the upper spine is flexed- and Janda's Lower Crossed Syndrome - the lumbar spine is rounded and the hips are flexed. This either contributes or is at least closely tied to the fact that many people carry their stress in their upper back and neck. Current breathing patterns reflect all of this - society has become a group of chest breathers and the diaphragm no longer functions.

In individuals where the diaphragm is no longer functioning properly (chest breathers) there is a great concern that their midline stability is compromised. If the diaphragm is no longer providing midline stability, the lumbar spine has lost one of the most important stabilizers. Many people are confused about "Core" stability- in fact, most people talk about the core, but cannot really describe what makes up the "core". From here forward, the term "core" is being abandoned.

Midline stability is the descriptor that best fits the task at hand. When looking at midline stability, the best way to see the pelvis and the trunk is as a cylinder. There is a top to the cylinder (the diaphragm), a bottom (the pelvic floor) and the wall (the thoracolumbar fascia, the obliques, the transverse abdominis, and the rectus abdominis). All have to function properly, or midline stability is lost. Another important feature of the diaphragm is that the fibers from posterior crura of the diaphragm and fibers from the psoas blend together as they attach to the lumbar vertebrae. If the diaphragm is not functioning correctly, this can carry into the psoas and all the way down into the lower extremity (Deep Front Line in *Anatomy Trains*).

Most programs address the wall of the cylinder and neglect the diaphragm and the pelvic floor. To quote Dan John and Pavel Tsatsouline (Tsatsouline 2011) :

> *"In a majority of athletic movements the spine does not move, and the back and waist muscles do not generate power but stiffen up the spine and in turn the torso into a 'transmission' for passing force through the body - for instance, from the feet to the hands. This 'tranny' must be stiff in order to maximize the transfer of force and protect the back."*

Scott Sonnon describes the function of the abdomen in a way that is slightly different than the standard view. Ask anyone what the "abs" do, and the answer will likely be spinal flexion. Sonnon's view on this area of the body is that from a functional view the "abs" restrict spinal extension.

In either instance, as either a transmission for forces or as a controller of spinal extension, the cylinder must be functioning properly. The diaphragm and the pelvic floor must be capable of their normal function. Dr. Kelly Starrett discusses how when the spine is in an overextended position the pelvic floor 'turns off' (Starrett and Cordoza). As soon as this happens midline stability is lost, the lumbar spine as at risk, and nothing good happens. In reality it is a multi-faceted problem. One of the key steps to correcting all of this is restoring breathing.

Like was briefly mentioned above, the diaphragm and the psoas are intricately connected. Therefore, the psoas has a direct tie into the ability to breath, which means that anytime there are psoas or anterior hip issues (really any issues involving the Deep Front Line), it is likely there is a change in the ability of the diaphragm to function normally. Couple this with the fact that many people spend a significant amount of time in a seated (hip flexed) posture which results in a psoas that does not like to allow full hip extension. This is a serious situation that has the potential to affect everything related to the NDS and movement. This fact, is why step one in fixing any movement dysfunction has to be to restore breathing back to how it is performed by an infant.

Grip is initially a reflexive action. In the world of primates, after the infant is born, it uses its hands and feet to "cling" to the mother. Grip allows the infant to survive as mom goes about her daily business. As humans, while there is no

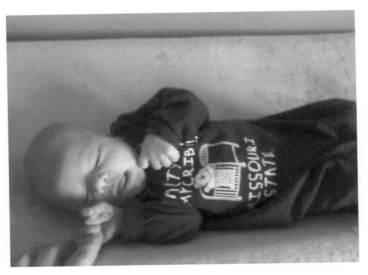

innate need to "cling" to mothers for survival, this primitive reflex is still present in infants and is seen all the way until around the 4 month mark. As the reflex blends into the conscious movement of gripping, several subtle but important changes are taking place. Every time the infant grabs something, the muscles of the forearm, upper arm and shoulder (specifically the rotator cuff) are activated to provide stability. Early in the NDS, specifically in the supine posture, there is no loading associated with this - the infant is holding onto and grabbing small toys/ items. The gripping action actually causes these muscles to fire *before* there is a load in the upper arm - it is the beginning of the reflexive stability in the shoulder, a feed-forward or proactive control of the shoulder. This reflexive stability generates stability in the shoulder to prevent any unwanted translation of the glenoid in the glenoid fossa which could damage several structures around the actual shoulder joint - it is protective in nature. Think about this: what would happen to the shoulder if someone grabbed a very heavy suitcase and the shoulder was not stable? Everyone has experienced this -picking up an object that was anticipated to be very light, and as it is picked up it becomes very apparent that we were not ready to receive the load. Or the opposite, expecting something to be very heavy, and then almost throwing the object as it is picked up because it is so light. The brain tries to anticipate and protect the delicate structures (shoulder, spine, etc) by using this feed forward stability in an unconscious manner. The entire upper body and trunk is involved in reaching for and grasping any objects (Cech).

Additionally, grip is an indicator of how well the entire body is *neurodynamically linked*. Meaning, if the body does not have a good foundation, and midline stability has not been reflexively "turned on" prior to an activity that requires gripping, grip will actually be decreased. Grip reflects neurological preparedness for an activity. Try this: tomorrow morning right after your alarm goes off and you are still groggy make a white knuckle fist as hard as you can. Later, after your first cup of coffee try this again. Likely your grip will be much stronger - but has there actually been an increase in strength?

Both breathing and grip are initially seen as reflexes. Like was mentioned before -at birth the infant only possess the ability to survive, barely. If breathing and grip are important enough from a survival standpoint for an infant to have these reflexes, they MUST be imperative to the development of that infant. In adults, if breathing and gripping are impaired, there is little likelihood that any further movement work will be affective. That is how important both are to movement.

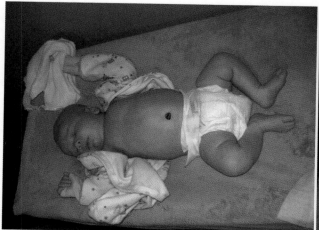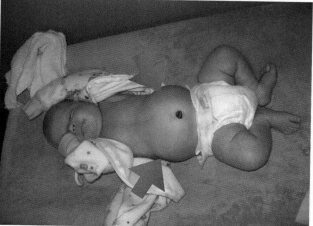

Notice the 360° - and especially the lateral- expansion of the abdomen during inhalation?

HEAD MOVEMENT and VISION

At birth, the visual system is neither fully developed nor fully functional. Newborns vision is 20/800 and they are limited to having a fixed gaze set at around 8 inches (Cech). Beyond 8 inches, and all they have is sound. They possess the ability to distinguish light and dark and to view objects that are very close to their face, but this is the extend of the visual system. The components of the eye are fully developed. The optic nerve is fully developed. Where the disconnect come from is within the brain itself - vision is not as essential to the newborns survival as those systems involved in breathing and the basic systems of life. In order to fully and normally develop, infants must be able to interact with both the environment that they are seeing and the individuals within their environment. As something is brought into the infants visual field, their attention is drawn to it. This innate action, coupled with the continued development of the vestibular system is what leads to the development of locomotion. Without it, motor development will be significantly affected.

> *"We used to think the motor system is hardwired, that people are destined to move in certain ways, but that is not so. You need to interact with the physical world to build normal body maps." (Doidge)*

Vision is an important sensory system that provides the developing infant with important -yet incomplete- information about their surroundings. Their interactions with their visual environment completes this information. If vision is compromised, or not functioning optimally, the input regarding body position and environmental information is decreased. This will cause movement or activities to be inhibited, because that infant is not able to get input at a rate that allows them to function or play at a normal level (Melillo). Between six and twelve months of age, infants will have developed full-color vision and have normal distance vision (Melillo).

The development of movement, and the NDS, is driven by vision, the vestibulocochlear system and gravity. Where the eyes look the head goes. Humans were designed to be in a state of homeostasis, meaning that the body is always making adjustments to level the visual field - from tilting the head, to shifting the pelvis, to developing a leg length discrepancy. For example, the pelvo-occular reflex is a reflex where, when the eyes look up, the pelvis subtly rotates posteriorly. When the eyes look down, the pelvis exhibits a subtle anterior rotation. This is one way in which the body attempts to subconsciously maintain a level visual field. The visual system helps to maintain both static and dynamic equilibrium - the body's ability to respond to sudden movements such as acceleration, deceleration, and/or rotation. Combined with input from the proprioceptors in the body and the vestibular system, the body is allowed to respond to the outside environment, interact with the world, and overcome gravity. The interaction of the three systems, in order of neural processing- visual, vestibular, proprioceptive- is what generates what is commonly described as balance.

When visual problems exist or when there are cervical restrictions, there is a high likelihood that other movement patterns will adjust accordingly to compensate for these issues. As infants are experiencing the NDS and as adults are controlling their environment they all need to see where they are going. Visual input is the dominant input that affects movement. Initiating movement with the eyes is essential to the development and the maintenance of efficient, effective movement.

Not surprisingly, but often overlooked, is the connection between the sub-occipital region and the visual system. The high number of visual nuclei and stretch receptors within these very small cervical muscles combined with their link to eye movement are essential in connecting vision to movement - this interplay effectively coordinates movements in the eye with the coordination of the firing of the muscles of the back (Myers). The text *Anatomy Trains* gives a great description of this relationship and how vision ties into what Myers describes as the Superficial Back Line (SBL). Essentially, the brain gathers the information from the high quantity of stretch receptors in the sub-occipital muscles and then organizes the entire SBL in a feed-forward manner to assist in maintaining a level visual field - a direct tie in to the Pelvo-Occular reflex mentioned above.

A 2014 thesis project by Missouri State University graduate student Tarah Trokey ATC looked at the connection between the sub-occipitals and the multi-segmental forward flexion pattern that is part of the Selective Functional Movement Assessment (Trokey). Her subjects performed a toe touch pattern, then underwent two minutes of a sub occipital release and then repeated the toe touch. What she found was a significant improvement in the multi-segmental forward flexion reach distance following a sub occipital release.

THE SUPINE POSTURE

Physiologic flexion - flexed knees, hips, lumbar spine, neck, arms, etc - is the dominant posture that newborns experience. In this posture, stability is provided by the ground - the entire backside of the infant from their head down to the pelvis is in firm contact with the ground. The entire spine is on the ground - the spinal curves have not developed this early on. This posture, requires the absolute least amount of stability from the infant. Keep in mind, infants are born with unrestricted mobility but no stability - the supine posture gives them this stability to begin their interactions with the environment.

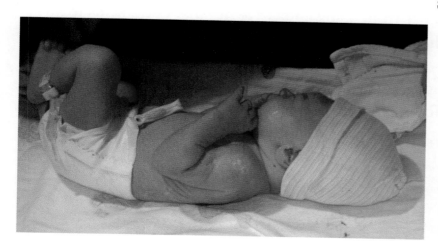

The first movements of the extremities are reflexive in nature, meaning they are not under the conscious control of the infant (Cech). These random movements are spastic, jerky and unrefined because at birth the brain has not developed movement maps for these (or any) gross movements. These spastic movements do serve a purpose - they begin to provide stimulus that is essential in the development of midline stability. As trunk stability is developed, and as movement maps are developed, then these movements are able to come under conscious control. Movement occurs in a cephalo-caudel direction and from mid-line to the extremities. As head movement is developed, from there the shoulders and upper extremities begin to come under conscious control followed by the pelvis and the lower extremities later.

Vision is very important to the development of the movement maps in a supine posture. As vision improves and the infant begins to see more objects, their head begins to follow the object. This requires the neck to develop stability. As the infant is able to track objects through a larger visual field, and as the spastic movement of their extremities develops some midline stability, they begin to develop enough stability of the upper extremity to begin to reach towards objects. Eventually, this leads to them being able to grasp the object, pull it towards them and then explore the item even more (touch, taste, smell, etc).

As these acts are repeated, they begin to become more coordinated, refined, and controlled. This is in response to the brain integrating the movement maps. "This is because the infant goes from using a massive number of neurons to an appropriate few, well matched to the task" (Doidge).

As infants begin to move their arms and legs more, they are continuing to develop more and more midline stability. Action requires a stable base (Cech). Early in the NDS, all of the reaching tasks occur from the stable supine posture. As

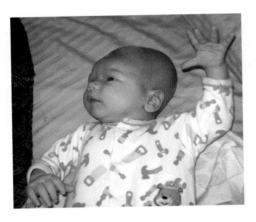 infants begin to expand the mobility demands of the limbs, they must continue to develop the stability and the strength components to match their mobility. Mobility precedes stability and strength 100% of the time (Many pathologies that are treated on a very regular basis occur due to the loss of this mobility- stability - strength relationship). Infants must develop this reflexive stabilization very early for further movements to develop. In essences, the body must prepare itself for movement *before* the movement actually occurs, and it must do this at a level below conscious thought. It must be anticipatory in nature. As this reflexive stability increases, the ability to pull objects towards the body increases, which leads to more sensory input of the world around them. When an infant is gently poked in the belly, one can see how this occurs - what they do is tighten their belly and make a very slight grunt.

As stability is increased, and more and more movement of the limbs is brought under conscious control the feet begin to gradually make their way to the floor - the pelvis begins a slight change in orientation out of its physiologic flexion (posterior rotation). This begins with, and contributes to the natural curves of the spine beginning to form. Bringing the feet to the ground is also an important aspect of the supine posture - although this occurs later on than what is seen in the early presentation of supine. This process is the beginning of lower body extension. As this forms, and as the prone posture develops, and as more control of the head and neck is gained the ability to roll from supine to prone, and from prone to supine develops. These (prone and rolling) will be discussed in the coming sections.

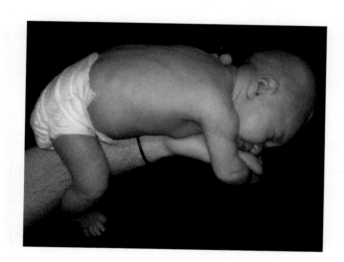

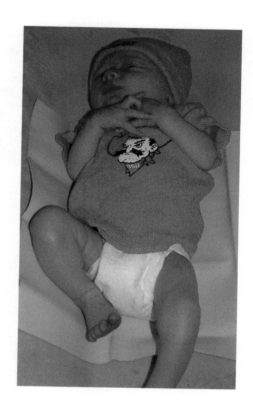

THE PRONE POSTURE

The prone posture is the fundamental extension posture. It is not just laying on the belly-certain things have to happen for true prone to occur. A newborn that is laid on their belly, will still exhibit physiologic flexion - there hips will stay flexed,

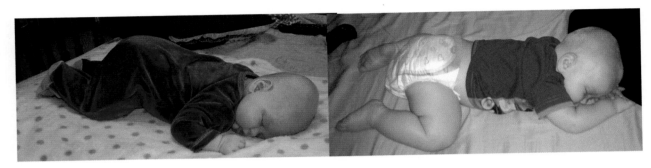

knees will be flexed, their arms will be flexed, and their spine will stay flexed. Midline stability in supine must be allowed to develop to the point that the curves of the spine begin to develop. This will then allow the pelvis and hips to "unwind" and move out of the way so that a true prone posture can be achieved.

With the heightened awareness of Sudden Infant Death Syndrome, the current standard is that infants spend a majority of time on their backs until they are able to roll over on their own. Prior to this, it is recommended that babies have adequate supervised "tummy-time" to appropriately develop. This tummy time allows for the first real activation of their posterior chain, but can be a very frustrating position for the young infant. Until adequate neck extension strength has developed, the infant will essentially be unable to raise their head - they will be "stuck" on the ground. However, while this position initially can be frustrating for the infant, the neck extension will develop in an effort to raise their heads and better observe their surroundings. As the head and eyes change their orientation, there is an increased demand placed on the trunk stabilizers due to the change in position of the vestibular system, the visual system and the change in alignment of the spinal column.

This neck extension is one of the earliest expressions of "strength" and strength development seen in the young infant. The prone position is one of the foundations of:

- Strength development (especially upper body strength and the entire posterior chain)
- Fine motor control of the upper extremities
- The development of speech.

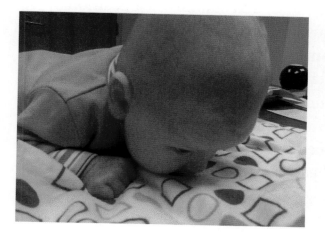 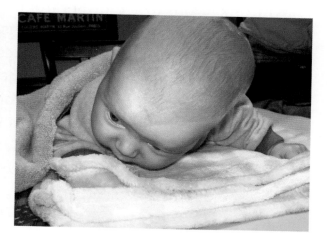

As infants develop the extension strength to lift their heads, they continue to try and lift their entire upper body off the ground by pressing their hands down into the ground. This weight bearing through the arms and shoulders provides the infant with a heightened sensory awareness (Cech). The increase in sensory feedback as well as the increased trunk and limb strength allows infants to move towards the quadruped posture and then gradually on to crawling/creeping.

Additionally, once the infants get more comfortable in the prone position - which allows neck extension strength to increase - they will begin to roll back and forth between prone and supine. Rolling will be discussed in greater detail in the next section.

Another benefit of the prone position is that this position and gravity allows for the anterior side of the body (or in Anatomy Trains language, the Superficial Front Line and Deep Front Lines) to "unwind" and elongate. That initial physiologic flexion begins to disappear. The pelvis is finally able to move out of its flexed (posteriorly rotated) position and move into a position that promotes hip extension and a normal lumbar curvature. Couple this with the tie-in of the psoas/diaphragm relationship mentioned earlier and the prone position shows itself to be crucial in establishing a normal breathing pattern in a "safe"position with the anterior hip structures in an elongated position.

As upper body strength begins to improve in the prone position, the head and upper trunk begins to get further from then floor, and stability in a position of thoracic extension is established. This is a very important development, since the loss of thoracic extension is a common compensation seen later in life. During the NDS, thoracic extension is established in a prone position by using the head and the arms to get the trunk off the ground, while the pelvis stays in contact with the ground for stability. This position allows the child to see more of the world and acts as a progression into the quadruped posture. "Moving from prone-on-elbows to the push up start position also has deep developmental roots from a sensory standpoint" (Cook 2010).

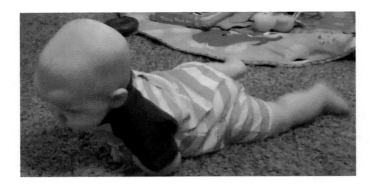
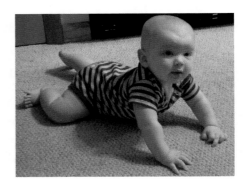

SEGMENTAL ROLLING PATTERN

Segmental rolling connects the supine and prone postures, and establishes the ability of the infant to reflexively stabilize (therefore protect) the spine AND to disassociate the hips from the shoulders. To put it in common terms associated with core stability, it is the ability of the inner unit to successfully provide stability to the spine as the spine rotates on an axis without a load. Segmental 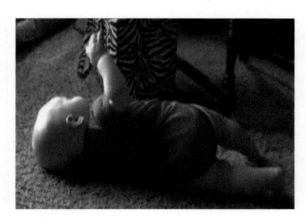 rolling is the first true locomotion based activity that allows children to expand their environment even further - this serves as the foundation of all single leg stance activities later in life. The prerequisites that the infant needs to roll are diaphragmatic breathing, eye and head movement, and the initial reflexive stability gained while reaching for objects in the supine posture - without these attributes having developed to appropriate levels, purposeful segmental rolling will not happen.

Segmental rolling is not the "first" rolling that infants demonstrate. Much earlier in the developmental sequence, infants will perform what is typically referred to as a log roll - or rolling where the pelvis and the shoulders are locked together. This initial type of rolling is a righting reaction and is not purposeful in nature. Segmental rolling and log rolling require two different activation patterns of the trunk muscles. Segmental rolling requires reflexive stabilization of the inner unit muscles, while log rolling requires the trunk muscles associated with gross trunk movements (the outer unit) to "lock" the pelvis with the shoulders. Log rolling involves minimal to no spinal rotation - this is one of the reasons that the log roll is the preferred repositioning technique used by Athletic Trainers when an athlete has a suspected cervical spine trauma.

Segmental rolling is driven by the visual system. When an infant sees "something" and that "something" leaves their field of vision, they will turn their head -which is very large and heavy in relation to their body size- in an attempt to continue tracking the "something" that captured their attention. As their head turns their body will be forced to follow along and this will result in them rolling over. Initially, this will be a random occurrence that will surprise the infant, but as their strength and stability increases it will progressively become more controlled and effortless. Once this is observed, the foundation of single leg stance has been established. The very simple act of getting one leg to cross midline begins a myriad of neurological adaptations and changes that begin to allow the two independently functioning hemispheres of the brain to communicate through the corpus callosum, which is essential for the rest of the NDS to occur. This is also the beginning of the cross lateralization - the development of the corpus callosum which allows communication between hemisphere of the brain to occur and for right side actions to be coordinated with left side actions.

Video Links:

Rolling - http://youtu.be/luMoohn7L34
Rolling 2- http://youtu.be/MS0QjEHMO5I

THE SEATED POSTURES

The seated postures and the quadruped posture begin to develop at roughly the same time, but in this text the seated postures will be discussed first. The seated postures are the first time the infant will experience a vertical posture away from the body of their caregivers - which usually is dominated by some carrying position. There are a variety of different seated postures that an infant can be in. Initially, supported sitting is seen as parents "prop" the infant up against objects. Supported sitting can also take place as the infant is in a seated posture with their hands on the ground, which provides added support. The infant does not possess adequate levels of strength or stability to maintain a vertical posture without the added support provided by their upper extremities or the object they are resting against. As trunk stability and strength are gained, unsupported seated postures will begin to be seen. The seated postures essentially allow for a "partially" vertical position - the ground provides stability to the hips and pelvis, so the infant is only responsible for establishing stability from the trunk up, it is a less challenging vertical posture for the infant.

The typical seated postures all have the hips placed into some end range motion - external rotation (ER), internal rotation(IR), or ER in one hip and IR in the other hip. This serves to in essence "lock up" the pelvis and further increase pelvic stability, but it requires the full mobility that infants are born with. This is one reason why adults tend to struggle with seated postures outside of a chair. The pelvis (and specifically the sacrum) needs to be vertical and stable in order for the spinal column to have a solid base to orient on. Without this, spinal positioning - and stability- will be compromised.

The commonly seen -but not only- seated postures seen in infants are:
- O-sit (ring sitting)
- V-Sit (wide base)
- Shin box (side sitting, cheerleader sitting)
- W-sit (both hips fully internally rotated, knees in front of the hips, and feet outside of the hips)
- OBLique sit (side propped position)

The various seated positions all allow for the lower body to be stable and the upper body to be free for the child to interact with their surroundings. This frees the hands and the upper body to begin to exhibit fine motor control and for fine motor skills to be established and improved. As postural/trunk stability and strength are improved in this vertical posture, the child begins to have the ability to move their trunk and upper limbs outside of their initial base of support and again further expand their environment. This also allows the child to transition into and out of the quadruped and crawling postures.

Oblique sit specifically serves as a bridge between the seated postures and quadruped. In fact, transitioning thru oblique sit can directly connect the supine and prone postures to the quadruped posture and on into the crawling pattern. Oblique sit allows the child to use their upper body to, in essence, drag their lower body out of their starting posture whether it is seated, supine, or prone. This is another instance where motivation serves as the catalyst to movement -

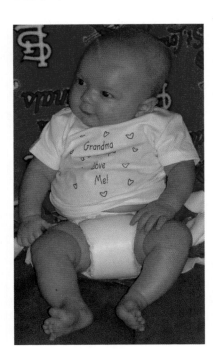 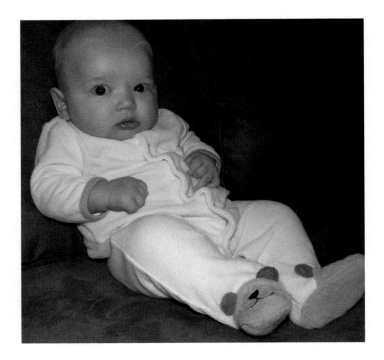

the child typically will see something they want and then reach for it. As their lower body and upper body progress to where they function together, the upper bodies reaching action serves to drag the lower body along and the child is able to transition from seated, supine, or prone into to the quadruped posture.

Supported Seated Positions

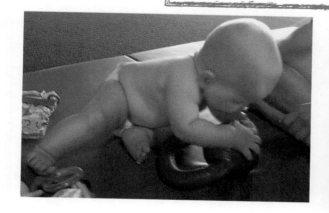
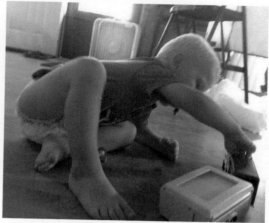
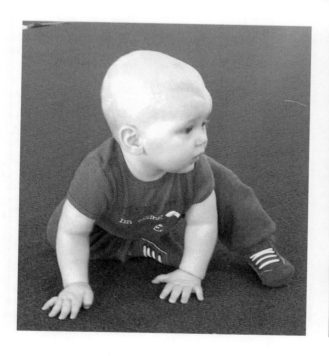
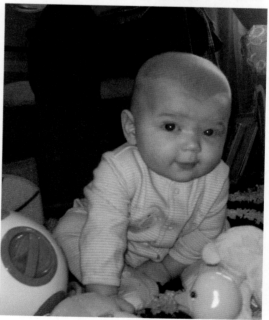

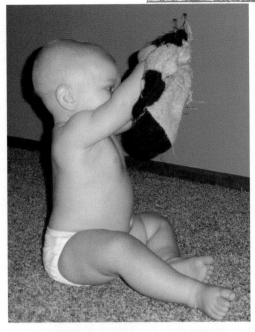

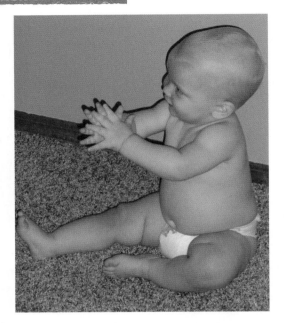

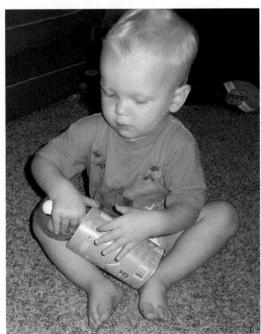

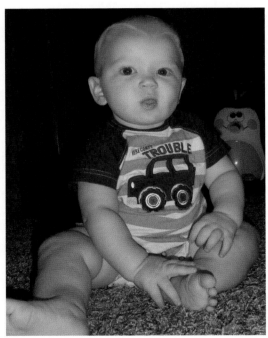

THE QUADRUPED POSTURE

In the quadruped posture the child has now moved up off of the ground and is supporting all of their weight on their hands and their knees. The hands are underneath the shoulders and are responsible for supporting the upper bodies load while the knees are under the hips and are responsible for supporting the load of the pelvis. In quadruped the orientation of the trunk is parallel to the ground. Additionally, the neck is now free to move into full extension on a loaded thoracic spine (in prone the thoracic spine has been supported by the ground). In quadruped, the pelvis begins to be loaded in a hip flexed position, which begins to lay the foundation for crawling to occur from both a strength and neurological standpoint.

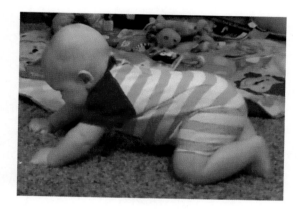

Because of the new posture, new strategies for stability and motor control will need to be established for the hip, shoulder, trunk, pelvis, and cervical spine. As these new strategies are learned, the infant will learn how to move from a position of six points of contact with the ground (two hands, two knees, two feet) to five points of contact as they lift one hand off of the ground and become more unstable, and eventually to four points of contact (two hands, two feet). This 4-point position is commonly referred to as the bear position and the child will actually elevate their pelvis above their shoulders.

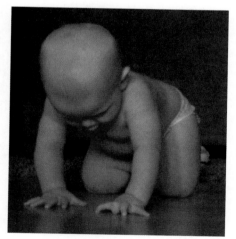

While the trunk is parallel to the ground in quadruped, the head will vary its position based on what has the attention of the child. Humans have an innate desire to maintain homeostasis, which results in children holding their heads "up" when in quadruped. This provides a level visual field, and positions the vestibular system in a vertically aligned position that resembles being held by the caregiver, sitting, or standing (which is seen later). While this serves to provide homeostasis to the child, it also increases their visual field - which again expands the environment of the child and allows for greater opportunities of interaction. The type and degree of vestibular input is both altered and increased in the quadruped posture. Since the head is no longer supported by the floor, there is an increase in movement and movement combinations of the head - cervical flexion/extension, rotation, lateral flexion, and many combinations of these movements. This increase in vestibular stimulation is essential for efficient and effective communication of stimulus to the brain and for strategies to be planned based on input from the vestibular system, the visual system and the proprioceptive system.

As mentioned in the previous section, the quadruped and sitting postures develop at around the same time. This allows for the child to transition back and forth between quadruped and sitting variations. These transitions between postures continue to further develop the stability needed for the higher levels of the NDS and serve as valuable motor learning opportunities for the child.

Once in quadruped the child will begin testing their stability boundaries by rocking back and forth as well as side to side. While at times this can be entertaining to the observer (specifically when the child goes beyond their boundary and falls over) it serves as a very important learning opportunity and training opportunity for the child. These rocking motions serve as the entry point to the crawling/creeping pattern - as the child rocks beyond their boundary of stability they will eventually move one arm out in front of them to catch themselves before they fall. As they figure this strategy out, crawling/creeping will develop.

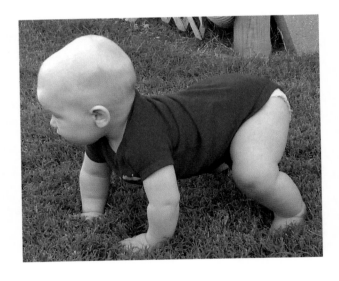

Sitting to Quadruped- http://youtu.be/PzIdN4I8x7Y
Rocking - http://youtu.be/fKSAojFsFK0

THE CRAWLING PATTERN

Depending on the text, crawling and creeping, while different, are often used interchangeably. Some texts refer to crawling in terms of an army crawl- the upper body dragging the lower body in a prone position - while they refer to creeping as a reciprocal pattern that occurs in quadruped. Other texts use the same terminology, but with the other definition. In this text, crawling will be recognized as the reciprocal pattern that is occurring in a quadruped posture. Crawling is a very complex movement pattern, in regards to both physical

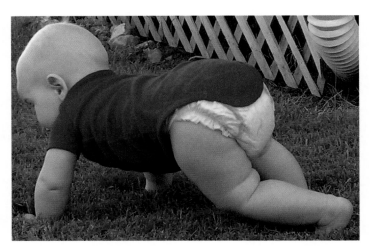

complexity and neurological complexity. Crawling builds off of the prior postures in the NDS and further establishes locomotion which began with the segmental rolling pattern. Crawling is a cross-lateral movement that requires all four limbs of the body, the trunk and pelvis, both hemispheres of the brain, both eyes, and both vestibular structures to communicate together in real time to adjust the movement strategy while actively moving.

> *"These activities work both sides of the body evenly and involve coordinated movements of both eyes, both ears, both hands and both feet as well as balanced core muscles. When both eyes, both ears, both hands and feet are being used equally, the corpus callosum orchestrating these processes between the two hemispheres becomes more fully developed. Because both hemispheres and all four lobes (of the brain) are activated, cognitive function is heightened and ease of learning increases." (Hannaford)*

Crawling is initiated by the rocking that begins in quadruped, and as the children begin to coordinate the movement between their upper extremity and their contra-lateral lower extremity, a very early crawling pattern is seen. When crawling finally happens, it is an asymmetrical, cross-lateral movement. It requires one lower limb to move into a flexed position while the opposite lower limb moves towards extension. The same is true in the upper body; however, the movements of the upper extremity limbs are matched to the opposite limb of the lower body - as the right leg extends, the left arm extends (extension in the shoulder is seen as the arm returning to the neutral position). The asymmetrical movement across the trunk begins to develop the foundation for the opposing movement that occurs during bipedal gait, and begins to set the stage for climbing patterns.

A 2014 study at Missouri State University by graduate student Kristian Stewart ATC investigated the relationship between the crawling pattern and fine motor control in children diagnosed within the Autism Spectrum Disorder (Stewart). She administered a test assessing fine motor skills followed by a period of crawling interventions. After administering the same test following the interventions, she found a significant improvement in fine motor skills both immediately after crawling and a week after crawling was performed. Crawling did improve the fine motor control in this group of subjects.

SIDE NOTE: *While crawling is important in the NDS, there is evidence that it may not be as pivotal as some want to believe. The NDS that is presented within this text, and the NDS that is commonly envisioned is based off of the development of children within the developed Western society. Within this model of the NDS, there is much evidence that shows if children miss the crawling stage of development there is likely to be far reaching effects that can present physically or cognitively. However, outside of the developed Western society a slightly different NDS has been observed. In undeveloped parts of the world where indigenous people still live and hold on to their traditions, crawling is not part of the NDS. In these populations, which can serve as a window into our past, crawling presents as a threat to the survival of the infant. Placing an infant on the ground places them closer to many threats - parasites, animals, dirt, etc. What has been observed by researcher Sara Wyckoff was that infants were held or carried around 90% of the time up until around one year of age (Wyckoff). At this point they were seated on the ground and developed a scooting pattern of movement where they kept their trunk vertical and used their arms to drag themselves around. Compared to a control group of children in Canada, these indigenous babies ended up walking significantly later - but they still progressed through the full NDS, minus the crawling. The unique butt-scooting locomotion they developed displays an alternative option to develop all of the physical and neurological benefits that are observed in crawling. What this leads to is the hypothesis that crawling is a relatively new step in the NDS that did not appear until around 200 years ago - or when dirt floors began to disappear from our living situations and placing infants on the ground was less of a threat to them.*

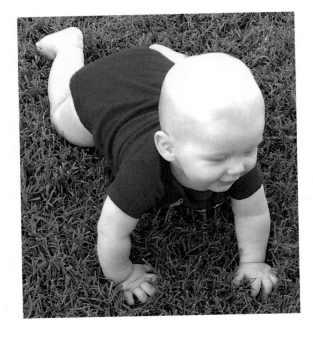

Video Links:

Crawling - http://youtu.be/wSODla4Lk3s
Sitting to Crawling- http://youtu.be/FhXF3hUklyo

THE TRANSITIONAL POSTURES

The NDS is fairly consistent up until the crawling pattern is seen, however, once children are able to crawl many options and variations are seen as the child transitions from the ground up to a fully vertical posture. This is often wrongly seen as "pulling up" onto objects. Regardless of what is happening, at this point the child is attempting to get their legs underneath them and stand up. This can occur through a variety of kneeling postures, the seated postures, or a squatting posture. The typically seen transitional postures are:

- Kneeling (symmetrical position of both lower extremities, with the trunk balanced above the symmetrical pelvis)
- short kneeling (both hips resting on the heels, knees fully flexed)
- tall kneeling (both hips partially or fully extended, knees flexed to around 90 degrees)
- Half kneeling (asymmetrical position of the lower extremities with the trunk balanced on an asymmetrical pelvis)
- short half kneeling
- tall half kneeling
- Squatting (both feet on the ground, hips below the knees)

These postures are seen as the transitional postures. Children are not able to fully and successfully control these postures in an unsupported manner until after their ability to control their center of mass is improved through practice and with the higher levels of vertical stance.

These postures serve as a bridge between the asymmetrical pattern of crawling and the asymmetrical pattern seen in bipedal gait, with the only difference being the orientation of the pelvis and trunk. As the position of the trunk is altered, other than strength, the biggest difference seen regarding core stability is the timing/sequence in which the trunk stabilizers fire. Stability is pattern specific, meaning good stability in one pattern does not guarantee good stability in another pattern.

The kneeling postures are the first expression of a hip hinging pattern seen in the vertical posture. This later presents itself as a deadlift pattern. The half-kneeling postures are the first time that the child loads an asymmetrically aligned pelvis in a vertical manner. This later presents itself as any position where the hips are working independently of each other as well as what is seen as deceleration. Squatting is the first time that the trunk is vertical and the knees are below the hips. This serves as a very important stage of developing the pelvic floor, which is the final piece in trunk and pelvis stability. Up to this stage, the diaphragm - which serves as the top of the "core"- has been established from the first breath the infant took after birth. The wall of the "core" - rectus abdominis, transverse abdominis, internal/external obliques, and thoracolumbar fascia- have all progressively developed throughout the NDS. Squatting establishes the finishing touches to trunk/pelvic stability (core stability as it is often referred to).

As the musculoskeletal system and the neurological system adapt to the new vertically aligned, unsupported postures, the child's ability to easily get into and out of these postures also improve. However, to get out of these transitional postures up into a standing posture requires some assistance. This assistance is seen -incorrectly- as "pulling up".

If this assistance were truly pulling up, when did the child develop the upper body strength to physically pull themselves up with enough force to allow their legs to extend? At this time period, the legs are not strong enough to allow the child to stand up unassisted, and the upper body is not strong enough to provide much assistance. However, the arms provide an integral component that allows the child to generate the required force to stand up. The pulling up is actually, and more correctly, pushing down. The child that wants to stand up, regardless of the starting posture, will place their hands at or above shoulder level on the 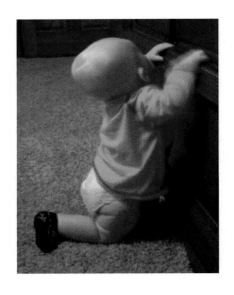 *object that they are using for assistance, and press their hands down into the object. This pressing down causes several reflexive activities to take place:*

- *The rectus abdominis fires to prevent trunk extension (Sonnon).*
- *The "inner unit" / deep spinal stabilizers are activated.*
- *The pelvic floor is activated*

- *The shoulder musculature (rotator cuff specifically) is activated.*

All of this combined with a temporary breath holding -valsalva maneuver- act synergistically to stabilize the trunk and pelvis to allow the strength that the infant does have to be expressed in a more efficient manner.

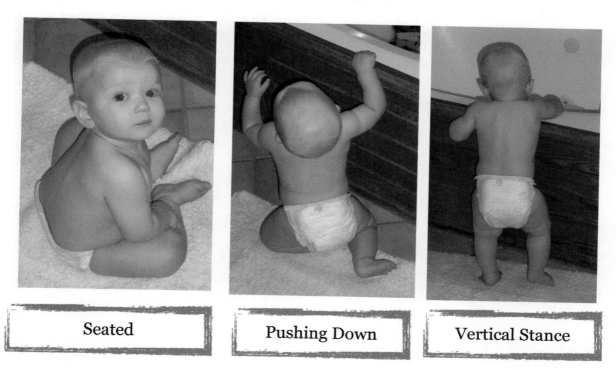

| Seated | Pushing Down | Vertical Stance |

Short Half Kneeling

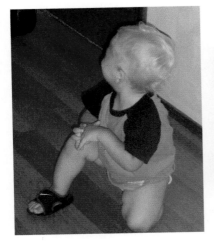 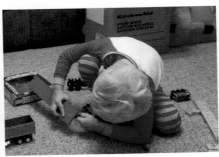 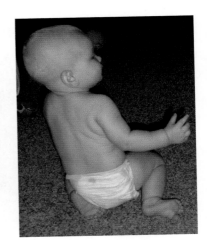

Short Kneeling

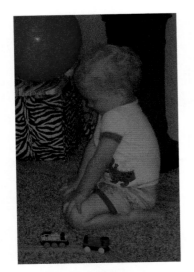 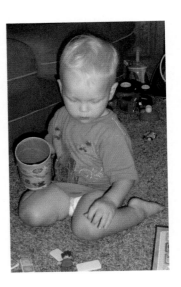

Tall Half Kneeling

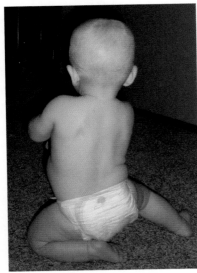

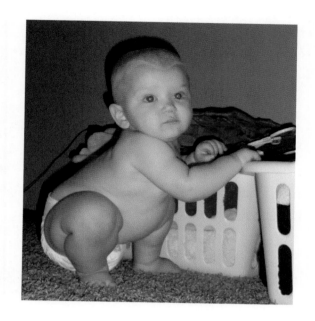

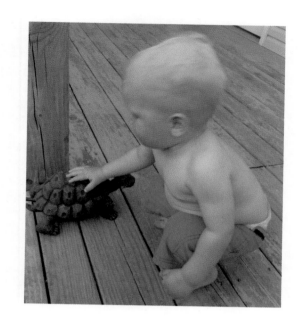

Squatting

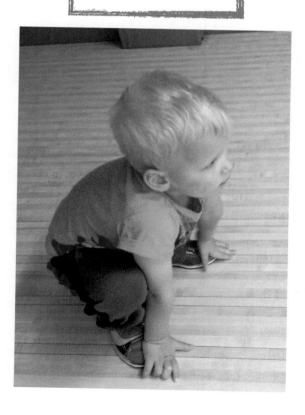

Video Links

Squatting - http://youtu.be/6KunTVAJfMs
Transitional Postures -http://youtu.be/XaUQieAA7b
Transitional Variations- http://youtu.be/Xcx01wZzEj8

VERTICAL STANCE

In vertical stance there are three variations:
- symmetrical stance - both feet in the same position (squat stance).
- asymmetrical stance - both feet doing something different (split stance).
- single leg stance - one leg on the ground, one leg off.

All three stances are different and require different stabilization and motor control strategies. In symmetrical stance, the pelvis is oriented the same on both sides - if one hip is flexed, the other hip is flexed; if one hip is extended, the other hip is extended. In asymmetrical stance, one hip may be extended while the other hip is slightly flexed; or on hip may be slightly flexed, and the other hip is in greater flexion. This difference at each hip begins to increase the stability required at the pelvis to maintain a level posture so that the spine can be balanced on a stable base. At this point, varying degrees of rotation are introduced into the pelvis. In single leg stance, one hip is bearing the entire load of the body. A Trendelenberg's sign (dropping 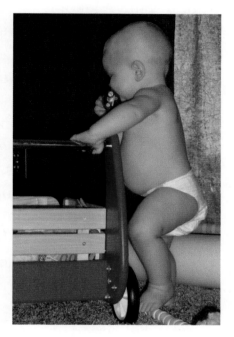 of one iliac crest) has to be counteracted in order to maintain a level atmosphere for the spine to be stacked on top of.

Vertical stance is a very challenging posture for the toddler - it requires stability at the lower extremities, pelvis, trunk and cervical spine in multiple planes in a vertically oriented position. Add to this the challenge of maintaining a vertical posture while the arms are reaching, grabbing, pulling, and pushing along with the head turning and moving as the toddler continually scans their environment. Vertical stance in a toddler is an example of perfect structural alignment - there are no compensation strategies at this age.

Once the toddler has progressed to vertical stance, there will be a period of supported stance followed by unsupported stance. The transition from supported to unsupported is similar to that seen in the seated postures - and the strategies they utilized in sitting will be employed once again to overcome this new challenge. The initial "wobbles" seen as the toddler begins vertical stance is their expression of motor learning. They are learning to find stability in this new posture; in essence, they are creating a new brain map for this new task. As their ability to stabilize improves and their strategies are refined, the wobbles will gradually lessen until they disappear. Vertical stance occurs as a speed bump prior to gait. A lot of falling happens as motor control in this posture develops - the "automatic butt centering device" (the diaper) gets used daily as the toddler loses their stability and collapses to the floor. As vertical stance is explored, and more time is spent here lower body strength in this posture begins to develop.

In adulthood, the expression of upright stance is far from perfect. Over time, adults have developed compensation patterns due to aches, pains, and injuries. Additionally, habitual daily tasks take a toll on the body structures - adults have built up lots of miles. Humans adapt to what is done on a daily basis. Habituation is the simplest form of learning - a slow relentless, adaptive act, which ingrains itself into the central nervous system (Key 2010). Unfortunately, in Western society, this involves an extended period of time in a seated position. All of this combines for an upright posture and bipedal gait that has strayed far from the perfect alignment that everyone began life with.

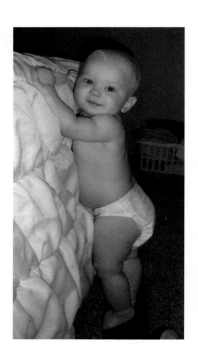

Video Links

Vertical Stance- http://youtu.be/etOFVnv_zxY

BIPEDAL GAIT

"We learn to walk by falling" - Gray Cook

Upright, bipedal gait - in addition to opposable thumbs - is one of the characteristics that separates humans from all other animals on the planet. The degree of mobility and stability, as well as the interaction between the mobility and stability and the nervous system, are on full display in bipedal gait. Bipedal gait is the culmination of all the prior developmental postures and patterns.

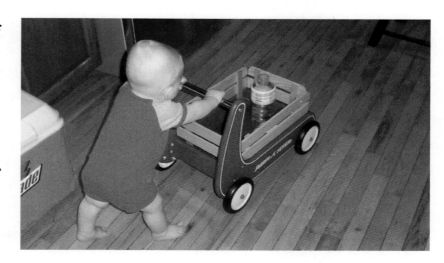

Normal bipedal gait is fully developed in 98% of toddlers by the age of four (Cech 2012). There is a very efficient and delicately balanced interplay between the opposite lower and upper extremities that allow bipedal gait to be successful. Just like the interplay exhibited in crawling, reciprocal movements of the arms and legs are seen in gait. This aids in the transmission of forces across the trunk. The efficiency of this energy transfer relies heavily on the timing of the trunk musculature and explains why historically humans have had the capacity to walk for extended distances and periods of time as new lands and territories were explored prior to the past 300 years. Napoleon is quoted as saying *"Wars are won on the legs of the foot soldier"*.

An important phase in the development of gait, and the requisition of lost gait, is the "cruising" phase. This is when toddlers have gotten their legs underneath themselves and are fully vertical, but are not quite stable enough on their own to confidently let go of their supporting object. They maintain contact with this object as they move around. Eventually, as confidence, stability, and strength improve the amount of contact needed lessens and the amount of movement freedom improves. Those first few steps every adult waits for their children to take is an example of this - one parent is the starting point and provides the needed assistance for the toddler to stand and the other parent acts as the motivation (and target) for the child to walk (or controlled fall) towards..

What is very unique to bipedal gait is the single leg stance period. The ability to shift the center of mass from single leg stance, to double leg stance, and over to single leg stance on the opposite side must be both effective and efficient. This continual dynamic reacquisition of the center of mass with every step is integral to the well being of the body. The degree of dynamic stabilization and timing/coordination of the musculature that contributes to movement is highly affected by posture. Any deviation from good static posture will inhibit this ability as we move into the bipedal gait pattern (this deviation is often seen in older children / adults in the presence of pain, injury or poor habituation).

Additionally, there has to be an unconscious ability to produce reflexive stabilization when going from single leg stance to double leg stance. With the upper and lower limbs functioning as opposing counterbalances, there needs to be a very high level of reflexive stabilization that takes place. If it does not occur, a less efficient gait strategy will be utilized, which will lead to a decrease in the efficiency of bipedal gait. In this scenario, the dynamic reacquisition of the center of mass will be affected, and the overall gait pattern will be negatively affected.

This less efficient gait pattern results in an increase in energy expenditure because the body will need to find a "work around" - since the most efficient pattern is not attainable. This results in compensations. Worse yet, those compensations have the potential to lead to either overuse injuries or insidious onset type injuries. Wolf's Law and Davis's Law - essentially that tissue will adapt to the stresses placed upon it- begin to cause the body to structurally adapt to these new compensations because of the habituation principle. This combination leads individuals down a path that is in a bad direction.

Note- The female winner of the 2014 Oklahoma City Memorial Marathon (Camille Herron) displayed a gait pattern that is far from text book. During the final few miles, the commentators and the race expert were discussing how some runners have gait patterns that look fluid and effortless while others (specifically Camille Herron) look much less technical and much more "painful". She has found a training method and a running technique that works for her. She also is a professional runner. Poor mechanics do not necessarily equal bad results - but it does increase the likelihood of problems.

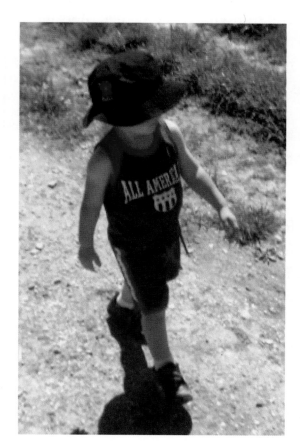
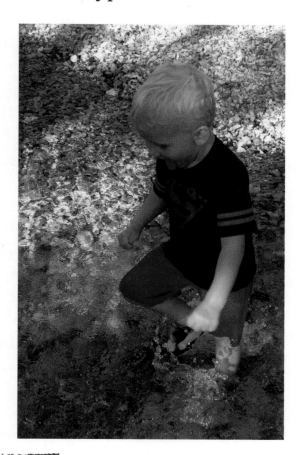

Video Links

Cruising- http://youtu.be/NfDhRcim7d4
Early Gait- http://youtu.be/ADes02x53BQ

BEYOND FUNCTIONAL PATTERNS

The NDS does not stop once a child reaches the walking stage. Walking is just the entry point to interacting and moving through the world in the most efficient manner possible. Bipedal gait and quadrupedal gate are distinctively different, and this is one defining characteristic of being human. Humans use their legs to get them to a location or into a position to use their upper extremities for a variety of purposes. Once the NDS moves beyond the functional level ("Beyond Functional") the complexity of the patterns utilized in the standing posture significantly increase in difficulty. These beyond functional patterns are:

- mature gait (98% display this by age four)
- running (emerges around age 3; mature running displayed between the ages of 6-10)
- galloping (43% accomplish this by age four)
- hopping (33% accomplish this by age four)
- skipping (14% accomplish this by age four)
- jumping (first displayed as jumping off low objects at around 22 months)
- throwing (begins between 2 and 4 years old)
- catching
- striking (initially vertical striking is seen; horizontal striking begins around age 5-6)
- climbing
- kicking (knee extended/little body movement around 2-3 years; knee flexion at 3-4 years; forceful kicking around 5-6 years)
- tumbling
- hanging

These patterns are developed because the healthy child continues to experience physical growth, improvement in coordination of motor skills and most importantly an energetic zest for play and activity. These patterns and activity allow the child to continue to refine how their body moves and responds and interacts with their environment; they continue to experience learning through these more challenging tasks.

The interesting part of how these patterns develop is how they affect what the child chooses to do as they get older and move into adolescence and even adulthood. These Beyond Functional patterns that initially are forms of learning, refinement, and play are truly the foundation of what is seen as "sport" or "athletics" in the older child. Any skill seen in any sport, is really just a combination of the Beyond Functional patterns. The biggest difference, is in sport implements (courts, balls, bats, sticks, etc) and more importantly rules. Jumping is jumping regardless of whether is is a 4 year old jumping in a puddle of water, an college football player jumping to catch a pass, a gymnast jumping to mount the balance beam, or a martial artist jumping to deliver a specialized strike. The act of leaving the ground requires the same things regardless of rules and age, what happens when the temporary flight is taking place determines the context of the jump.

This is important in regards to "Sport-specific" and "functional" training and rehab. Sport-specific and Functional are more reflective of successful marketing terms than successful training plans. They sell very well. Their effectiveness is best left to be judged by the number of athletes that are injured (or remain injured) and that receive scholarships to play at higher levels. But they generate a significant cash-flow from parents looking to get their child the edge they need to retain the title of Little League MVP. The problem, is that often times these philosophies are applied to adolescents. Based on the development of the typical child, the following stages of development serve as great arguments ***AGAINST*** sport specific or functional training and support focusing on these basic developmental skills:

- Children do not master running, throwing or catching until the ages of 6-10 years old. (Bertoti 2004, Cech 2012)
- Reaction times remain fairly constant in children until the ages of 8 or 9 years old, and do not reach adult levels until 16-17 years old. (Bertoti 2004)
- Mature depth perception is not present until the age of 12. (Cech 2012)
- Children do not develop the ability to accurately track moving objects until 5-10 years of age. (Cech 2012)
- Spatial awareness does not begin to develop until the ages of 6-12. (Cech 2012)

- Adult levels of vestibular function relative to postural control in standing do not reach adult levels until the age of 15. (Cech 2012)

Unfortunately, well-intentioned adults get in the way of normal development by instituting adult rules, to their child's play much too early. No T-ball team is "Elite" or "Select" no matter how good they are. Kids need to play, kids need to make the rules of their play. Adults need to sit back, watch, learn from, and enjoy what is occurring in front of them when their children are taking part in play. Surprisingly, a large group of kids around the same age left alone will develop their own games with their own rules.

At the same time every high school, collegiate, and adult athlete should be able to effectively and efficiently display these beyond functional patterns. However, years of specializing tend to degrade the ability to perform these basic, foundational skills. Just like the NDS from breathing to gait can serve as a roadmap to restore lost movement, the beyond functional patterns can serve as a roadmap to restore lost sport skills and improve athletic performance.

Climbing

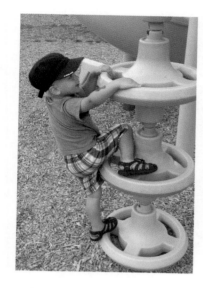 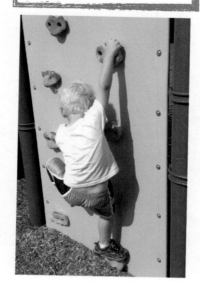 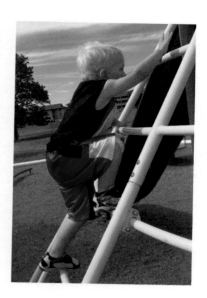

Running

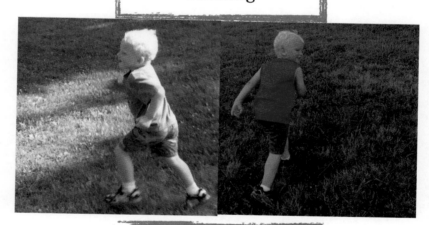

Carrying

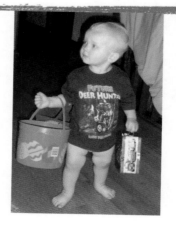

Throwing

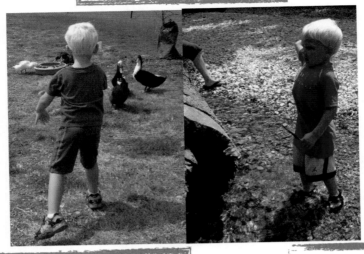

Jumping - Down First

Jumping

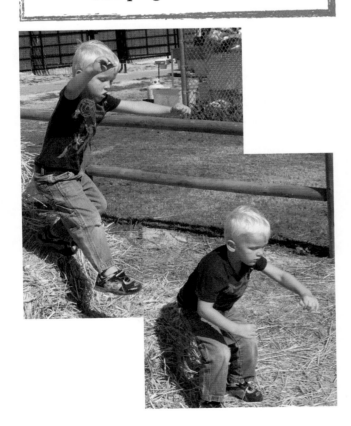

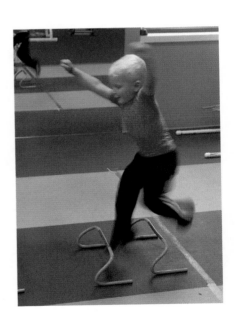

Striking

Striking

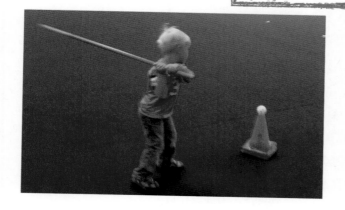
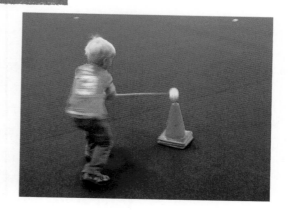

Hanging

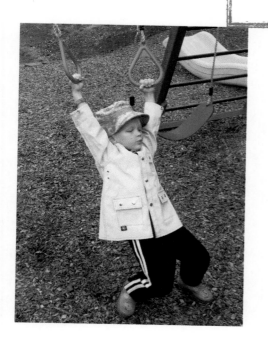
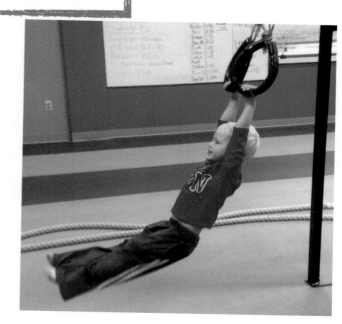

Video Links

Climbing- http://youtu.be/7NOubCrZjDA
More Climbing- http://youtu.be/rORErsevMDE
Even more Climbing- http://youtu.be/ZxFUUt9VT7Q
Brachiation/hanging- http://youtu.be/DLFX0-CVQAc
Jumping- http://youtu.be/DUA1wobJjL4
Catching/Throwing- http://youtu.be/3KqXw3uVFA0
Carrying- http://youtu.be/MzmOWhL8EZQ
Running- http://youtu.be/x0-gD-IR8a0
Balance Beam- http://youtu.be/QXQtCcvtvYM

NDS WRAP UP

The neurodevelopmental sequence continues all the way into the second decade of life, however the final 18 years of development pale in comparison to the first 2 years. Never again will the degree and level of changes - both physically and neurologically - be comparable to everything that takes place in the first 2 years of life. The first 2 years establish the foundation that all cognitive learning, motor learning, social skills, language skills, and athletic skills are built upon.

With all of this in mind, the NDS acts as an overlooked -but consistent- roadmap to restore lost movement. Movement can be lost due to several factors:

- injury
- stroke
- trauma
- illness
- habit (or poor habits)
- aging
- training errors

Two pertinent quotes that apply specifically to the treatment of injury and pain come from the text Musculoskeletal Interventions:

> *"The developmental sequence has provided the most consistent base for almost all approaches used by therapists" (Voight, Hoogenboom et al. 2007).*

> *"Since motor control is acquired during the developmental sequence, when motor control is adversely affected, a recapitulation of the sequence may be the most effective means of reestablishing control" (Voight, Hoogenboom et al. 2007).*

When the NDS is allowed to progress normally or is restored after movement patterns are lost, the functional skills and sport-specific skills are able to be successfully and safely layered on top of this solid movement foundation. When there are alterations or restrictions within the NDS that are not addressed or ignored, and "functional rehab" is performed, this solid base of movement is not present. "Functional" and "Sport Specific" rehab and training have grown exponentially in popularity over the past few years without the same level of growth, respect, or education within the therapeutic and training communities. This approach, in the absence of a solid foundation rooted in quality movement only leads to further problems.

One emphasis here is to redefine the term "Functional". Functional is purposeful. Therefore, the true meaning of functional movement is essentially movement with a purpose - not what is erroneously referred to as "functional" by those in the world of marketing. The purpose here is to as efficiently as possible restore movement and then restore strength and finally restore "function". To do that, the assessments outlined later in this text are focused on establishing a functional classification (or diagnosis for the medical professionals). This functional classification can then be utilized to establish a corrective strategy once quality movement has been established. This functional classification can aid in the efficiency of the strengthening philosophy. One avenue of this that will be addressed in greater detail later is the idea of addition by subtraction - improving strength by temporarily removing those activities/lifts that cause more harm than good.

> **Video Link**

NDS Transitions: http://youtu.be/K-_HGFqcT_g

For Medical Professionals

A medical diagnosis is physiologically or anatomically based, which leads to rehabilitation protocols that are time based. The medical diagnosis is valuable in determining contraindications to the therapeutic protocol, but not in guiding the choices within the protocol. A functional diagnosis identifies the primary dysfunction that the rehabilitation protocol needs to be geared toward correcting (Voight, Hoogenboom et al. 2007). For example, the medical diagnosis patellofemoral compression syndrome (PFCS) does a great job in identifying the irritated structures. But, how does someone treat this? There are easily 15-20 different reasons why this area of the body can be irritated. Without a functional diagnosis, randomly picking which of the 20 causes gives the clinician a 5% chance of selecting the actual cause - not the greatest odds, especially in the world of ever rising healthcare costs.

Understanding the NDS allows the clinician that has identified the functional diagnosis to know where their interventions need to be focused in order to restore foundational movement. Without understanding the NDS, the framework on which the interventions are based is likely to be flawed, which will have a negative effect on the clinical outcome.

For Non-Medical Professionals

Establishing a functional classification for clients with training goals is vital to the success of that client. The primary concern is to determine if a client has health problems or fitness problems - to determine if they are in pain or if they are pain free. The first layer of the Screen that will be discussed later in this text is to filter out pain and direct it appropriately to a medical professional. Pain always indicates a health problem and in many cases is outside of the scope of almost every coach, trainer, and fitness professional. Having a client address their health problems first will ensure a better experience for everyone involved.

Establishing a functional classification also determines a great starting point for every client. Quality movement improves efficiency of all higher level movements. Good quality movement can make strength training much more effective and result in better outcomes just by the fact that addressing movement problems will get that client out of their own way - it will take the parking break off.

The NDS in Adults

The progression of the NDS occurs in children regardless of what parents' or caregivers' do to speed it up or slow it down. Certain environmental triggers can alter the rate of the NDS (nutrition, atmosphere) and the caregivers can be very influential in the rate the NDS proceeds - more from how they provide stimulus and learning opportunities for the children than anything else. But, how does the NDS affect, or influence adults? Recently, a shift in the thought process of the ability of the brain to change has taken place (Doidge 2007) (Blakeslee 2008) (Ramachandran 2011). This shift in thinking has opened the door to understanding that the brain remains plastic (open to permanent changes in structure, and function) for the entire life span. This characteristic of plasticity is very important for understanding adults capacity for dramatic changes in many areas.

Adults have a lifetime of compensations that result in drastic changes in movement from when they were children with authentic movement patterns. The freedom of mobility that children are born with disappears in most adults, and positions that are simple for children to get into are impossible for adults to match. Once mobility changes occur, changes in stability happen, changes in motor control take place, and movement takes a turn for the worse. The result is adults with basic movement problems that are trying to function at very high levels.

The NDS can serve as a roadmap for those individuals that have lost movement quality and lived a life of stacking movement quantity on top of a poor base. Unfortunately, this describes most people, regardless of activity or athletic level. Quantity has always trumped quality, until recently. Functional Movement Systems introduced the Functional Movement Screen (FMS) to the world in the late 1990's. This was the introduction of assessing movement quality in a manner where there was actual objective data. This will be discussed in greater detail in a later chapter. Regardless of age, training level, activity level, or anything else movement is universal. How movement develops is universal. Unfortunately, many professionals in the fitness and medical industry have attempted to develop their own "greatest" way to fix and teach movement. A quick observance of the US general population will show how successful this has been. The framework for fixing and restoring movement has been with everyone from birth - it has just been pushed to the back of the mind. The NDS is the framework in which movement originally develops, and can serve as the framework to restore poor quality movement. The NDS is -regardless of age- a hierarchy of movement sequence that can be traveled on in both directions. In the infant, movement difficulty progresses. In anyone that has poor movement quality, movement difficulty can be regressed. The NDS is not a one way street - it flows in both directions. The thing to keep in mind when considering the NDS in those beyond the age of 5 is that movement quality has likely been adversely affected by life - the mobility everyone was blessed with has likely been lost to some extent, which then alters the entire Mobility/Stability/Motor Control spectrum.

The Mobility / Stability / Motor Control Spectrum

Developmentally, mobility precedes stability and stability comes before motor control and strength. Infants are mobile from the onset, and gradually develop the ability to stabilize which then leads to the performance of purposeful movement as motor control is established. In terms of progression, development occurs from the head to the toe, the spine to the fingertips, and deep to superficial. This directly correlates with the development of the Central Nervous System and the myelination of the peripheral nervous system.

Elements of mobility and stability interact continuously to produce movements. It is not an either / or scenario - both need to work together seamlessly to produce the desired outcome. Mobility and stability are dependent upon limb length, joint architecture, soft tissue quality, passive restraints and the level of motor control that is present. Mobility can essentially be thought of as the freedom, or degree of movement. Stability is how one uses or controls the mobility they possess. Motor Control is the constant interplay between mobility and stability in the presence of purposeful movement. The sequencing of the NDS is about developing stability in different postures (the mobility is already present) which then allows motor control to be established in different patterns. To quote McGill (McGill 2004):

> *"The muscular and motor control system must satisfy the requirements to sustain postures, create movements, brace against sudden motion or unexpected forces, build pressure, and assist challenged breathing, all while ensuring sufficient stability. Virtually all muscles play a role in ensuring stability, but their importance at any point in time is determined by the unique combination of the demands just listed. Training a single muscle, or at least focusing on the activation of a single muscle leads to dysfunction."*

The motor control continuum requires mobility and stability to be balanced - adequate stability must be present to control the mobility that is present. Some activities will require more of one or the other, but there must be a finely balanced interaction between the two in order for smooth, effortless, efficient movement to occur. Individuals need enough mobility to move through the fundamental movement postures and patterns uninhibited, and they need sufficient stability to move through the fundamental postures and patterns under control.

The balance between mobility and stability is dictated and controlled by the nervous system. Having full mobility does not just allow for a greater range of motion, but it insures adequate quality sensory input to be present. Keep in mind, movement is a behavior and the quantity and quality of input into the system is what dictates the output from the system - in this case movement. When sensory input is diminished, the resulting movement will also be adversely affected. Think of how hard it is to talk, eat, or drink after visiting the dentist when you have had a shot to numb the pain from the filling they put in. The shot was an analgesic medication - it decreased the sensory input from the area, and had not affect on the ability of the muscles to contract. Not having any sensory input from the area, makes those simple activities quite hard. The same principle applies to movement - without adequate sensory input, spatial awareness is affected, the sense of body awareness is affected, and movement becomes even more challenging.

The same progression - mobility precedes stability which leads to motor control - applies to movement restoration There cannot be barriers, or mobility restrictions, to the movement patterns without there being stability and motor control problems. Barriers to optimal mobility can come in many forms: pain, capsular restrictions, tissue adhesions, inadequate muscle length, hyper-tonic muscles, or scar tissue can all impede mobility. The presence of mobility restrictions require resetting optimal mobility before reinforcing the movement with stability. Notice here the descriptor chose was 'optimal' not perfect. To quote Brett Jones again, "Better is better". Chasing perfect mobility in most people will be a never ending chase.

Once optimal mobility is reset, stability is reinforced and motor control of the movement pattern can be reloaded. Infants are born with mobility, but must gain their stability. In adults, mobility has to be restored before stability can be gained. Then the stability has to be established from head to toe and midline out. This is a key principle of the NDS that applies directly to the Movement

Restoration philosophy: re-establish the deep spinal reflexive stabilization in order to establish a solid base for well-coordinated movements. Stable postures provide the base for all movement patterns.

Final words on the NDS

The NDS is **THE** roadmap for establishing and restoring movement. The principles that allow the NDS to occur in the manner in which it does are the same principles that can be utilized once quality movement is lost:

- Mobility before stability before Motor Control
- Head to toe, midline out progressions
- Stable, sequential postures for patterns to operate off of
- Movement is a behavior
- Breathing is the Keystone of Movement
- Grip is an indicator of the CNS and influences everything
- Simple to complex
- Ground up control
- The Ground and Gravity are very influential

Leonardo Da Vinci is credited with the saying *"Simplicity is the ultimate sophistication"*. The NDS is a very obvious expression of this - it results in a high level of movement competency, but is very basic and very simple. The complexity and the application of the NDS have virtually gone unnoticed by all but a very select few. In a recent grant proposal submitted to the NATA that was designed to investigate the NDS and the aging process in regards to fall prevention, grip was one of the measures that was going to be measured. To quote the expert reviewer, that recommended this proposal be denied because of its limited relevance: "Not clear why grip is done". They go on to state:

> *"The same sequence in which an infant explores, discovers, and interacts with their environment to develop movement is present in every person regardless of age* (from the proposal). *However, the elderly are not 'learning' the movement, it is not novel to them. This is a theoretical flaw* (reviewers comment)."

What this unknowing expert is missing in regards to classifying this as a theoretical flaw is the process of plasticity. Humans are always learning - humans ability to learn is another aspect of survival. Like was mentioned before, every movement either reinforces a good pattern of movement or strengthens a bad pattern of movement - over time this is habituation. While in one breath the expert reviewer states that the "elderly are not learning movement" in the next he states "it is not novel to them". The definition of novel is "new or unusual in an interesting way" (Merriam-Webster Inc. 2005). The reviewer is slightly misguided in their understanding of development, every day everyone is learning movement for their entire lifespan - the elderlies movement is new to them everyday. It is a progressive decline that every day gradually gets worse; it is a regression of the NDS. Reviewing the principles outlined earlier in this section can be life changing when applied to the elderly population.

PART 2
Assessing Movement Quality

Historically, clinicians have used a symptom and impairment focused approach to injury assessment and treatment. This approach is based on the belief that the painful tissues and local impairments are the source of the problems. The goal of this type of evaluation is to identify the anatomical tissues that are symptomatic and collect objective measurements of the resulting impairments. Treatment plans are then directed at resolving the problem by relieving the symptoms and impairments associated with the medical diagnosis. From the perspective of a strength coach, having a medical diagnosis gives little direction or clarity in what can or cannot be done from a training perspective. This results in a overall restriction from activity which is frustrating for everyone involved. Two separate languages are being spoken.

There are established standards or normative numbers for range of motion at every joint. Strength measures are a little different and less able to be truly standardized (due to age depend, sex, training age, sport, etc) but even here coaches typically have norms for their athletes based on all these factors. In either instance, it is easy to see when someone is where they need to be, or if they are doing poorly. Looking at movement has typically been much more subjective. A running joke -that bears quite a bit of truth- is "I don't know what good is, but I do know what bad is". There are so many variables within any movement, that making it objective can be quite challenging. In the mid 1990's the Functional Movement Screen (FMS) was developed. It is a screen made up of seven basic movements and three clearing tests that begins to objectify movement based on a 4 point scoring system (0-3) and objective minimum criteria for each movement. It is a simple screen that is beginning to finally be supported by research - until recently, those opposed to the FMS pointed out flaws with the screen that revolved around reliability and a lack of clinical research studies. There are several other tools out there that have been developed to assess movement - the National Academy of Sports Medicine has developed their own assessment tool that looks at different large movements and incorporates goniometer measurements. Certain individual practitioners have established their own set of assessment tools (Craig Leibenson's Magnificent 7, Stu McGills Back assessment) that all work well and have been successful for them. The key point is that there needs to be a concrete way to asses movement.

The rest of this text will relate movement to the FMS, and the SFMA (the clinical version of the FMS for medical practitioners). The simplicity of each tool and the reliability of each, along with the philosophy behind each tool serve as the reason for these being the tool of choice moving forward. With the traditional approach, focus has been placed on the involved anatomical structures and the immediate surrounding area. Some will take the liberty of looking at the joints above or below, which is a great way to expand the vision of what is going on but why stop at 1 joint distinct? Why not two or three? Why limit it at all? Little or no attention is directed towards the rest of the body and its involvement to the injury situation.

Pain

Before moving any further, there needs to be a section on pain. Pain changes everything - from a movement perspective (this is one of Gray Cooks most famous sayings) but also from an intervention perspective. Pain serves as the line in the sand. When pain is present, further testing is needed by medical professionals. What exactly is pain is typically the next question. The International Association for the Study of Pain defines pain as *"an unpleasant sensory and emotional experience associated with actual or potential tissue damage, or described in terms of such damage"*. They take the explanation even further, going on to state that pain is ALWAYS a subjective psychological experience (Delforge 2002). Pain obviously has its physical components, but there is always a deeper layer of subjectivity associated with it that can blur the entire picture. It truly is not as simple as it appears on the surface. Because of this, only those medical professionals specifically trained in treating pain (MD's, ATC's, PT's OT's, DO's, DC's) and licensed by the State they practice in should treat pain. Everyone not listed has both a professional and ethical (and in most States a LEGAL) responsibility to refer those in pain to qualified medical professionals.

Pain is most often viewed as the primary problem in western medicine: eliminate the pain and the problem will be eliminated. The traditional rehabilitation efforts have been directed at eliminating the symptoms of pain. Pain, however, is not the problem - it is the "check engine light" that alerts us to problems that should be addressed. The biggest shift in looking at pain, is that because of the intricacies in what makes up pain it needs to be looked at as an output from the brain - not input to the brain. In many cases, an individuals pain is caused by compensations or impairments elsewhere in the body that results in excessive stress being placed on the structures that become painful - unless there are actual, acute structural problems (ACL tear, lateral ankle sprain, fractures, etc). The focus of most efforts to relieve pain is placed on identifying and addressing the painful structures. Pain following injury typically arrises out of one or more factors:

1. Pain that is site-specific to the injured part, as a result of trauma and the associated inflammation that ensues. Typically, this results from the

chemicals associated with the inflammatory phase of the healing process as well as the actual tissue trauma.

2. Pain generated by mobility restrictions in outlying regions, leading to movement barriers that force compensations and poor movement patterns (shoulder impingement, anterior ankle impingement, etc).

3. Pain generated by stability defects in outlying regions, leading to barriers that causes compensations and poor movement patterns which leads to altered stress on tissues (anterior knee pain, low back pain, etc).

4. Pain generated because of physical, structural, or functional limitations (scar tissue formation, trigger points, changes in tissue quality).

5. Pain generated by faulty alignment of joints (habitually changed posture)

6. Pain generated by limited or changed structural alignment (habitually changed posture).

Of these six reasons that pain can exist in the body, only one (number one above) is the result of actual or real tissue damage. The other five result from the compensatory strategies that the body takes to meet movement needs presented to it each day - NOT ACTUAL TISSUE DAMAGE. In *The Brain That Changes Itself (Doidge 2007)*, there are two fascinating quotes in regards to pain:

> *"Pain is an opinion of the organism's state of health rather than a mere reflexive response to injury"*

> *"...the prawn preempts the mistaken movement by triggering pain the moment before the movement takes place. What better way for the brain to prevent movement than to make sure the motor command itself triggers pain."*

Changing Focus

Human behavior can be boiled down to two very basic desires - Seek pleasure and avoid pain. Pain avoidance is vital in everyday life, it serves a larger point. Pain avoidance in movement may prevent pain in the short term, but will always led to more pain later on. Finding pain, addressing the behavior that leads to the pain, and then correcting this behavior (READ THAT AGAIN - it does not say 'fix the pain') will begin to lead to resolving the true source of pain. The ability to to do this is extremely dependent on being able to subjectively assess movement.

Over the past two decades, more emphasis has been placed on taking a "Functional" approach when resolving pain and/or fixing movement. While this has been a step in the right direction, it has essentially taken place without a well thought out plan or a map to guide the journey. There are well established quantitative norms for most physical measures, but like mentioned earlier movement has been left out of this. The attempt to take functional approach with activities was done without having a means to assess the quality of the individual function to begin with and more importantly without there being a true understanding of how those "functional" movements develop. A recent article discusses the importance of how higher levels skills are taught and acquired based on the NDS outlined earlier in this text.

> *"It is important to understand that development is sequential in nature, and this sequence of maturation and development should be the basis for developing a training strategy" (Myer, Kushner et al. 2013).*

The moat obvious mistake that has been made with the functional approach is that the emphasis has been placed increasing the challenge, level of difficulty, or similarity to the activity without any consideration for the fundamentals. Higher level skills are based on lower level proficiency. Remember back to the NDS sequence - walking will never be accomplished without adequate time in prone, supine, quadruped, seated, and standing postures. Functional will never be accomplished without basic movement skills- skipping, galloping, hopping, etc, and this is assuming that the fundamental skills have set the stage for these higher level activities to develop.

The FMS and the Selective Functional Movement Assessment (SFMA) provide a standard or assessing fundamental movement based on basic and fundamental movement patterns. This allows for a broad view of the individual to be established and to use a global assessment strategy to determine the overall picture of the individual. Instead of coming to, and treating a medical diagnosis a functional diagnosis can be determined. Emphasis is not placed on identifying the anatomical location of the symptoms, but rather is placed on identifying and addressing the cause of these symptoms. This approach requires accepting and believing that the body is one functional unit where everything must work together well in order for the body to function correctly. Thomas Myers text *Anatomy Trains* is a great example of how the body should be viewed under this new mindset.

"Where do I start?"

Answering this question must first begin with an understanding of where the end point, the final goal, is. The end goal of any Movement Restoration Program should be to optimize they individual ability to move, control their body, produce force, and reduce force during their chosen activity. Arriving at the end point is accomplished by improving the individuals ability to move through and control basic movement patterns. The question of "where do I start" is answered by the simple, yet profound statement of "wherever you are". In other words, where is the individual in the NDS? Specifically, in what postures and patterns are they having problems? The appropriate place to begin is the earliest point at which problems within the NDS are seen. How is that determined? This is reason number two why the FMS and the SFMA were chosen as the Movement Restoration assessment tools. The FMS does have a direct correlation to the NDS:

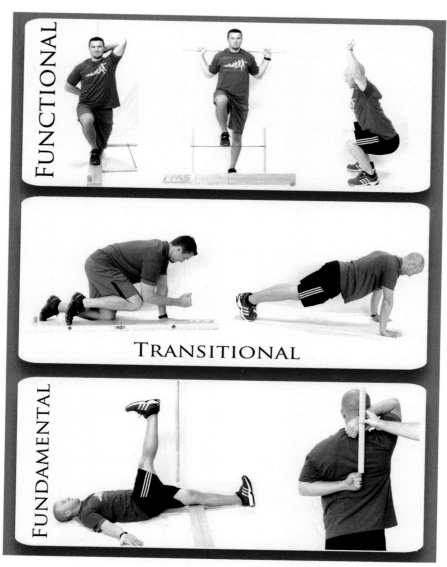

FIGURE 2.0 - THE FMS

FMS Movement	Postural Level	NDS Posture	NDS Pattern
Active Straight Leg Raise	Fundamental	Supine	Reaching of the limbs
Shoulder Mobility	Fundamental	Prone	Reaching of the limbs
Rotary Stability	Transitional	Quadruped	Reaching of the limbs, rolling, crawling
Trunk Stability Push up	Transitional	Prone	Pushing down
Deep Squat	Functional	Symmetrical Stance	Squatting
In line Lunge	Functional	Asymmetrical Stance	Pushing down, crawling
Hurdle Stance	Functional	Single Leg Stance	Reaching of the limbs

FIGURE 2.1 - THE FMS AND THE NDS

The SFMA is not as clear-cut in how it ties into the different postural levels as the FMS is. In essence, the entire movement must be considered - while the Multi-segmental flexion test occurs in the standing posture, the test is looking at the ability for gross flexion and hip hinging to occur. This is best seen developmentally during the transitional phase of development.

Back to the question of where to start - starting from wherever you are is always the appropriate option. However, as strength coach Dan John quickly points out - "Everyone seems to know where their point B (their goal) is. Not many people know where their point A is." Knowing where the starting point is, and what obstacles or speed bumps may lie in the way is the key to determining the plan of care - or the training plan - for each person. The absolute best way to do this is with the FMS or the SFMA.

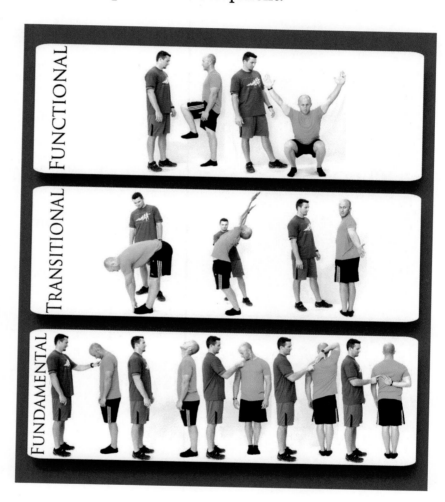

FIGURE 2.2 - THE SFMA

Just like the FMS, the SFMA does have a direct correlation to the NDS:

SFMA Movement	Postural Level	NDS Posture	NDS Pattern
Cervical Flexion	Fundamental	Supine	Head control/ Flexion
Cervical Extension	Fundamental	Prone	Head control/ Extension
Cervical Rotation	Fundamental	Prone/Supine	Head control/ Rolling
Shoulder patterns	Fundamental	Prone	Reaching of the limbs
Multi-Segmental Flexion	Transitional	Supine	Hinging
Multi-Segmental Extension	Transitional	Prone	Hinging
Multi-Segmental Rotation	Transitional	Prone/supine	Rolling
Single Leg Stance	Functional	Stance	Rolling
Deep Squat	Functional	Stance	Squatting

FIGURE 2.3 THE SFMA AND THE NDS

The "Protocol"

This entire project began with the task of creating an ACL and Shoulder surgery protocol for a group of physicians so that every rehab clinic they sent their patients to could have the same clinical outcomes as Mercy Sports Medicine. They wanted a global protocol to cover everything that was easy to follow and guaranteed everyone would achieve the desired outcome. This was a daunting task, that lead to what has to be the simplest and easy to apply protocol ever - Assuming those applying it have the requisite level of needed education. The process to determine specifically where each persons 'Point A' is, is as follows:

1. Assess and identify the Movement Problem(s) using either the FMS or SFMA.
   a. Is it a Mobility / Stability / or Motor Control Problem - or is it all of the above.
   b. What is the appropriate Postural Level to begin with.
   c. What is the appropriate Pattern to target.
   d. Is the beginning point Static or Dynamic.

Once the beginning point is determined, based on what has been gathered through the assessment, moving forward with interventions can begin:

2. **Reset** the NDS Postures by removing mobility and/or soft tissue restrictions.
3. **Reinforce** the NDS Patterns by improving the stability at each NDS Posture.
4. **Reload** the appropriate NDS patterns at the appropriate NDS posture by layering on strengthening drills.
5. Strengthen the new movement patterns.

The Three Levels of Posture
"Good movement control requires good postural control."

Development of purposeful movement in a gravity-rich environment proceeds through three distinct levels of postural requirements that have been mentioned previously. As an infant moves through the NDS, he or she progressively develops strategies for stability in progressively more demanding postures. Each postural level requires more complex and coordinated programing on the part of the central nervous system, further adding to the stability and motor control demands of the particular movement. The three levels of posture are:

1. **Fundamental** - This consists of supine, prone, and side-lying. In the fundamental posture, the body is supported by the ground with minimal postural stabilization demands placed on the CNS. It is in this postural level that the infant - born with full mobility and freedom of movement but no way to control it - begins to explore their environment and develop stability. As stability develops, less support from the ground is needed.

2. **Transitional** - This entails all the postures after the fundamental level, but before the functional level. This includes progressively more challenging postures, where less stabilization is provided by the ground and more demand is placed on the CNS to overcome gravity. Transitional postures include a wide variety of positions including quadruped, sitting, and kneeling.

3. **Functional** - These are the vertical, weight bearing postures that give rise to bipedal gait. These are the variations of vertical stance - symmetrical stance (the feet are aligned in the same positions), asymmetrical stance (the feet are NOT aligned in the same positions), and single leg stance (one foot is off the ground).

Both the FMS and the SFMA were designed -either with intent, or by accident- to screen and assess movement in each of the three levels of posture. If defects are seen in the fundamental levels, it stands to reason that these problems will exist to some degree in the higher levels of posture. However, stability is posture specific. This means that within each postural level, the strategies to establish a stable platform are different due to differing body positions, differing influences of gravity, and a different orientation of the head. Because of this, stability that is established in one posture CANNOT be assumed to fix stability problems in other (either higher or lower) postural levels, but it can serve as a foundation to progressively establish stability across all three postural levels. For example establishing stability for someone in a supine posture will not likely affect their bad squatting pattern, even though the supine posture is the starting point of the squat. If that gained stability in supine is then trained in quadruped and then trained in the kneeling or sitting postures, and then addressed in vertical stance the likelihood that the squatting pattern will be improved is much higher - assuming the protocol from earlier is followed as the guide to the interventions.

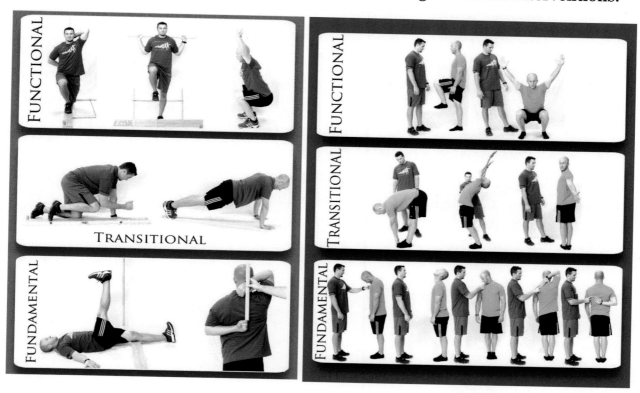

FIGURE 2.4 - THE FMS AND THE SFMA POSTURAL LEVELS

The Assessment Process Explained

The goal of the assessment process is to establish the individuals 'Point A' and for the clinical/strength coach to gather the most complete perspective on the quality of the individuals movement *capabilities* (not movement *capacities* - these are tested with traditional performance based test: vertical jump, 40 yard sprint, strength tests, etc). In both the clinical world and the performance world this requires a shift from the traditional process of evaluation where the goals have been:

- Clinically - Determine the Structure that is affected
- Performance - Determine the performance weaknesses

This "shift" begins with assessing the movement quality prior to any further testing. This altered approach begins with determining what movement patterns are problematic which then allows the rest of the testing to dig deeper as to why they are affected (if needed. In certain worlds, the 'why' is not as important, especially if the goal is to get stronger or move faster and pain is not part of the equation). Once the FMS or the SFMA (if pain is present) is performed, further testing (either clinical testing -ROM, MMT, Special testing, etc.- or performance testing can be performed as is appropriate based on the movement quality of the individual).

In short, the FMS alerts the tester to the presence of mobility or stability issues, and determines the need for further evaluation (as needed). The SFMA directed the clinician towards the location of the mobility, stability or motor control issues that are causing the pain or compensations that are discovered.

FMS - A deeper explanation of how to use it in the Clinical Setting.

This section is specifically targeted at the clinical individuals who can legally treat pain. However, the information is good for everyone to understand how the clinician is utilizing the FMS so that a common language can be spoken once a referral network has been established between providers.

The FMS was designed to be used in the healthy population to identify movement pattern impairments that can be predictive of injury. In the hands of the properly trained individual, the FMS can be invaluable in guiding exercise prescription. In the hands of a properly trained clinician, the FMS can effectively be used within the clinical setting where the ultimate goal is to return an injured athlete/ individual to their sport. **HOWEVER, once again this distinction will be pointed out - treating pain, and resolving pain are legally left to those Healthcare professionals that are educated, trained and *licensed to practice medicine*.** In selective clinical situations, when used appropriately, the FMS is a very helpful first step in the evaluation process. These select clinical situations are:

- When the patient is not complaining of pain at the time -meaning, they present for their evaluation but are not complaining of pain currently but have pain with certain activities only.
- When the patients pain is "chronic" or has an "insidious" onset of pain.
- When any patient is being returned back to activity.

The FMS is not appropriate in these clinical situations:

- When the patient is complaining of pain at the moment.
- In acute injury situations (ankle sprain, etc).
- When swelling is present.
- Following a surgical procedure - until full ROM is restored and pain is resolved.

Using the FMS allows the clinician to determine how the individual moves through the fundamental movement patterns and begins to clarify whether the patients complaints are based on mobility or stability issues. The things to keep in mind for the clinician using the FMS is that the FMS only answers the following questions:

1. Are there mobility issues?
2. Are there stability issues?
3. Is there pain present with the movement or the clearing tests?

It is important to understand that the FMS does not attempt to answer the question of WHERE or WHY the individuals have mobility or stability issues. Those questions can be answered later with the SFMA or the clinically indicated impairment tests that may be needed. Clinically, another thing to keep in mind is that if the FMS is going to be performed, all of the FMS needs to be performed as it is described. Meaning, do not modify the FMS. The beauty of the FMS is in its simple sophistication - the FMS has built in redundancies that will pick up issues that may have been subtle or missed on one portion, but are obvious in others. Modifying the FMS or changing the FMS means that it is no longer the FMS. The redundancies built into the FMS include looking at movement patterns in many different ways.

Movement Pattern Redundancies		
Hip Extension	5 tests	DS, HS, ILL, RS, ASLR
Hip Flexion	4 tests	DS, HS, ILL, ASLR
Shoulder Extension	3 tests	ILL, RS, SM
Shoulder Flexion	4 tests	ILL, DS, RS, SM
Knee Extension	3 tests	DS, HS, ILL
Knee Flexion	4 tests	DS, HS, ILL, RS
Elbow Extension	3 tests	DS, TSPU, RS
Elbow Flexion	3 tests	SM, TSPU, RS
Ankle Dorsiflexion	3 tests	DS, ILL, HS
Wrist Extension	2 tests	DS, HS

FIGURE 2.5 - FMS REDUNDANCIES (COOK 2010)

Clinicians utilize the FMS with a broader background in anatomy, assessment, impairments, and injury physiology than most individuals who utilize the screen.

This is actually the BIGGEST problem when using the FMS in the clinical setting. While the FMS is not designed to be a diagnostic tool, when placed in the hands of a healthcare provider that treats pain, the line gets blurry. When used by someone trained in how to assess injuries, a "diagnostic mindset" often gets applied to the FMS. This does not mean that diagnostic thinking should be applied to the FMS, or that clinicians can get more information out of the screen. No matter who uses the screen, it only gives information on mobility, stability, and pain with movement. What this means is that the clinicians should have a deeper understanding of the information it does give them. Most importantly, it sheds light on the individuals movement patterns and provides a first glimpse into what needs further assessment. What must be in the forefront of the mind is that a **screen** *(the FMS)* is used to determine if further **assessment** *(the SFMA)* is needed, and an assessment is used to establish which specific **tests** *(diagnostic in nature)* warranted. To put it simply - use the screen as a screen.

If pain is discovered during the FMS, the situation changes slightly. The FMS algorithm directs any pain towards further evaluation by a medical professional. If a medical profession is applying the screen, the next step is a more specific assessment. Ideally, this is the SFMA, but can also be whatever clinically relevant diagnostic tests may be appropriate for the situation - this is left to clinical discretion.

The FMS and the SFMA: how do they work together?

"It's lack of clarity that creates chaos and frustration. Those emotions are poison to any living goal." -Steve Maraboli - Life, Truth, and Being Free.

Functional Movement Systems has done an excellent job of creating a standard operating procedure for assessing movement. They have essentially provided a tool to assess movement in any setting, situation, or instance - they bring clarity to the chaos of movement. But, just like any collection of tools there can be some confusion as to which tool is the best choice for the given situation. Situational appropriateness becomes an issue-which movement assessment is the most appropriate for the given situation. Unfortunately, the only one that can 100% answer the question is the person asking the question.

Often times, people disregard the FMS or the SFMA because of the confusion that develops from the gathered information (the FMS scores, or the SFMA classifications).

Gray Cooks text Movement (Cook 2010) established a framework to clarify this confusion, the *Six P's of Corrective Exercise:*
   4. *Pain*- is there pain with movement.
   5. *Purpose*- what is the target outcome.
   6. *Posture*-which posture is the best starting point (see the FMS/NDS or SFMA/NDS chart).
   7. *Position*-what position(s) demonstrate compensations.
   8. *Pattern*- how is the pattern affected by the corrective exercise.
   9. *Plan*- how can you design a corrective plan around the information you have.

Pain is the dividing line that establishes the distinction between the different movement tools - **if there is pain, the SFMA is _ALWAYS_ the correct tool.** When pain is present (unless it is pain from an acute injury), the only acceptable answer is to perform the SFMA (or refer out to someone qualified to do the

SFMA). The FMS or the Y-Balance Test are inappropriate to use. **If there is no pain, then either the FMS or the Y-Balance test are appropriate**. Rarely is it ever appropriate to intermix the FMS and the SFMA (meaning using both at the same time to determine a corrective strategy).

Often though, the SFMA and the FMS are used in sequence with each other with the line continuing to be pain. The SFMA will be the starting point for an individual presenting with pain, but at some point (when pain resolves) a transition to the FMS is warranted. Confusion occurs when clinicians try to fix a dysfunctional-painful pattern on the SFMA while concurrently trying to fix an asymmetry on the FMS. What results is frustration in the tools -the FMS and the SFMA- when the real problem is the fact that the clinician used the wrong tool.

The Y-Balance Test is also a great tool in the movement assessment tool box when the goal is performance training only (no injury, pain, etc). The beauty of the YBT is that it is extremely user friendly and requires no interpretation. It only identifies asymmetries from side-to-side and from normative values. If no asymmetries are present, move on to training focused on improving conditioning levels. If asymmetries are noted, at that point in time performing an FMS is the appropriate step to determine the best plan for corrective exercise.

Once the correct assessment tool is utilized, identify the most obvious movement problem first and place the individual into the most appropriate posture to start their corrective exercise. Progress them through the Movement Restoration Sequence until the targeted pattern has been improved. Reassess and continue to move forward with the tool that is the most correct for the situation, knowing that once pain is no longer an issue it is okay to move to the FMS. HOWEVER, if pain returns, moving back to the SFMA is also perfectly okay, and the responsible thing to do.

PART 3

The Movement Restoration Sequence

In the Movement Restoration Sequence, the interventions occur from the ground up and the head down/midline out - regardless of whether the FMS or the SFMA was utilized as the assessment tool.

"I never deal directly with the affected part or articulation of the body before I bring about improvements in the head-neck relationship and in breathing. In turn, improvement in the head and neck and in breathing cannot be achieved without correcting spine and thorax configuration. Again, to do this, the pelvis and abdomen must be connected."

Moshe Feldenkrais (Feldenkrais and Beringer 2010)

The FMS/SFMA Tie-in to the NDS

The creation of the FMS and later the SFMA was not directly based upon the principles of the NDS, but surprisingly follow those basic principles extremely well. Both tools have a basic fundamental mobility component, a transitional stability component, and a higher level motor control component. This allows the information that is gained from either assessment to be applied to the NDS to utilize from a decision making standpoint. All three areas (the NDS, the FMS, and the SFMA) are based on a hierarchy sequence of movement, which then serves as a roadmap to the direction that corrective exercise need to take place. The definition of corrective is "meant to correct a problem; intended to make something better" (Merriam-Webster Inc. 2005). The goal of the assessment is to determine what corrective strategy can best be utilized to make the individuals movement problem better - the ability to see the FMS and the SFMA from the perspective of the NDS serves as the best way to apply a corrective strategy in a sequential, hierarchical manner.

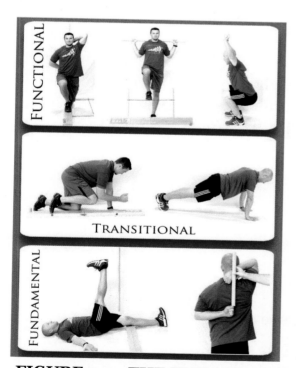 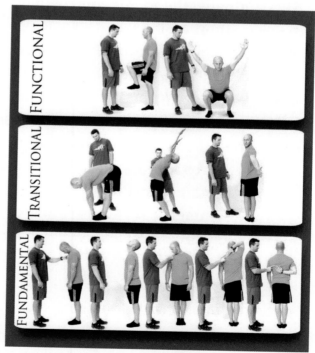

FIGURE 3.0 - THE FMS AND THE SFMA BASED ON THE NDS

The FMS Corrective Strategy

Recall the Protocol listed earlier in the text - this section will address specifically how to navigate through the process of restoring movement based on using the FMS as the assessment tool. The corrective hierarchy based on the FMS is (Cook 2010):

1. Active Straight Leg Raise (ASLR)
2. Shoulder Mobility (SM)
3. Rotary Stability (RS)
4. Trunk Stability Push up (TSPU)
5. In-Line Lunge (ILL)
6. Hurdle Step (HS)
7. Deep Squat (DS)

This relates back to the NDS - priority is assigned based on the mobility/stability/ motor control continuum and the postural levels. Top priority is given to the mobility tests and to the Fundamental postural levels (ASLR and SM). From there, priority goes to stability and the Transitional postural levels (RS and TSPU). Finally, the motor control and Functional postural levels (ILL, HS, DS) are given attention if needed. To determine which areas to target, the scoring of the FMS must be considered. Overall scores reveal little when determining a corrective strategy - a score of 14 can be achieved in many different ways. Looking at the individual scores is what reveals the most information and allows a better corrective strategy to be established (Loudon, Parkerson-Mitchell et al. 2014). The order of scoring importance is:

1. Scores of 0's need to be referred.
2. Asymmetrical 1's
3. Symmetrical 1's
4. Asymmetrical 2's
5. Symmetrical 2's

Based on all of this, the following score will serve as an example:

Test	Left	Right	Total
Deep Squat			1
Hurdle Step	2	3	2A
In-Line Lunge	2	2	2
Active Straight Leg Raise	1	3	1A
Shoulder Mobility	2	3	2A
Trunk Stability Push up			2
Rotary Stability	2	3	2A
TOTAL SCORE			12

FIGURE 3.1 FMS EXAMPLE 1

This screen would result in the ordering of correctives being:

1. ASLR
2. DS
3. SM
4. RS

In this instance, the general acceptance would be that there is a mobility problem with this person (even though the ASLR is not 100% a mobility test, and stability is a large component of the drill). Correctives would need to begin in the supine-quadruped postures that target the patterns of head control and reaching of the limbs and sequentially progress to the fundamental postures. There may be problems in the Fundamental or Transitional levels, but everyone will walk away from their session and live in the Functional level, therefore the NDS needs to be applied from whatever level is the starting point all the way to standing. To maintain the corrections, establishing sound movement in the Functional postures is vital (that is where life happens).

However, once a score is improved - in this example that would be improving the ASLR score of 1/3 to a score of 2/2- the entire screen needs to be re-administered. After changing the fundamental ASLR, the higher movements (DS, SM, RS) all have the potential to be changed.

But what if the scoring were to be a little less obvious:

Test	Left	Right	Total
Deep Squat			2
Hurdle Step	2	2	2
In-Line Lunge	2	2	2
Active Straight Leg Raise	2	2	2
Shoulder Mobility	2	2	2
Trunk Stability Push up			2
Rotary Stability	2	2	2
TOTAL SCORE			14

FIGURE 3.2 - FMS EXAMPLE 2

This screen would result in the ordering of correctives being:

1. ASLR
2. SM
3. RS
4. TSPU
5. ILL
6. HS
7. DS

With this, the first question would be are corrective drills really necessary because this person meets the minimum movement quality standards across the board. Depending on the situation correctives may not be warranted, but should it be decided that they are needed (some times meeting the minimum movement standards may not be adequate for certain individuals) the corrective strategy would begin with the ASLR and progress to SM, RS, TSPU, ILL, HS and finally DS. Any FMS score can generate a corrective strategy.

Often, the next question turns out to be "But, how do you navigate multiple problems on the FMS?" This can be done, however, it is much more complicated. If someone has asymmetrical 1's on the ASLR, RS and ILL how do you navigate all three simultaneously? There are two trains of thought on how to address this:

1. Perform drills for the ASLR, then drills for the RS, and finally drills fro the ILL. This is a viable option, but that is three sets of drills which will take three times as long. If time is valuable, this might not be the best option.

2. Filter the corrective exercise choices using the ASLR, RS, and ILL as the filter. Using the ASLR as the first filter leaves, for example, 100 correct exercises and 100 incorrect exercises (the numbers are to show how this works and are not reflective of the actual number of ASLR corrective exercises that are wrong or right.) Take the 100 correct exercises based on the ASLR and apply the RS filter and that

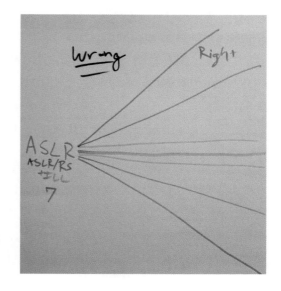

number is reduced to 50 correct choices, but now 150 wrong options. Apply the final filter, the ILL, and now the pool or correct corrective drills drops to 25, but the pool of bad choices has grown to 175. There are MANY drills out there that will address the ASLR, RS, and ILL individually, but only a few that can have a positive impact on all three areas. Choosing the correct exercise here can be more challenging, but if the correct corrective is chosen the payoff can be dramatic. Developing this ability comes from clinical experience - a nice way of saying clinical mistakes.

Don't forget that pain changes everything on the screen - that is why pain automatically warrants a score of zero if it is encountered during the screen. The only professional way to treat pain that is uncovered during the FMS is by referral to the appropriate medical professional.

In any instance, once the screen is performed and pain is not part of the equation, the next question: "Is this a mobility,stability, or motor control problem?" If the weakest areas of the FMS are the ASLR or SM, then mobility is a component of the problem. If the weakest areas are the RS or TSPU, then stability is likely a component of the problem. If the weakest area is the ILL, HS, or DS, then motor control plays a role. Notice the wording that was used - "...a component of the problem". Mobility, stability and motor control are present and working together in every portion of the FMS and movement in general. The steps to restore movement are:

1. **RESET** the mobility restriction(s).
2. **REINFORCE** the new range of motion by improving stability.
3. **RELOAD** the pattern and improve motor control.

"Reset"

Developmentally, mobility precedes stability therefore from a corrective standpoint mobility needs to be established prior to stability. Movement is a sensory experience, having restricted mobility reduces the volume of sensation that contributes to the experience. Improving mobility will always increase sensory input to the CNS due to the proprioception system that is stimulated by the new range that has been established. Typically, areas of mobility restrictions that affect movement patterns include the cervical spine, the thoracic spine, the hips, and the ankles. Mobility restrictions can result from:

- accessory joint motion/capsular restriction
- soft tissue restrictions
  - ▸ neural tension
  - ▸ trigger points
  - ▸ muscle shortening
  - ▸ hypertonicity
  - ▸ scar tissue
- insufficient stability
- emotional stress
- postural stress
- physical stress
- a poorly managed injury

Address the mobility restrictions with appropriate manual therapy and mobility activities. *Appropriate manual therapy* can be anything from a foam roll to very specific trigger point release. This brings up the topic of trigger points. Trigger points can be either active -producing clinical complaints (pain)- or latent. Latent trigger points produce the other affects characteristic of trigger points: increased muscular tension or muscular shortening. Latent trigger points do not, however, produce pain (Simons, Travell et al. 1999). This is important. Everyone has trigger points, and enough time on a foam roll will find many trigger points that were not even painful. Addressing each and every trigger point is much too time consuming, and often times will cause problems. Functional trigger points (trigger points that are latent but result from a need to maintain daily functions) are like crutches that allow everyone to make it through the day with their dysfunctions but with less pain from their dysfunctions. If these 'crutches' are removed, the pain of the dysfunction increases. Only the trigger points associated with the movement dysfunction need to be addressed. These can be determined from the FMS. The FMS has been shown to have direct tie ins with the NDS. What has been held back until now, is how the FMS has direct tie ins to the fascial lines that are described in Anatomy Trains. The FMS reveals which movement patterns are affected, this can then be used to identify the fascial lines that will likely have trigger points that are directly connected to the dysfunction.

FMS Test	Primary Fascial Line	Secondary Fascial Lines
Deep Squat	FL	DFL
Hurdle Step	LL	AL, FL, DFL
In-Line Lunge	SPL	SPL, AL, FL, DFL
Active Straight Leg Raise	SBL	DFL, SPL
Shoulder Mobility	AL	SBL, SFL, DFL
Trunk Stability Push up	FL	DFL, SFL, AL
Rotary Stability	DFL	SPL, FL, AL

FIGURE 3.3 THE FMS AND THE FASCIAL LINES - SUPERFICIAL BACK LINE (SBL); SUPERFICIAL FRONT LINE (SFL); LATERAL LINE (LL); ARM LINE (AL); DEEP FRONT LINE (DFL); SPIRAL LINE (SPL); FUNCTIONAL LINE (FL). (MYERS 2014).

Using the first FMS from above (Total score of 12; ASLR 1/3, DS 1, SM 2/3, RS 2/3) the starting point for the manual therapy would be somewhere along the course of the entire Superficial Back Line. This could be anywhere from the sub-occipitals down to the plantar fascia.

Once mobility has been improved, there is a window of opportunity to begin working on stability within the affected area. To maintain the added mobility, this window of opportunity must be fully utilized before it is lost. Any added mobility requires stability drills.

"Reinforce"

Stability is only warranted after mobility has been improved. Stability drills in the presence of poor mobility are a waste of time, so taking the time to address any mobility problems prior to is always needed. Stability is all about timing and activation, not strength - training stabilizing muscles to be strong will not result in improved stability. Stabilizers need to turn on prior to larger movement - they need to 'anticipate' movement and fire before the prime movers turn on otherwise the prime movers will overshadow the stabilizers every time. Stability is only posture specific, so beginning in the lower levels of the NDS the(Fundamental or Transitional) requires transitioning the stability into the functional postural levels. Identifying the appropriate postural levels for the stability activities is vital for the success of the stability interventions. Again, the FMS can serve as a guide to determine the appropriate postural level (see Figure 2.1) to begin the interventions in. The chosen posture should be moderately challenging but allow for ultimate success without any change in breathing patterns or other compensations.

Static stability needs to be addressed prior to dynamic stability There are many ways to accomplish this without closing the eyes -this tends to be most common way individuals choose to challenge stability. Keep in mind, vision plays a major role - in fact it is the primary source- in stability and balance. Finding other ways to challenge stability through various NDS postures and patterns will generate better outcomes than just taking away a persons visual input.

Breath holding should also be avoided at all costs when addressing stability. The diaphragm is a significant contributor to midline stability via the trunk cylinder. If the breath is held via a valsalva maneuver, intra-abdominal pressure will increase and generate stability. However, this stability is not an appropriate strategy for stability in corrective drills. Using the valsalva maneuver to increase intra-abdominal pressure and stabilize the spine is a higher level option of spinal stability that can be used as a performance skill. What needs to be developed at this time is a strategy where the diaphragm can contribute to spinal stability but still function appropriately for respiration. If corrective exercises are dosed to the point that a valsalva maneuver is necessary to maintain a stable posture, then the dosing of that specific drill is being applied inappropriately.

"Reload"

After mobility has been improved and has opened the window of opportunity for stability to be layered on, the next step is motor control. The new pattern of movement needs to be given the appropriate level of stimulus -in this case challenge- to in essence cement the new pattern. Loading the pattern will increase the physical demand within that pattern and controlled repetitions will increase the stimulus to the CNS. This repetition will allow a new motor pattern to develop, and/or replace the faulty pattern, based on Hebb's Law (Muscles that fire together, wire together). Repetition allows a new pattern to become a permanent pattern (Varier, Kaiser et al. 2011).

This "Reloading" is often the part of the equation that is the most underutilized. Layering in strength and repetition allows a targeted pattern to fully utilize all the gained mobility and stability that has been established up to this point. Just like in the reinforcing stage, choosing the appropriate postural level and pattern to begin and continuing through the NDS to the functional postures must occur for the overall success. This also serves as the transition point into formal strengthening, which will be covered in the Strengthening section of this text.

Red/Yellow/Green Light

The other avenue of the FMS Corrective Strategy, that is probably even more powerful than what has been discussed so far, involves Addition by Subtraction - improving movement by removing the movements/lifts that cause problems. This is the Red Light/ Yellow Light / Green Light List. Originally, this was popularized by Brett Jones and Gray Cook at the CK-FMS Workshop series. The Movement Restoration Project has taken this list and expanded upon it to include barbell, bodyweight, and athletic related drills. These complete lists can be seen in **APPENDIX 2**. They simply work by filtering out drills/movements/exercises that do not directly strengthen the impaired movement patterns. Each FMS test has a list of red light, yellow light and green light drills that is based on the following philosophies:

- **Red Light Drills**- These drills will directly challenge a movement pattern that has already been established as being dysfunctional or asymmetrical and should be avoided. These will only make things worse.
- **Yellow Light Drills**- These drills do not directly challenge a dysfunctional or asymmetrical movement pattern, but should be implemented with caution and direct supervision since they may or may not have a positive impact on the targeted patterns. If drills in this category do not have a positive impact, those drills become Red Light Drills.
- **Green Light Drills**- These drills do not challenge the dysfunctional or asymmetrical movement pattern and may actually be helpful in correcting the targeted movement pattern.

Keep in mind, these are not corrective exercises. These are drills that often are utilized as the supplementary training for an athletes sport, and likely are being supervised and prescribed by their sport coach or a strength coach. While following this list does limit the exercise selection for the individual, this is **_only temporarily the case_**. Once the individuals FMS score changes, their R/Y/G list of exercises will change accordingly. This is one of the most overlooked avenues of communication between the coaching world and the medical world when dealing with and handling athletes that are injured and restricted from injury.

The SFMA Corrective Strategy

The SFMA is designed to identify the most dysfunctional link and sometimes the painful link in the fundamental movement patterns. The key to corrective exercise based off of the SFMA as the assessment tool is to address the most dysfunctional, non-painful patterns. The non-painful, functional patterns are essentially normal; the painful, dysfunctional patterns cannot be addressed due to the pain; and the painful, functional patterns cannot be addressed due to the pain also. Keep in mind once again that pain changes everything and will only cloud the decision making process of the corrective exercises if it is not avoided (or addressed first).

Just like in the FMS Corrective Strategy, utilizing the SFMA to establish a treatment plan requires that mobility issues (JMD- Joint Mobility Dysfunctions- and TED -Tissue Extensibility Dysfunctions in SFMA language) be addressed before fixing the stability problems (SMCD - Stability/Motor Control Dysfunctions). The beauty about the SFMA, is that where the FMS gives general recommendations to the problem (mobility or stability only, but not more specific) the SFMA gives specific recommendations (a weight bearing hip fundamental extension problem).

The SFMA begins with a Top -Tiered assessment, and then based on what is observed here is followed by a series of breakout assessments that will ultimately direct the clinician to the specific problem (JMD, TED, SMCD). If a top-tier assessment is performed, the corresponding breakouts **MUST** be used to follow up - just performing a top-tier assessment does not reveal any true information as to the cause of the problem. The tip-tier allows for refinement and/or better localization of where the actual problem is hiding, but it does not reveal the problem. The breakouts further strip down each movement pattern to help zero in on the specific problem within the problematic pattern.

Selecting the correct corrective exercise based on what the SFMA reveals follows the same philosophy as the FMS. Is the problem one of mobility, stability, or motor control? Reset mobility, reinforce stability, and reload the movement. The

SFMA corrective strategy is identical to the corrective strategy employed following the FMS: Mobility first, stability next, and motor control to wrap things up. The only differences are that within the SFMA strategy, pain may come into play and the information regarding the problematic areas will be more specific.

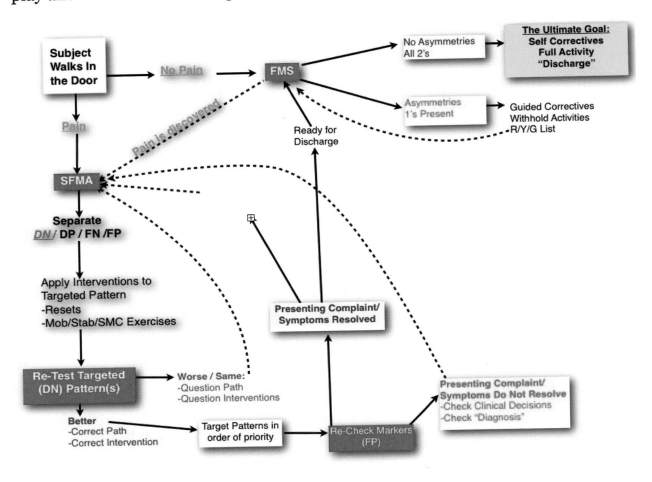

FIGURE 3.4 - THE FMS/SFMA FILTER PROCESS

What Happens with the selected corrective strategy does not fix the problem?

In this instance, there has likely been a mistake or a problem within the assessment. Most likely the incorrect pattern was targeted for intervention. This often occurs because of a lack of precision within the chosen assessment. Assess tight, train loose - meaning, during the chosen assessment be extremely precise and picky but during the correctives allow a little wiggle room. The information gained by the assessment is only as good as the assessment was performed. If the FMS is applied in a sloppy manner, the quality of the information will be in question and the corrective exercises are likely to be chosen based off of bad information.

If the problem does not improve, the first option to salvage the situation is to re-assess the individual. Do this with an open mind. Do not try to outsmart the FMS or the SFMA - both have redundancies built into them as a sort of checks-and-balance system. Both the FMS and the SFMA are just tools, which means they are only as good as the individual applying them, interpreting the information from them, and applying that information towards a corrective strategy. The main reason that this is done is to confirm that the previously identified dysfunctions were done so correctly and that nothing was missed in the assessment process. When performing a reassessment it is often helpful to have another individual serve as an extra set of eyes - *"We don't see things the way they are, we see them the way we are"* —Talmud. Bringing in another person brings in another perspective that might shed light on the situation. If an individuals symptoms or movement problems do not resolve after the reassessment and what that leads to, then there is sufficient reason to believe that something else might be going on. At this point, there should be a discussion with the individual regarding their activities and, for the healthcare professionals, if they were seen by a physician a discussion with the physician regarding the plan of care needs to take place.

The Corrective Exercise Continuum

Using the NDS for corrective exercise selection is a sequential model that follows how every person originally learned to move. This information is nothing new; the key difference is blending of this model with the FMS, the SFMA, and the fascial lines and knowing where in the NDS to place each person based on their FMS scores or their SFMA data. The key with this continuum is that each person must progress to the end of the NDS - regardless of where they start, everyone must finish in vertical stance. Age, conditioning level, injury, and surgical procedure all need to be considered when developing a corrective exercise plan but should not affect the sequence of exercises. If anything it will affect the timing of the appropriate exercises.

Appropriate sequencing might not seem too important, but can be vital to the outcome of the corrective strategy. Mobility comes before stability, and stability comes before motor control. Choosing the correct level of the NDS to begin is important, but then the sequence needs to be followed in regards to patterns and postures. Static drills need to precede dynamic drills, and body weight should always be mastered before external loading occurs. Navigating through all of this is once again referred to as Clinical Experience. Additionally, knowing when the fascial lines develop during the NDS can aid in corrective exercise selection - especially, if the FMS has been performed and the problematic fascial lines have been identified.

Fascial Lines	NDS posture where the lines develop	NDS Patterns where the lines develop
Superficial back line	Supine	Flexion
Superficial front line	Prone	Extension
Deep front line	Quadruped, Sitting	head movement, crawling, pushing down, squatting
Arm Lines	Prone, Quadruped, Sitting	reaching of the limbs
Spiral Lines	Half kneeling postures	rolling
Functional Lines	Kneeling postures	crawling, squatting
Lateral Line	Single leg stance	rolling, gait

FIGURE 3.5 - THE NDS AND THE FASCIAL LINES

Knowing the affected fascial line(s) gives insight into which NDS posture can be exploited to get the most benefit out of the corrective strategy and which patterns will address the fascial lines the most efficiently. Knowing that someones Spiral Line is their problematic fascial line can guide them towards a half kneeling intervention that involves the principles of rolling - chopping or lifting would fit perfectly here, assuming the mobility/stability/motor control continuum has been followed to that point in time.

Putting it all together.

How does all of this get applied to a real person in real time? The FMS example from figure 3.1 will be used. Laid out together, all of the information would look like this:

	Fascial lines affected	Postural Level	Patterns
1/3 ASLR	SBL	Supine	Reaching of the limbs
1 DS	FL	Symmetrical Stance	squatting
2/3 SM	AL	Prone	Reaching of the limbs
2/3 RS	DFL	Quadruped	Rolling, crawling

FIGURE 3.6 - PUTTING IT ALL TOGETHER EXAMPLE

This information reveals that there will likely be trigger points that directly affect the movement situation within the SBL, FL, AL, and DFL, with the SBL taking the top priority in the corrective sequence. It also directs the interventions to begin in the Supine posture with reaching of the limbs. There are many drills that can fall under "Supine, reaching of the limbs" - the ASLR series from the FMS world is a great example, as is the Leg Lowering series. The postural progression would occur in this manner:

1. Supine
2. Prone
3. Quadruped
4. Symmetrical Stance

The patterns that will be introduced would occur in this manner within the appropriate postures:

1. Reaching of the limbs
2. Rolling
3. Crawling
4. Squatting

An example corrective protocol for this situation would be as follows:

1. **RESET** - Soft tissue
   a. Lacrosse ball work
      i. sub occipitals
      ii. erector spinae
      iii. popliteal fossa
2. **RESET** - Mobility work
   a. Supine Wall ASLR crocodile Breathing
   b. Supine ASLR Series
   c. Arm bar
   d. half kneeling windmill
3. **REINFORCE** - Stability work
   a. Supine Front hip series
   b. Prone to Quadruped transition
   c. half kneeling chop
4. **RELOAD** - Motor Control
   a. half kneeling hip hinge
   b. elevated dead lift
   c. Goblet squat
5. **RESTRICTIONS** - Red/Yellow/Green Light List
   a) ASLR Restrictions
      i. Deadlifts
      ii. Cleans
      iii. Snatches
      iv. Sprinting
      v. KB Swing, Clean, Snatch, Deadlift, Windmill, Overhead swing
   b. DS Restrictions
      i. Overhead pressing
      ii. Snatch
      iii. Clean
      iv. Squats
      v. KB Press, squats, clean, snatch, swing

This serves as just an example - there are many different corrective exercises that can replace those listed here. Knowing the person needing the corrective drills allows for better and more appropriate exercise selection.

Applying the Corrective Exercise - The Finer Points of Instruction.

People instinctively want to help each other, especial those attempting to help another person move or perform better and those in the healthcare industry that are helping an individual rehabilitate from an injury. Often times, this eagerness gets in the way and actually causes problems. No one instructs or coaches a child through the NDS. The NDS just naturally occurs - it is sensory driven and controlled by gravity. All caregivers can really do is get in the way and cause problems. Often times, though, applying corrective exercises often is dominated by verbal instructions and the other senses (vestibular, tactile, visual, etc) are often ignored. Movement is a complete sensory experience- not just one sense. Typically, an academic approach is taken when teaching movement where over instruction full of big words dominate the sensory experience. This flaw is based on the perception of how one person sees movement, the perception of how the second person feels the movement and how this person interprets the instructions that the first person verbalized to them. Throw in the feedback from the visual, vestibular, and proprioceptive system fighting against the individuals desire to please the person giving them instructions and the result is a "hot mess" of awkwardness and frustration. The best instruction and feedback is non-verbal. The person moving must feel the movement and interpret ALL of the sensory input; movement is a behavior, not just a response.

An overlooked key to teaching movement lies in what is known as the "mirror neurons." Mirror neurons lie in several regions of the brain and have become more and more understood since their discovery in the 1990's. These neurons have been referred to as "the neurons that shaped civilization" (Ramachandran 2011). Mirror neurons have been ascribed a wide variety of functions: imitation, language processing, embodied simulation, empathy, emotion recognition, intention reading, language acquisition, language evolution, manual communication, sign language processing, speech perception, speech production, music processing, and aesthetic experience (Cook, Bird et al. 2014). The portion of the mirror neuron functions that directly affect instructing movement is the imitation portion. Automatic imitation is said to occur when observation of an activity involuntarily leads to the performance of a topographically similar action (Cook, Bird et al. 2014). What this means is that when an activity is seen by an individual, corresponding areas in the observers brain are stimulated similar to how the performers brain is stimulated by actually performing the activity. Humans learn movement by mimicking movement via the mirror neurons. Mimicking results in the ability to transmit knowledge through example.

> *"When a normal subject watches another person performing any action - say, squeezing a tennis ball with the right hand- the muscles in the subject's own right hand will register a tiny uptick in their electrical "chatter". Even though the subject doesn't perform a squeezing action herself, the mere act of watching the action leads to a tiny, but measurable increase in the action-readiness of the muscles that would contract if she were performing it. The subjects own motor system automatically stimulates the perceived action, but at the same time it automatically suppresses the spinal motor signal to prevent it from being carried out - and yet a tiny trickle of the suppressed motor command signal manages to leak through and down to reach the muscles"* (Ramachandran 2011).

Taking advantage of the ability of the highly efficient mirror neuron system to teach movement takes two steps:
1. "Watch me"
2. "Be my reflection"

In the "Watch me" stage, the individual watches the movement being performed for as long as they need. In the "be my reflection" stage. they get to practice the movement by mirroring the individual leading the movement. Essentially, the person learning the movement is being the mirror image of the person leading the movement. Very few -if any- verbal cues are used; the vast majority of cuing is visual, tactile, and proprioceptive based. After the person learning the movement has begun to display an basic level of imitating the movement, then small sensory stimulus can be applied to make the movement better.
1. Limited verbal instruction - "eyes up"; "don't hold your breath".
2. Tactile feedback to make a error worse - the basis of Reactive Neuromuscular Training (RNT), where movement is made worse in an effort for the individual to perceive the movement flaw.

3. Speed of movement instruction - adjusting the speed of the movement to maximally allow the proprioceptive system to be stimulated.

The best way to improve retention and awareness of a drill is through immediate feedback - was the movement successful or unsuccessful. Allowing the individual the opportunity to feel the movement gives immediate feedback - either feeling and recognizing movement errors, or feeling correct movement gives immediate feedback to their chosen movement strategy.

PART 4

Strengthening

"How we do something is often more important than what we do."
Moshe Feldenkrais.

In this instance, the something is "getting strong". The 'how' of getting strong (the philosophy) is much more important than the 'what we do' part (the tools/ lifts). Dr. Mark Cheng recently posted a picture of a kettlebell and an FMS kit with the caption *Strength with Integrity*. The previous sections have all been about establishing movement integrity, why would it be any different moving forward? The answer is never, unfortunately, many in the strength world lose sight of this and move into the "by any means necessary" mindset.

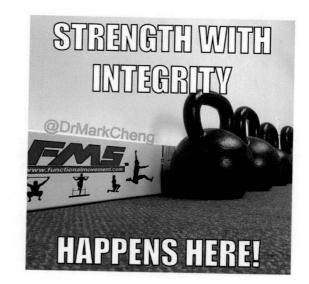

The definition of strong is: *"having great physical power and ability; not easy to break or damage; not sick or injured"* (Merriam-Webster Inc. 2005). While getting strong is often associated with the first definition and is solely focused on physical power, the last two components of the definition of strong are what truly round out and define real strength - not easily broken, sick or injured. How often is strength associated with broken, sick, or injured? How often is getting strong associated with relieving any of those problems?

StrongFirst Instructor Nikki Shlosser made the following observation:

> *"I have a theory that very small children instinctively seek strength by picking up or moving relatively heavy things - but is it because it's just a challenge like any other challenge, or is it because their bodies are just supposed to get stronger?"*

This is a great observation and one that poses the question of how does strength fit into the development of children? Rarely do children seek to get stronger on purpose; it is the side effect of their curiosity.

Children are born without preconceived notions, ideas, or assumptions about anything. A Child's first months are about sensations - the richer the sensory environment, the faster and larger their developing brains grow. Everything is new to them. Adults see a plain cardboard box, and the toddler sees a fort to hide in. An adult sees a rock on the floor, a child sees something to put in their ear. Their innate curiosity is the gift that allows them to develop both mentally and physically. Thomas Edison is quoted as saying "The greatest invention in the world is the mind of a child." Every object and task provides a new sensory opportunity to learn something - curiosity thrives, and so does the rate of both physical and cognitive development. Iron is no different - every training session provides a new sensory opportunity as well as a new movement opportunity to get better and stronger.

Strength is the forgotten attribute to successful movement. Corrective movement, functional movement, and sport specific movement have garnered the most attention over the past few years. Strength has been described by Brett Jones and Dan John as the physical attribute that improves all other attributes. Brett describes strength as a glass. The bigger the glass (or the more strength that is present) the greater you can fill the glass with the other attributes - whether it be sport skills, power, durability, etc. Without strength, everything else is limited. Another very similar way to view strength is as a 'buffer'. In sports, as well as normal daily activities, when things go wrong (a mis-step, a sudden change in needed movement, etc) possessing a higher degree of strength can serve as that buffer and prevent things from going from bad to worse. For example - a sudden change of direction during the game for that football player that is strong may result in a sore ankle the next day - for a weak athlete, this same situation may result in some degree of ankle sprain. The weak athlete has less wiggle room to account for the rapid change in movement strategy and therefore has no successful strategy to get out of harms way.

Everyone wants to do what the professionals do - weight vests, skilled lifts, agility drills, speed work, whatever the newest and fanciest "thing" is. What is missed is the level of strength that that athlete or individual possesses to be able to do the fancy advanced drill. In the rehab world, corrective exercise often time morphs into a similar role - many people get caught up in only doing correctives and forget to move on. Overall, strength has suffered. In the youth athlete world every kid is playing for a scholarship - weekend tournaments in Podunk USA are given the same level of importance to the little leaguers family as the McDonalds All American Game. Only, no scholarships are on the line in either - in the former no one really cares about the outcome, and in the latter scholarships have been signed already. Because of this focus on sports participation, the very sound recommendation of actually preparing for the sport is ignored - there is no glory in training. Two months of preparatory training are the recommendation for all youth athletes (Myer, Kushner et al. 2013). In the geriatric population, where maintaining strength is paramount to survival (Dodds, Denison et al. 2012) strength is relegated to only activities that are deemed "safe" from a facility liability standpoint - everything is done in a seated machine. Fall prevention programs are put into place that have little outcome on falls and have no outcomes on strength. Getting strong and staying strong are vitally important, but relegated to the dusty corners of most facilities. Looking at the typical fitness facility will reveal the publics misplaced love affair with cardio. The attributes of health and resiliency have been completely forgotten and removed from what is seen as strong.

"I pick things up and put them down" is a line in a commercial promoting a gym franchise that attempts to make light of those that are in the pursuit of strength. The skill of getting strong is anything but simple or easy. Referring back to the NDS again reveals the methods to develop strength - progressive resistance in a manner that gradually increases in difficulty due to motor control. Strength, like movement, develops from the midline out which reflects the primary need to protect and stabilize the spine, and then develop movement and strength in the extremities.

Bodyweight is the initial resistance program for everyone - every toddler is an excellent bodyweight athlete. Dr. Moshe Feldenkrais described the newborn as "tabula rasa"- a clean slate. Unlimited and unrestricted mobility. Not many adults - or even kids past puberty- are a clean slate. Many people looking to get strong are much like a 10 year old car with 10,000 miles; everyone has racked up miles, has gotten some dents, and are not as clean as when they were younger. Everyone brings their own issues to the table. Many people are "fit" but very few are "healthy". Trying to add strength to this equation without the appropriate prep work is a recipe for disaster. Gray Cook often says "Move well, then move often." That could be expanded to "Move well, move often, then move a lot."

Mobility, stability and strength are woven together like a braided rope. Individually, each is good, but when they are woven together in a balanced manner they become much more resilient than their individual parts. Too much or too little of any will have negative effects on the overall well-being of an individual, which will negatively carryover into everything else they are attempting to do. The key is to develop these qualities in the same manner in which they were originally developed: mobility, stability, motor control, strength. When life, sport, habits, or injury impair any of these three, the other two will also show negative affects. Maintaining a balance in life and in sport while looking to reduce the likelihood of injury is a fine balancing act that everyone must maintain.

Developmentally, strength development progresses in unison with the NDS. This is primarily because until stability is present, conscious deliberate movement with the intent of overcoming gravity cannot take place. This subtle fact is a key to tying corrective exercises to strength training - mobility and stability must be present to reach full strength potential in any individual. This is not saying that those with mobility restrictions cannot be strong, it is just stating that they are likely not reaching their full potential. Full range of motion is a requisite to develop the highest levels of strength. Additionally, this helps to maintain adequate mobility which insures a quality sensory experience during strength training. The range of motion discussion tends to revolve around the movement of squatting the most, with proponents of full range of motion squatting on one side and proponents of mini-squats (90° of knee flexion or less) on the other. In North America, Europe and Australia 120° tends to be adequate knee flexion for normal activities of daily living (ADL's). However, in the Middle East and Asia, 120° is far less than the 165° of knee flexion needed for ADL's. In this region of the world deep knee flexion serves as an important component of prayer, socializing and eating.   The point of this is that squatting below parallel is necessary.   Ranges of motion that are necessary should be strengthened.   A 2003 study (Spanu and Hefzy 2003) looked at the biomechanics of deep knee flexion and revealed some important information:

- The anterior fibers of the ACL only carried a load from 0-5° of knee flexion. The posterior fibers of the ACL carried forces in the first 36° of knee flexion and became unloaded from 36 to 100° of knee flexion and then began to carry forces again as the knee went into deep flexion.
- The oblique fibers of the MCL carried no load at any degree of knee flexion. The posterior fibers carried a very small load only from 0-5° of knee flexion.
- The greatest level of hamstring co-contraction with the quadriceps occurs at 30° of knee flexion, and decreased with greater knee flexion.
- The PCL carries a high load as the knee is flexed. At 90° of flexion, roughly 203kg (450 lb) of force is placed upon the PCL. The highest levels of force on the PCL are seen between 105-120° degrees of flexion. Flexion angles deeper than 120° saw this level of force rapidly decrease.
- The highest levels of tibio-femoral contact force occur from 0-5° of knee flexion and then progressively lessen thru full flexion.

Sufficient strength through an unrestricted range of motion that allows for the desired ADL or sport activity is required for optimal health. When strength deficits are present, the body will find a way to accomplish the desired task in a manner that often times results in problems. Strength alone can serve as a great corrective exercise- assuming quality/symmetrical movement is present. At a 2013 workshop, Pavel Tsatsouline described strength and corrective exercise in this manner:

> *"Strength is like steak. Correctives are live vegetables. You must have both, and cannot live on only one."*

Strengthening errors

Open any rehabilitation text and there will be a chapter dedicated to the latest "Functional" and "Sport-Specific" exercise to fix whatever is broken. Watch any late night TV and there will be a plethora of fitness infomercials promoting the latest and greatest tool, product, or method to get ridiculous results in no time at all. In both worlds, there are hundreds of exercises to target every minute muscle that could possibly be weak and every muscle that might be tight. Isolationism at its finest. If these approaches worked (which they should since they are published in professional text books and are aired on public TV), then why are the top three predictors of injury still prior injury, asymmetry and motor control? Sore arms are common in overhead athletes; runners live with shin splints; sprinters fear the common hamstring strain; low back pain affects almost everyone everyday. If sports were truly the cause of these widespread injuries that are often viewed as part of the sport, then why doesn't every athlete playing the sport suffer these problems?

The problem is that rehabilitation and training professionals have moved too close to the problem. To see the Grand Canyon from the rim is amazing; to see the Grand Canyon from a helicopter is awe inspiring. The human body and its problems are the same way. The professionals need to take a step back to see the entire picture. The days of 3 sets of 10 thera-band exercise needs to be relegated to the past. Strengthening must be a part of the larger picture that includes mobility, stability and motor control; it must be part of a higher purpose. Getting stronger is not a purpose - it is a goal. The purpose of strength training must be balanced with quality movement - rarely does the strongest competitor win; it is usually the strongest competitor that moves the best and is injury free. This is the heart of being athletic - strong, mobile and resilient.

Strengthening has been attempted to be simplified incorrectly. Instead of devising tools, equipment, and devices that make getting stronger easy (machine weights, etc), the goal should have been to simplify the application of the exercises to get strong. Gaining strength is simple. Physiologically, it has been known what parameters must be met to increase the strength of a muscle or muscles. "Simple" and "easy" were confused; easy ways to get strong have dominated the market and texts for many years with little to no success - look at the injury rates in sport, the failure rates of the physical requirements in the military; not to mention the trend of obesity rates across all age groups.

Schmidt's Theory of human movement reveals seven basic patterns of movement: push, pull, squat, bend, lunge, rotation, and locomotion. McGill (McGill 2004) describes six basic patterns of movement which vary slightly from Schmidt's: squat/lunge, push/pull, lunge, gait, twist, and balance. In the Movement Restoration Sequence, the patterns of movement that need to be strengthened are based on the way that strength originally develops as part of the NDS:

1. **Pushing** - characterized by moving a load away from the body. This can happen vertically (overhead) or horizontally (over the chest) or at many angles in between. Pushing is one of the first developmental patterns to emerge, and is assessed directly with the FMS Trunk Stability Push Up.

2. **Pulling** - the opposite of pushing; the resistance is pulled into the body, or the body is pulled towards a fixed object. Again, there can be a vertical component, a horizontal component, or any angle in between. Pulling is a very important portion of the developmental sequence and is actually what allows standing and walking to occur due to the initial "pushing down" component of pulls that generates midline stability.

3. **Rotation** - the act of rotating about an axis, typically in the transverse plane. Here the rotation my occur around the mid-line of the body or the mid-line of a limb, or in some cases of a joint. Twisting, or rotation, is the first form of motivated locomotion within the NDS and is assessed several times during the FMS. Equally, the ability to resist rotation is very important from a movement standpoint and an injury reduction standpoint.

4. **Hinging** - typically hinging or bending is viewed as "a movement with maximal hip bend with minimal knee bend" (Bolton and Tsatsouline 2012), and is the act of lifting something off the ground. While it is subtle portion of the developmental sequence during the transitional phase, it is not specifically seen on the FMS. It is a precursor developmentally to squatting.

5. **Squatting** - a symmetrical stance where the movement of the hips and knees bend maximally (Bolton and Tsatsouline 2012) at a very similar rate. Squatting is a portion of the transitional postures and is assessed directly with the Deep Squat on the FMS.

6. **Lunging/stepping** - an asymmetrical stance pattern where one leg is doing one thing, while the opposite leg is doing something different. Typically one hip is staying neutral or extending slightly, while the other hip is flexing while both knees are flexing to some degree. This is precursor to bipedal gait and deceleration and also is assessed with the In-Line Lunge on the FMS.

7. **Carrying** - the act of carrying an object from point A to point B. This type of carrying should not be mistaken with the style of carrying seen in strongman type competitions - any changes to optimal positioning or posture negates the benefits of this style of carrying.

8. **Hanging** - the act of grasping an object and hanging from it, which results in a fractioning of the body. Like pushing and pulling, hanging can have a vertical, horizontal, or angular component. The key here is that there is no (or limited) contact with the ground and the body is in some manner of suspension. Dr. Ed Thomas has stated that the body cannot fully develop without some degree of brachiation. While hanging occurs later in the NDS and is not assessed in the FMS it does play a significant part in the development of normal movement.

Every beneficial strengthening drill can be classified into one of the above categories. Balance is not included in the strengthening sequence because from a developmental standpoint balance (which is a combination of the visual, vestibular, and proprioceptive systems working together) contributes to the formation and refinement of all the other patterns and is truly a foundation or precursor to strengthening.

Strengthening as part of the NDS

The order in which strength develops as part of the NDS is:
1. Pushing
2. Pulling
3. Rotational
4. Hinging
5. Squatting
6. Lunging / Stepping
7. Carrying
8. Hanging

Often times, randomly prioritizing strength is based on the goals of the athlete (as referred to earlier their point 'B') without knowing their actual strength needs (their point 'A'). Neglecting to assess their strength levels prior to beginning any strength building programs is a recipe for slow progress. Upper body strength is pivotal in lower body strength exercises. Vice versa, lower body strength is pivotal in upper body strength exercises. As an example - it is common knowledge that female athletes tend to have a noticeably higher rate of anterior cruciate ligament (ACL) tears than their male counterparts in almost every sport. Many reasons have been proposed by many experts and researchers, including hormonal variance, differing pelvic structures, and decreased lower body strength levels. A systemic review of literature on ACL injury prevention programs show very little effects of any ACL injury prevention programs that incorporate lower body strengthening, jumping, and technique training. This meta-analysis investigated 5 studies and determined that, based on the results, in order to prevent *just one non-contact ACL injury*, 89 athletes would need to take part in a preventative program for an entire season (Grindstaff, Hammill et al. 2006). Figuring there are 15 athletes per basketball team, that would require 5.9 teams to take part in a season long preventative program to keep 1 athlete from tearing their ACL. Not the most practical or efficient use of time for the other 88 athletes. In all of this, there is one glaring commonality - no documented ACL injury prevention program has incorporated or even considered the role of upper body strength on the likelihood of ACL injury. From a developmental standpoint, lower body strength cannot develop without sufficient upper body strength - why would it be expected to be different in those past puberty?

The other side of the coin is the typical male that lifts weights - either recreationally or as part of a strength program. Typically, the male training program is devoted to getting the attention of the females - a "Suns out, Guns out" or "Curls for the Girls" type program where 95% of the time is devoted to the muscles that can be seen when posing for the fitness center mirrors. Little time is dedicated to the lower body and little, if any time is dedicated to anything that the mirror does not show. The result? The stereotypical male that is bound up and unable to move freely - their myopic focused training has neglected balance and progression which results in a loss of much needed mobility. In both instances, poorly aligned programming dictates the final product.

As part of the Movement Restoration approach to strength training, several principles must be applied:
1. Safety First
2. Strengthening is a behavior.
3. Strengthening starts and ends with the brain.
4. Every repetition matters - each rep is either re-enforcing a bad pattern or strengthening a good pattern.
5. Strengthening occurs in response to a rich sensory environment.
6. Isolation does not exist anywhere in the body - the brain has a tendency to favor patterns.
7. Shoes restrict sensory input, and therefore interferes with the re-acquisition of movement.
8. Progressive increases in difficulty are required through full ranges of motion (sufficient mobility for the desired lift is required).

Other than #1 and #8, these should be familiar - they served as the principles to movement and were described earlier. Once resistance of any kind is added to a movement (bodyweight, barbells, kettlebells, sandbags, dumbbells, milk-jugs, rocks, etc) the level of attention to the movement *should* automatically increase. The issue of safety has several points:
- Respect for the implement is inherent for the safety of the movement.

- Insuring optimal postural alignment is necessary (especially in regards to the feet, spine and the pelvis).
- The surrounding environment should be clear and viable for a quick exit should things go wrong and an emergency exit/bail-out is required.
- Planning for a lift gone wrong is much better than hoping that a lift will go right - adequate spotters on appropriate lifts and a safe/clear area to drop the weights on appropriate lifts will result in being able to lift another day.
- Breathing that matches the lift.

In regards to #8, progressive increases in difficulty - this progressive increase in difficulty encompasses much more than just loading options. The difficulty of any lift can be altered to a level that is appropriate for each individual. For example, a kettlebell windmill can be performed in the following manners:
- Standing with a kettlebell overhead
- Standing with a kettlebell held down low
- Open half kneeling with a kettlebell overhead
- Open half kneeling with a kettlebell held down low
- Standing with the front foot on a low box, and a kettlebell overhead
- Standing with the front foot on a low box, and a kettlebell held down low
- Standing with a barbell overhead
- Standing with a barbell held down low
- Open half kneeling with a barbell overhead
- Open half kneeling with a barbell held down low

There are many other variations of the windmill, but hopefully this displays the point that within any exercise, lift, or drill there are many different variable progressions and regressions that can be applied.

Footwear when lifting is another point of contention. First and foremost, any facility rules should be followed. However, using the logic of shoes will protect the feet is flawed. A 45 lb plate will break any foot that it is dropped on - all a shoe will do is keep any mess in a confined space, leaving less clean up for the facility staff. Running shoes and even most cross training shoes typically have an elevated heel and a lot of cushion. This does two things - diminishes the sensory input from the feet and pitches the center of mass forward. Both of which have a dramatic effect on movement quality and experience. Shoes that have no sole

(Merrel's, New Balance Minimus, Vibram's) all avoid this. All are better options than the popular, fashionable shoes that dominate the market.

Breathing for Strength

Diaphragmatic breathing is essential for the NDS to progress normally because of everything that appropriate breathing develops (see the **DIAPHRAGMATIC BREATHING AND GRIP** section above). These same benefits carry over to strength training in regards to both efficiency and safety. Various authors have detailed strategies for breathing during lifts. The two that line up the best with the Movement Restoration Approach are Pavel Tsatsouline's *Simple and Sinister (Tsatsouline 2013)* and Scott Sonnen's *Primal Stress* (Sonnon 2012). The keys for breathing during strength training:

- On the inhale, the mouth is closed and the tongue is resting gently on the roof of the mouth leaving the inhale to occur through the nose. The inhale occurs during the eccentric portion of most lifts.
- The breath is drawn deep into the pelvis - the belly is actively pushed out anteriorly AND laterally against braced abdominals.
- No shoulder and/or upper back movement should occur. Typically if this is seen, breathing is occurring in the chest which can lead to movement of the thoracic spine.
- The exhale should be scaled to the level of effort being exerted. The exhale should occur through pursed lips, with extra attention being placed on any sticking point that may occur during the concentric portion of the lift.
- On certain lifts, a grunt will initiate the concentric portion of the lift.

In all instances the breathing should match the movement - this is referred to as biomechanically matched breathing. The breathing matches the movement -on the eccentric phase of a lift a braced inhalation occurs; on the concentric phase of a lift a forced exhalation occurs.

The FMS and Strength

The FMS serves as an excellent guide for appropriate strength training activities. It does this through the Red/Yellow/Green light recommendations (**See the attached appendix**). The earlier section of the Red/Yellow/Green Light explains the importance of this "Addition by Subtraction" approach and how it can be applied to training. The main point of that section was on what lifts could be removed or avoided in order to improve movement quality. The other aspect of this is that a list of "safe" lifts/drills can also be established through the green light exercise and some of the yellow light exercises. This list can be combined with each individuals goals and a program can easily be generated that is made up of only exercises/drills/lifts that improve movement quality in addition to making individuals strong.

The Lifts.

Pushing up (Pushing I)
Red Lights: SM, RS, TSPU, OHS

Pushing up from the floor begins to build both strength and stability (trunk, pelvic, and shoulder) for more complex and challenging tasks. To do this, normal thoracic spine mobility and anterior hip elongation is needed. When it comes to pushing up for strength, the trunk and pelvis must function as one functional unit - the glutes and the lats (the Back Functional Line in Anatomy Trains) must work appropriately for the movement to occur efficiently. Additionally, the Deep Front Line needs to function at a level that allows the entire Functional Line to do its job. As Tsatsouline stated: *"Tensing the glutes amplifies any exertion."* Shrugging the shoulders up to the ears or moving them forward is "disconnecting" the arms from the powerful torso muscles (Tsatsouline 2004). This also displays a lack of scapular stability which has a negative impact on overall motor control of the movement. To keep the shoulders connected, gripping the ground is essential - this facilitates scapular stability. This subtle act increases the neural drive of the movement and along with spiraling the arms (corkscrewing) increases the extent of which the shoulder and arm display stability and reduces the energy 'leaks' of the movement. Tsatsouline discusses this detail in his book *The Naked Warrior (Tsatsouline 2004)*. In *Easy Strength*, Tsatsouline and Dan John describe the push up in this manner:

> *"Although the push up is as basic as it gets, don't touch it until the plank is on the level. It makes me cringe to watch kids - and adults - do the 'hungry cow' push ups, with the lower body sagging and the scapulae sticking out. Gray Cook insists that stability must come before strength, and he knows what he is talking about"* (Tsatsouline 2011).

The importance of this lies in the ability to maintain a rigid, firm base (the trunk, pelvis, and entire lower body) while generating force through the arms - pushing is less about being able to push and more about being able to develop a firm base to push off of. The stability created and controlled in the trunk, pelvis, and lower extremity serves as a precursor to generating strength in these regions during other lifts and drills outlined later.

Pushing Overhead (Pushing II)
Red Lights: SM, RS, TSPU, OHS

Pressing a load overhead is an activity that is discouraged by MANY healthcare professionals. Like many things pressing overhead is not a bad lift - *HOW* someone presses overhead can make this a bad lift. Pressing overhead is bad when not done properly, which, by current fitness standards, happens most of the time. Pressing is a mindful movement - if an individual is not invested 100% in the movement, they will not get the full benefit of the movement but they will get all of the problems associated with it. When done properly, pressing overhead promotes shoulder packing, grip, proper breathing, proper balance, the upper extremities working with the lower extremities, and the the core functioning to transfer energy up and down the fascial lines.

Proper pressing ties the latissimus dorsi (the lats) of the pressing arm to the gluteus maximus of the opposite hip via the thoracolumbar fascia (the back functional line) Improper pressing leaves the shoulder alone on an island to complete the task, which also leads to many problems. Contrary to the popular fitness mentality that believes pressing is all about the arms and shoulders, pressing actually begins in the feet - the feet press into the ground to initiate the upward movement (very important note-no downward movement actually takes place).

Because of this, pressing overhead should not occur until the individual is proficient at the deadlift. The deadlift will initiate in teaching the back functional line (lats and glutes) to work together, and serves as a great way to teach the shoulder to stay stable while loaded. All of this allows the arm lines to continue the press off of what the lats and glutes initiate - a great press requires the functional lines and the arm lines to work seamlessly together.

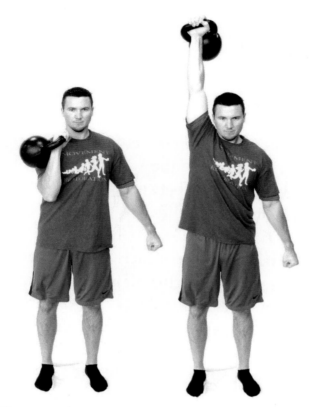

ILLUSTRATION 4.0 - THE KB PRESS

Pulling
Red Lights: SM, TSPU, OHS

Pulling can happen in any plane of motion, but is generally classified as either vertical (pulling up) or horizontal (rowing). In any variation, either a load is pulled towards the body (as in a kettlebell row) or the body is pulled towards a fixed point (as in a pull up). In any variation of rowing, the Back Functional Line and the Arm Lines dominate the movement but are dependent upon the balance between the Superficial Front Line and the Superficial Back Line (Myers 2014). This interplay creates much similarity between pulling and the hinging that will be discussed later, specifically the deadlift.

When pulling the body towards an object, there is an aspect of hanging (to an extent) that will occur, either fully hanging off the ground or bearing a significant portion of body weight through the upper body. Anyone who is not a kid will likely have some developed compensations that will affect their ability to safely, efficiently, and effectively hang. The specific technical points that need to be considered in these individuals, specifically to insure safety are:

1. **Head Position:** The head remains neutral for the duration of the movement, regardless of the plane of motion in which the pulling occurs. Because of the direct connection between the head and the pelvis (through the Superficial Back Line), moving the head out of a neutral position can alter pelvic position which then potentially can alter mid-line stability.

2. **Shoulder Position:** The shoulders need to stay "packed". This means that the scapulae need to be oriented in a manner that prevents the head of the humerus from translating anteriorly. The easiest way of thinking of this is that each scapula needs to be kept in the opposite side back pants pocket. This seems like an active retraction motion, but in reality it is accomplished by setting the scapulae into a good position prior to initiating the movement by staying tall and keeping the shoulders away from the ear - and then maintaining this alignment for the duration of the movement. At the same time, pinching the shoulder blades together is not recommended, there is a fine line between the two.

3. **Mid-Section (Abdominal region):** The recommended position for pulling is one that allows for proper stability and energy transfer to occur. The easiest way to describe this is as a gymnastic hollow position. This is not the hollow position taught in rehab that is seen as a way to activate the transverse abdominis. The torso must stay rigid enough to resist extension and rotation, but not so rigid that it makes the movement inefficient. The ribs need to be pulled downward, which will engage the lateral aspect of the core cylinder (internal and external obliques as well as the Quadratus Lumborum) as well as the anterior of the cylinder (rectus abdominis). This should be accomplished without any loss of height, and with a slight posterior tilt of the pelvis

4. **Hips:** In short, the hips need to stay fully extended. The slight posterior tilt needed to accomplish the hollow position above sets the stage for the glutes to be clenched, which further stabilizes the pelvis and mid-line region. This action, through reciprocal inhibition, also serves to lessen the ability of the psoas and the iliacus to dominate the spinal stability strategy, which is important to re-pattern in those that are anterior hip dominant.

Pulling can be accomplished in almost all of the postures from the NDS. The goal of pulling dictates which posture will be best served as the base to pull from. Sitting, quadruped, kneeling, a squat, and prone all serve as excellent postures to pull from if the goal is to improve midline and/or pelvis stability. Vertical pulling from supine is a great pulling variation to develop upper body strength (this posture is the dominate posture that pulling within the TRX system takes place). Horizontal pulling from a vertical stance will develop stability and upper body strength while vertical pulling from this posture will tend to favor upper body strength. In short, any variation of pulling can be applied to any posture - as long as all the points above are followed - to achieve the desired outcome.

Rotation
Red Lights: SM, RS, TSPU, ILL, HS

Many different versions of rotation training can be employed. The one that will be discussed the most in this text is the turkish get up. The degree of rotation that is occurring at each individual limb as well as around the midline make this an excellent drill in training for rotation. Additionally chops, lifts, windmills, and a variety of medicine ball and/or sandbag drills may be utilized to train for rotation. The reason the turkish get up (TGU) is preferred is because it requires appropriate levels and timing of total body tension and emphasizes that the body work as one functioning unit. In order for rotation to occur anywhere in the body, adequate mobility, stability, motor control and the ability to resist rotation must exist and be demonstrated in many other areas of the body at the same time. Isolated rotation does not occur in actual purposeful human movements. Rotation can be isolated to individual sections, but the benefits of this are limited - a great example is the thera-band shoulder exercises every throwing athlete does to prepare to throw. What is the incidence of shoulder or elbow pain in throwers that follow this? These exercises do have a purpose, but that purpose is not how they are actually utilized.

The TGU utilizes many components of the NDS. Supine, rolling, crawling, seated, half kneeling, and all of the stance patterns (symmetrical stance, single leg stance, and asymmetrical stance) are exhibited during a TGU. In addition to training for rotation, the TGU also has the following benefits:

- promotes cross lateralization
- promotes upper body stability
- promotes lower body stability
- promotes midline stability
- promotes reflexive stability of the trunk and extremities
- ties the right arm to the left leg, and the left arm to the right leg
- gets the upper extremities working reciprocally
- stimulates the vestibular system
- stimulates the visual system
- stimulates the proprioception
- promotes spatial awareness

- develops front/back weight shift
- develops upper body strength, trunk strength, and hip strength

The TGU allows the body to develop mobility, stability and strength thru a variety of angles, postures, and stances by moving around (under) the load instead of moving a load, which is typically what is performed with most drills.

Teaching the turkish get up is well beyond the scope of this text. Many resources are available to learn the turkish get up and how to properly instruct the turkish get up. Anything seen on YouTube™ is likely not in this category. The preferred method of learning the Turkish get up is through a qualified kettlebell instructor, preferably one within the StrongFirst™system of instructors.

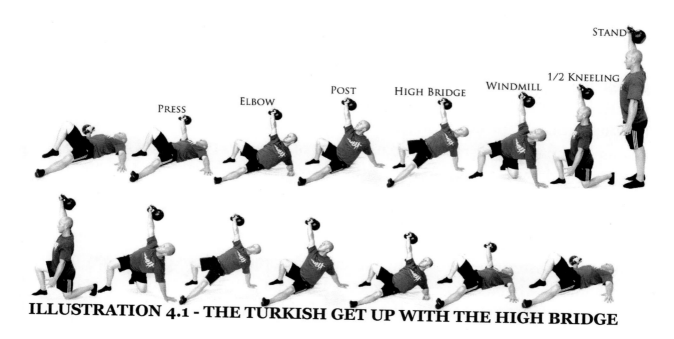

ILLUSTRATION 4.1 - THE TURKISH GET UP WITH THE HIGH BRIDGE

Hinge (Bending)
Red Light: ASLR (Swings)

Bending over (hinging) is a pattern of exploration. Children bend over something to explore it, and then will squat down to investigate further or pick it up. This pattern is important because it teaches the upper body and the lower body to function together in a manner that is safe and efficient. Unfortunately, most people have lost the ability to bend from the hips (moving the pelvis on the femur) and have developed a pattern where the bending occurs in the lumbar spine. The key to the hinging pattern is in the anterior-posterior weight shift that occurs. Possessing this ability is paramount to spine safety and every hinging variation that occurs. The ability to hinge at the hips while keeping a rigid and neutral lumbar spine requires a posterior weight shift to occur, which forces the entire Superficial Back Line and Back Functional Line (most importantly the glutes) to dominate the movement. Minimizing lumbar motion - in fact, preventing ANY lumbar motion - while hinging at the hips is the goal with the hinging pattern. The ability to generate pelvis on femur flexion is actually a very challenging pattern for most people because of the posterior weight shift and keeping a rigid and neutral lumbar spine. However, it is vital for performance and health (remember, strength has a greater purpose and one of those is health) that this be mastered in many different postures - standing, kneeling, half-kneeling, and quadruped. Additionally, hinging serves as the entry point into a squat - that posterior weight shift, and unlocking the pelvis to move freely on the fixed femur is what allows a squat to be initiated in a manner that drastically improves the safety and health of a squat.

While this may seem elementary to most people, it is anything but simple to restore for an individual that has lost their hinge and spends many hours in a habitually hip-flexed posture (sitting at work, school, commuting, recreation, watching tv, eating, etc.). All of this time spent in a seated posture with our back supported by a back rest leads to a pattern in which there is no reflexive mid-line or pelvic stability. This then leads to lumbar flexion replacing hip flexion as the preferred pattern of hinging - even though the long term ramifications of this are drastically bad; the body will always choose an immediate pattern of ease over a pattern that promotes long term health.

The initial goal of hinging is to teach the hip hinge and the individual to consciously separate hip flexion from lumbar motion. Once this goal is achieved, the next step is to introduce the deadlift to the individual and begin to aggressively load this new pattern. This can be achieved via a barbell, kettlebells, sandbags, dumbbells, or anything else that can be picked up from the floor. Adequate strength must be developed in the hinge pattern - this cannot be overlooked. Teaching the hips to move a heavy load in the presence of a stable spine has carryovers to not just athletics and occupation, but everyday life which leads to a healthy back. Occupationally, everyone has been hearing the mantra "Lift with your legs, not with your back" for a very long time, but little has truly been done to equip employees with a real strategy or plan to do this. The plan is - 1)establish a hip hinge at the hips and not the lumbar spine, and, 2) deadlift. Once adequate strength in the hinge is established the next step is to do this dynamically (*No guidelines for what "adequate" is, is being outlined here because that is really individually dependent based upon multiple factors. In the StrongFirst™ world, a double body-weight deadlift is expected for the guys, and a one-and-a-half times body-weight deadlift is expected for the girls. In some circles, this number is low, while in others those numbers will never be touched. The key is to get to a point on the deadlift where the training is* **supplementing** *the performance - both too little and too much can cause problems.*)

The dynamic hip hinge translates to being able to hinge at the hips -under an outside resistance- and maintain a stable and neutral lumbar spine. This specifically has carry over into the world of sport and athletics - keeping a stable spine while moving the hips is a key component of many sports. Doing this safely tends to be problematic. Enter the kettlebell swing. The kettlebell swing and swinging a kettlebell are two completely different activities. Picking up the kettlebell with a purpose, and then performing a movement that incorporates total body tension and power development is 180 degrees from picking up a kettlebell and mindlessly letting it swing up an down. There are vertical forces (from the ground up) and horizontal forces (forward and behind the body) that require deceleration and acceleration. Moving to a single arm swing variation

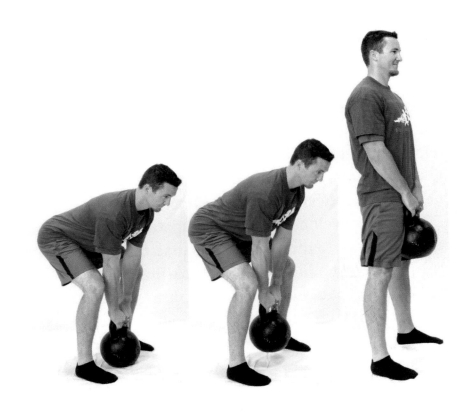

ILLUSTRATION 4.2 - THE KB DEADLIFT

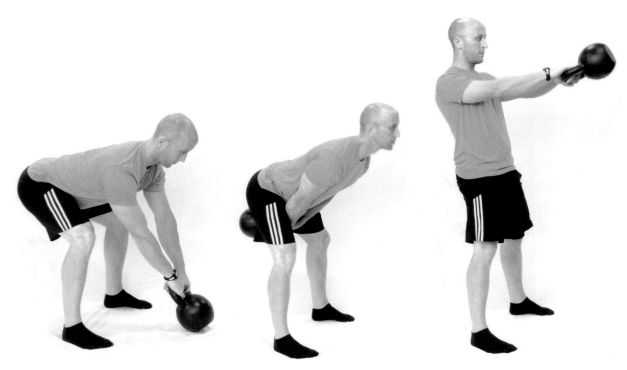

ILLUSTRATION 4.25 - THE KB SWING (A BALLISTIC HIP HINGE)

adds in rotational forces that must be controlled across the shoulder girdle, trunk, pelvis, and lower extremities. All of this must happen in the presence of a stable lumbar spine and perfectly functioning and timed hips. The swing is a lesson in cycling tension and relaxation; at the hips, the trunk, and the shoulder. To quote Pavel in his latest book, *Simple and Sinister:*

> *"Drive with your hips and let it (the kettlebell) freely pendulum. On the upswing the arms and shoulders only transfer the hips' power; but they do not lift the kettlebell. The arms must be straight and loose to do the job - like ropes. If your technique is correct, the kettlebell will form an extension of the arms"* (Tsatsouline 2013).

In the barbell world, the dynamic hinge that follows the deadlift progression can be seen in a properly executed barbell clean. Being able to move into a triple extension position under a load is a beautiful expression of power, and is seen in the properly executed barbell clean. This is followed up by a deceleration phase where the bar is caught in the rack position on the shoulders while the hips move into slightly flexed position. Again, the common thread between the barbell clean, the kettlebell swing, the deadlift, and the hip hinge is that the spine must stay rigid and neutral while the hips create and absorb the forces. Jeff O'Connor teaches a barbell progression for athletes that progresses through a sequence of lifts that connects the overhead squat to the bench press in five lifts. This seemingly unconnected progression:

1. Overhead Squat
2. Back of Neck Press
3. Deadlift
4. Muscle Clean
5. Back Squat
6. Bench Press

This is part of a much larger progression of barbell lifts that he teaches where each lift sets the foundation for the subsequent lift. The beauty of the barbell clean is the twist on pelvis stability that it teaches when the bar is caught in the rack position. The anterior loading of the bar on the shoulders often leads to the pelvis dumping forward (anteriorly tilting) under a load. Being able to counter this and maintain a neutral pelvis while receiving the load of the barbell is one caveat that other forms of loading cannot address.

Squatting
Red Lights: ASLR, OHS

"Squats are bad fer yer knees!" How often has this proverb been spoken by personal trainers (sad), strength coaches (very sad), or PT's/ATC's/MD's/DC's (disheartening). Squatting without the needed mobility, stability and motor control pre-requisites *is* bad, and makes for bad squats. However, if adequate mobility and stability is present and good motor control has been established via a posterior weight shift from the deadlift, then squatting is a great movement. Studies have shown that the greatest stress on the ACL occurs approximately during the first 5 degrees of knee flexion (Spanu and Hefzy 2003). Stress on the PCL is the greatest at 110 degrees of knee flexion (Spanu and Hefzy 2003). If anterior knee pain is present during a squat (or even low back pain, hip pain, etc.) the problem is more then likely not their squat; chances are it is a stability or mobility problem elsewhere that just presents itself as knee pain during a squat. The easiest way to find out? Refer out for an SFMA - remember, pain is warranting follow up which directs the path toward the SFMA and not the FMS.

Before squatting takes place, one additional pre-requisite is having the ability to touch the toes. Not because of the "flexibility", but because of the anterior-posterior weight shift and the ability of the Superficial Back Line to elongate adequately. Without these two aspects of the toe touch, good squatting cannot happen. This does not mean someone that cannot touch their toes cannot squat, it means that this person will achieve a squat through a series of compensations that over time are not healthy.

One of the best ways to introduce the squat from a teaching standpoint is with the kettlebell via the Goblet Squat. Dan John describes the goblet squat like this:

> *"Then I moved to holding the horns (of the bell). I have this notion that the body thrives on a balance point, so for years, I've either used a finger or had the athlete touch their skin while doing a movement. It seemed natural to have the kids touch their elbows on their knees"* (Tsatsouline 2011).

The goblet squat allows the upper body and spine positions to be maintained while the individual squats down between their heels. The elbows to the inside of the knees is a great learning opportunity and provides immediate feedback on the movement - plus it prevents a lot of valgus collapse at the knees.

From a barbell standpoint, the squat can be loaded either on the back of the shoulders (back squat) or the front of the shoulders (front squat). Both have their benefits and their drawbacks. In both, and with the goblet squat, the spine must stay motionless while the hips and the knees flex as the hips drop towards the heels. Where the load is held (in front of the body, on the front of the shoulders, on the back of the shoulders or overhead) dictates the actual angle that the hips drop towards. Creating an appropriate "shelf" for the bar to rest is vital to the execution of the squat and the stability that is initially generated for the movement. StrongFirst™ teaches a Barbell certification course that utilizes a powerlifting approach to creating this shelf. Jeff O'Connor teaches barbell squats from the perspective of applying the lifts directly to performance athletes, which leads to a slightly different teaching progression to establish good squat technique. How the NSCA (National Strength and Conditioning Association) teaches the squat varies greatly from both of these approaches. The commonality is in the attempt to maintain a rigid and neutral spine in the presence of hip and knee flexion/extension.

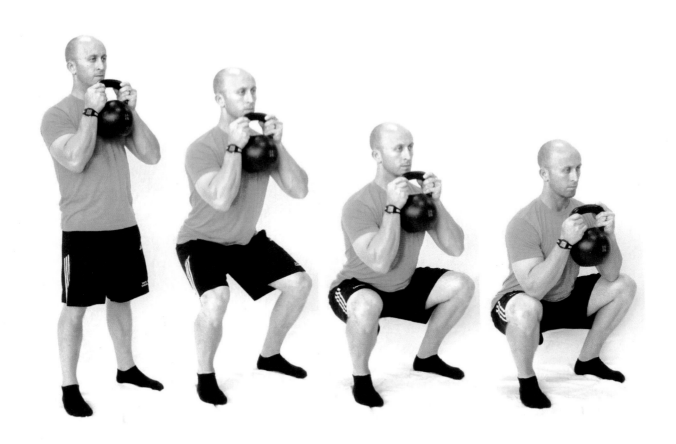

ILLUSTRATION 4.3 - THE GOBLET SQUAT

Lunging
Red Lights: ILL, RS, ASLR

Training in an asymmetrical stance is much needed, especially for those that spend a lot of time in an asymmetrical stance pattern (running, etc). Lunging can consist of actual lunges (where the body travels forward), as well as split squat and elevated split squats (either leg being elevated). Having one hip in flexion and the other hip extension drastically changes how the pelvis generates stability in the presence of movement - the motor control strategy changes immensely from symmetrical stance. There are several expressions of an asymmetrically oriented pelvis in the NDS: crawling, half-kneeling, short half-kneeling, sitting, and asymmetric stance. All of this requires the pelvis to stay level in the presence of the femurs doing differing motions so that the trunk position can be maintained. Anytime asymmetry is introduced into the system, there is a level of anti-rotation that must occur during movement. During athletics, running, cutting, decelerating, and changing directions all occur in the presence of asymmetric stance. Training for this environment is vital for performance, health, and reducing the risk of injuries.

Being able to decelerate and control a load in a lunge position can be very beneficial to most athletes. This can be accomplished beyond the standard eccentric portion of a lunge in a few different ways. A kettlebell jerk or a barbell jerk where the final stance is a split stance are two examples of force absorption in asymmetric stance that can be easily taught once the individual can front squat and overhead press.

Another important area of strength training that needs to be addressed, but does not fall directly under the lunging category is single leg training. Single leg stance requires even more stability and motor control to maintain a stable pelvis than asymmetric stance because now there is the additional requirement of strength to maintain single leg stance. Single leg training is very important for any athlete in any sport that requires running, planting, cutting, and decelerating. Step ups, single leg deadlifts, and single leg squats (pistols) are all varieties of single leg stance training that contribute to single leg strength as well as single leg stability and motor control that every athlete must incorporate into their training at some point to some degree.

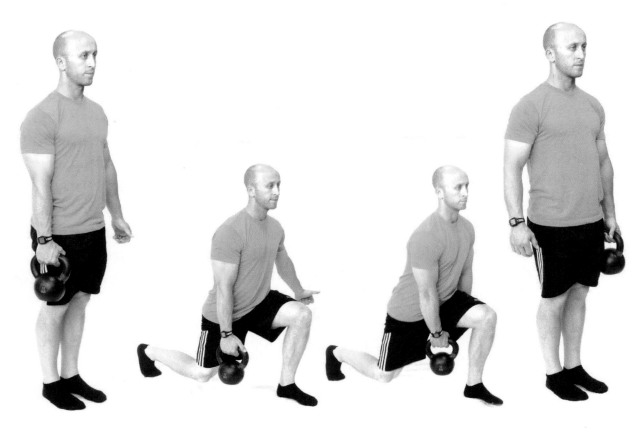

ILLUSTRATION 4.4 - THE TACTICAL LUNGE

Carrying

Red Light: HS, SM (overhead only), TSPU (OH only), RS (asymmetric loading only).

The act of carrying begins with children as soon as they gain the ability to walk freely. Once they are able to get from point A to point B without assistance, their hands are free to carry toys from point A to B. Carrying an object while walking seems simple, but, the impact that it has on the ability to maintain shoulder, trunk, and pelvic stability is enormous. Maintaining a stable pelvis, spine, and shoulder while carrying a load in any position while transitioning between single leg stance and asymmetric stance can be a significant challenge, and can be quite taxing but is also quite beneficial. Carrying a heavy load can be both corrective and instructive - finding the proper alignment to efficiently carry the load can not be accomplished through verbal instruction, it has to occur through trial and error. The key to carrying is that no spine movement can take place, which places a unique load into the Lateral Line and the Deep Front Line - and specifically the Quadratus Lumborum (QL). The QL plays a significant role in stabilizing the lumbar spine onto the pelvis due to its attachment points on the lumbar vertebrae and the pelvis.

There are many different carrying variations - 1 arm, 2 arm, arms down by the side, arms overhead, arms in the "rack" position (elbows tight to the body, hands in front of the shoulders, upper arm in contact with ribcage). Additionally, these five variables can be mixed to get the desired outcomes - 1 arm overhead + 1 arm in the rack; 1 arm down by the side + 1 arm overhead; etc.

A quick note on carrying - this is not the strongman style of carrying objects. This variation of carrying requires proper structural alignment that should not be altered - once technique degrades, the carrying needs to be concluded. In the strongman style of training, the goal is on quantity - the goal here is quality. Breathing should be maintained, but will be challenged depending on the style of the carrying option chosen. For the overhead carrying option, an optimal overhead position is required - which also means that on the FMS any SM and/or

TSPU asymmetries, 1's, or zero's will restrict this option. Ideally, the overhead position will consist of:

- Neutral pelvis (no anterior or posterior tilting).
- Neutral (not flat) lumbar spine.
- No rib flair.
- Full shoulder flexion (Biceps next to the ears).
- Full elbow extension.
- Cervical spine in a neutral position - no forward head posture.

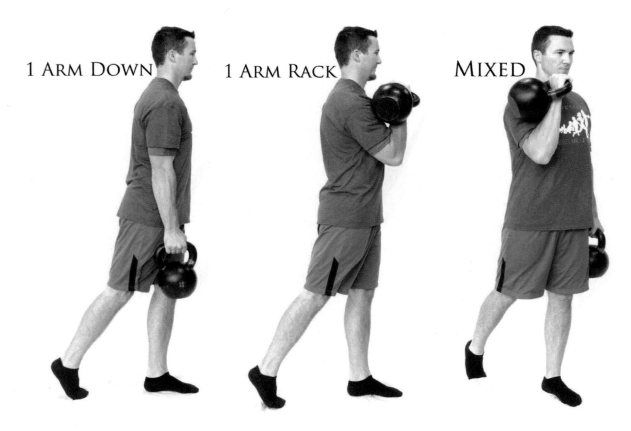

ILLUSTRATION 4.5 - KB CARRY VARIATIONS

Hanging
Red light: SM

Hanging (or brachiation) from the limbs occurs in children at many points within the NDS, but fully unsupported hanging only occurs once the child has developed adequate strength to maintain the load of their body off the ground (typically after vertical stance is achieved). Dr. Ed Thomas stands by the fact that humans cannot fully develop without brachiation. In his article *"Children of Clay"* (which can be found at www.energycenter.com/grav_f/inver_clay.html) Dr. Thomas highlights all of the benefits of brachiation.

From a fascial line approach, hanging allows for various fascial lines to develop - specifically the arm lines (AL) and the functional lines (FL). Hanging allows these lines to be oriented in a manner that alters the force transmission through the lines. Suspending the body by the arms also allows for the connective tissue to handle stress in a manner that is very unique. Compression of the joints accounts for one type of loading, which, due to gravity, is also the most common way in which joints are loaded everyday. Tensioning joints and their surrounding soft tissue is the other way in which joints can be "loaded", however this loading does not require compressing the joint itself.

Other benefits of hanging deal with grip and breathing. Grip strength and endurance is taxed by suspending the body off the ground. Various levels of unloading can occur with hanging - either fully unloaded brachiation, or various levels of unloaded brachiation (like what occurs when using a TRX™Suspension system). The degree of unloading directly influences the level of gripping that is required. Once the body is suspended, breathing becomes more difficult, since many of the accessory muscles of inspiration now are unable to assist with breathing because they are assisting with maintaining the bodies load. This requires the diaphragm to function as a muscle of inspiration, which for many people can be quite a challenge. For those that can diaphragmatically breath, doing so while suspended can enhance this ability.

Various forms of brachiation can occur; already pull ups and rowing varieties have been discussed. The simple act of hanging from a bar is the entry point to brachiation. From this point, there are many progressions that can occur. One simple progression is:

1. Hanging diaphragmatic breaths
2. Hanging Cervical Patterns (Flex/Ext; Rotation)
3. Side to side weight shifts
4. Side to side traveling
5. Single arm hang

A Note on Strengthening Movement Patterns

"Strengthen movements, not muscles" is a saying that has been around for over a decade, yet has not been actually executed in most situations. The philosophy is embraced, but the actual implementation is of an old-school, isolationist approach - there is a disconnect between what is actually being done and what is said is being done. The concept is great; the application is lacking.

Most people cannot define what strength is, or what it takes for someone to be considered 'strong'. Strength is the attribute of athletics that is the easiest to improve - lift a heavy enough weight repeatedly over a long enough time period and strength will improve. Strength can only be built upon quality movement patterns, otherwise performance is being layered upon dysfunction. Unfortunately, the fact is that many therapists and coaches have very limited ways to measure strength and never measure movement quality (with the FMS). This leads to the mindset of blindly increasing strength - anything is better than nothing. The result is an individual who looks like Tarzan, but plays like Jane - their numbers in the gym are impressive, but their numbers on the field do not reflect this.

Strength is a valuable asset in the world of performance, athletics and occupation. The ability to apply this strength to the chosen field of play (or occupation) is invaluable - and very often overlooked or neglected. Having an offensive lineman with a 500 lb bench press means nothing if they cannot set their feet appropriately to apply that force into the defensive player. Every system in the body contributes to this ability: the musculoskeletal system, the CNS, the visual system, the vestibular system, the proprioceptive system, and the cardiovascular system. To get to the point where one looks *AND* plays like Tarzan requires a well rounded program that emphasizes **Strength with Integrity**.

Strength is the most important attribute when it comes to athletic performance, and is one that the majority of people are lacking the most in. However, strength alone will never guarantee success in athletics - if that were the case every sport would be dominated by powerlifters or body builders. Strength is the building block that is stacked on top of quality movement, and strength serves as the building block that performance and skill are stacked upon. Strength must be built upon for success outside of the powerlifting to occur - speed, agility, power, deceleration, quickness, reaction, spatial awareness, depth perception, visual tracking, auditory cuing, and coordination all must be developed in the presence of adequate strength.

Tying it all together:
Bridging the Gap between everything.

A lot of information has been presented in the prior 170+ pages that encompasses rehab, fitness, performance, corrective exercise, the neurodevelopment sequence, assessment, pain, and several other topics. But now to address the 800 lb gorilla in the room - how does it all fit together? Seems like it would be a complicated answer, but to quote Di Vinci - "Simplicity is the ultimate in sophistication." How this all fits together is actually quite simple - it does not. Saying that it all does would be an egregious error that would truly be driven by the marketing side of things. However, there are some commonalities that do bind all of these topics together. These common threads are:

1. The Neurodevelopmental sequence
2. Movement progression/regression
3. Finding what is appropriate for the person standing in front of you.

This text could have easily been written from an angle that focused on exercises and drills - in that aspect we have a library of unique drills that expands daily. However, that angle only results in an exercise manual that any monkey could pick up and mimic. We did not want to do that.

This text could have easily focused on one type of drills - bodyweight, mobility, strength, TRX™, Sandbags, Kettlebells, Bands, etc. Those products are already out there, and if they truly were successful in what they did there would be no need for this text.

How Movement Restoration ties this all together is from the perspective of order and efficiency. This is what we call the "North Carolina Drill", because the first place we did this (completely unrehearsed in a room of 150+ individuals) was in North Carolina. Put this list of exercises in order:

Zercher Squat
Crawling
Clamshells
Supine knees to chest
1/2 kneeling ankle mobs
Cat/Camel
Step up
Step down
KB Press (1 KB)
Arm Bar
Pull up
KB Swing
Farmers Carry (2 Dumbbells)
TRX Row
Barbell Clean
Brettzel
Plank (on elbows)
Foam Roll T-spine mobility
Toe Touch Progression
Life line leg lowering
jump rope
Barbell Military press
Cable half-kneeling chop
Goblet Squat
Single leg stance with opposite leg reach
Pistol

Now, you may think some information is missing. Specifically "in order based on what?" That is our point exactly. This list entails corrective exercise, various strength drills/tools, mobility drills, soft tissue work, etc. It could be applied to an individual with rehab goals that is seeing a therapist, or it could easily be applied to a person with fitness goals, or even sports performance goals. Does not matter. The **_only_** assumption that is made is that these drills are 100% appropriate for the individual. Back to that 800 lb gorilla. How did **YOU** order these? Any thing like this?

	North Carolina Drill Answer:		
1	foam roll t-spine	14	Pull up
2	Brettzel	15	toe touch progression
3	1/2 kneeling ankle mobs	16	Barbell Military press
4	life line leg lowering	17	Goblet Squat
5	supine knees to chest	18	Zercher Squat
6	arm bar	19	step down
7	clamshells	20	step up
8	plank	21	SLS w/opposite leg reach
9	Cat/Camel	22	pistol
10	crawling	23	Farmers Carry (2 DB)
11	cable half-kneeling chop	24	Barbell Clean
12	KB Press (1KB)	25	KB Swing
13	TRX Row	26	jump rope

The safe bet is no; the order you selected was different. 'Different' based on your background and your bias. But, when all bias and opinion is removed from exercise selection what is left is the NDS. Mobility first, then adding stability and strength while progressing through the developmental postures (applying the order of the patterns within each posture), followed finally by loading (speed of movement, loading sequence, etc). The NDS shows that sequence and order are of utmost importance, and can be paramount in the success of skill (and strength truly is a skill) acquisition.

Gray Cook is quoted as saying, *"The language of movement is feel."* Aristotle stated, *"For the things we have to learn before we can do them, we learn by doing."* Both happen as movement is learned - at any age. The problem is most people are more concerned about how they feel *after* a training session, and have little self-awareness to what they are feeling *while* they are performing the drills and exercises during their training session. Quantity has been glorified and popularized to the point that quality has been lost. This only strengthens the argument for correctively ordering everything in a training session based on something larger than the training goals set forth in the daily workout. People will not -no matter how much we try to give them the benefit of the doubt- be attentive to a majority of what they do in the gym. Those that do, are reading this text. Applying this sequence for success to their training ensures that each drill is sequenced to build off of the prior drill.

Will this build hypertrophy? Who knows, but form typically follows function. Will this ensure success in a sport? Alone, it is unlikely. Will this provide "Fat Loss"? Depends on the activity level and the diet going into it. It *WILL* improve movement quality, which in turn will allow strength to be improved and will have a positive impact on the overall health of the individual. Beyond that, it will depend on the situation.

The neurodevelopmental sequence provides the order for almost everything movement related. Should we strive to all move like children? Maybe, but that alone will not do anything but provide another set of unrealistic exercises for people to attempt to do and ultimately abandon. Striving to apply the principles that allow children to move like, well, children is the goal. Children's only goals are to play and have fun - not bad by any means. Adult life complicates these goals, but the principles to how children move can (and should) be applied in any instance - mobility before stability; acquiring movement from the head down and the midline out; moving from the ground up; a sensory rich environment; and a progressive increase in challenge all are the building blocks of success in any chosen task.

We hope you have been moved!

Appendix 1

The <u>forgotten</u> benefits of the Turkish get up.
This article was originally published on the StrongFirst™ website
(www.strongfirst.com/blog/the-forgotten-benefits-of-the-turkish-get-up/)

"As above, so below" - Unknown

We like what is new. Look at how well Apple has benefitted every time they release the latest iPhone, iPad, or Mac. The followers of Apple are fiercely loyal. The nice thing about Apple and this craze over their products is that they are continuously pushing the technology forward. The downfall is the marketing craze they generate surrounding the release of their latest and greatest product. Is the need to push the industry forward generating their drive, or is it the all mighty dollar?? I would like to think it is mostly an internal drive to be better than they were yesterday, but in reality they are a for profit business that is selling products that no one else on the planet can create. If we look at the technology that Apple has popularized, they weren't the first to actually come up with some of their most popular products - Sony had MP3 players on the market well before the iPod exploded. What Apple did was popularize and market it in a manner that the public had to have it. Big mistake for Sony.

When Pavel introduced kettlebells to the West several years ago, the Turkish get up was reintroduced. Pavel didn't "create" the get up, he just dusted it off and pulled it out of obscurity. Brett Jones and Gray Cook shed new light on the get up as a wonderful mini-assessment and corrective drill with the CK-FMS, Kalos Thenos, and Kalos Thenos 2. Dr. Mark Cheng added the high bridge to promote hip extension and the get up was forever changed - and controversial. To high bridge or to low sweep, that is the question. The answer is always going to be: it depends on your goals. The popularity of the get up soared! The get up was a rock star - everyone was doing get ups, get up variations, get up breakdowns, and heavy get ups. YouTube loved it! The pendulum had swung to the overexposure side of the board. But like it has been said before, after every peak is a valley - we are in that get up valley.

Let's take a deeper look at why the get up is so powerful and so diverse in its application. Before we do that, let's look at crawling. Crawling, much like the get up has been around for a while - no one invented it and no one entity owns it. It is a powerful but small part of the entire neurodevelopmental sequence (the progressive development of movement patterns and strength that begins at birth and continues until we are vertical).

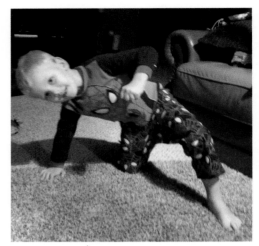

The earliest I can find that it was used clinically was in the early 1970's by Moshe Feldenkrais. I watched Gray Cook drop the IQ of an entire room several years ago when he asked people to crawl. Why is it so beneficial? Here is a list of the reasons:

1. Promotes cross lateralization (getting right brain to work with left side)
2. Promotes upper body stability
3. Promotes lower body stability
4. Promotes reflexive stability of the trunk and extremities
5. Ties the right arm to the left leg, and left arm to the right leg
6. Gets the upper extremities working reciprocally (legs too)
7. Stimulates the vestibular system (1 of the 3 senses that contribute to balance)
8. Stimulates the visual system (the second of 3 senses that contribute to balance)
9. Stimulates the proprioception system (3rd oft he 3 systems that contribute to balance)
10. Promotes spatial awareness
11. Develops a front/back weight shift
12. Develops upper body strength, trunks strength, and hip strength

Quite a few things, that essentially make crawling kind of awesome. But, it's biggest limitation is that the orientation of the body never changes (crawling is always done on all 4's with the he trunk parallel to the ground) and loading it (volume, resistance, etc) defeats the purpose of crawling. Crawling's biggest gift to the world of movement is the neurologic adaptations it promotes. That is pretty much it. During the NDS once an infant is proficient at crawling and has developed adequate strength and stability, they move up the sequence to walking. Being vertical is a much better posture to develop strength, power, metabolic loading, etc. Developmentally that is where a majority of those attributes are developed. All that being said, every person I see is likely to crawl. Once they have nailed it, we only revisit it as a quick assessment. I also recommend everyone brush their teeth - this gives you a shiny grill and is good for cardiovascular health (huh?). After meals for about 2 minutes at a time is adequate. I don't recommend they brush for 10 minutes, or with a heavier brush, or brush too hard.

Back to the get up. Why is it so beneficial? Here is a list of reasons:
1. Promotes cross lateralization (getting right brain to work with left side)
2. Promotes upper body stability
3. Promotes lower body stability
4. Promotes reflexive stability of the trunk and extremities
5. Ties the right arm to the left leg, and left arm to the right leg
6. Gets the upper extremities working reciprocally (legs too)
7. Stimulates the vestibular system (1 of the 3 senses that contribute to balance)
8. Stimulates the visual system (the second of 3 senses that contribute to balance)
9. Stimulates the proprioception system (3rd of the 3 systems that contribute to balance)
10. Promotes spatial awareness
11. Develops a front/back weight shift
12. Develops upper body strength, trunks strength, and hip strength

Does that list look familiar? Unlike the limitation of crawling (only occurring in one posture) the get up works thru several postures of the NDS - Supine, Rolling, Crawling, Asymmetrical stance, Single leg stance, and Symmetrical stance.

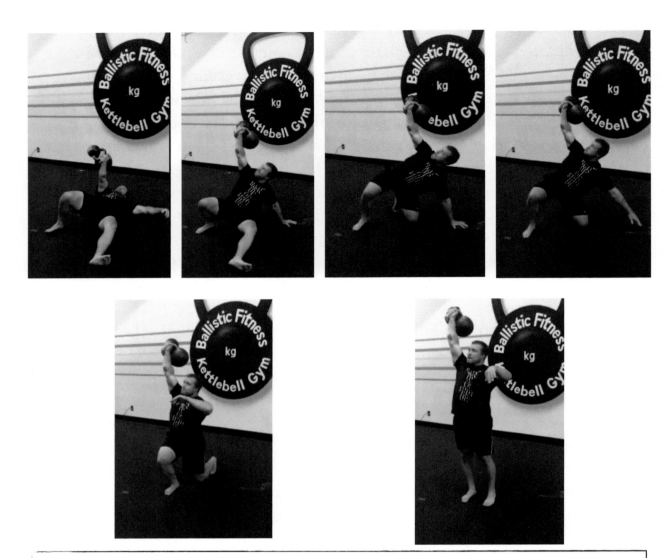

Derek Miller SGF II performing a 68kg get up at Ballistic Fitness Kettlebell Gym in Fayetteville Ark. A heavy get up is very "corrective". Symmetry, strength, and neurological coordination are in FULL display here. A perfect display of pressing down to get up. Very Strong.

Additionally, as a lift you can proceed to adding substantial load to the get up to magnify the strength and stability components. So, even though we are in The Valley of get up popularity, the get up is just like crawling - only much better.

One of the overlooked benefits of the get up is a misconception that the name presents. The "up". How does an infant rise to standing from either a seated, quadruped, or kneeling posture? I'll bet you answered with "they pull up". You, my friend, are wrong. It appears that they pull themselves up - but they are infants and lack the upper body strength to physically pull themselves up. What appears as pulling up, is them placing their hands above shoulder level and pressing down. This pushing down activates several trunk stabilizers which allows them to push their feet into the ground to rise up. So, in essence what they are doing is pushing down to get up. The get up is the PERFECT representative of this overlooked developmental feat - one that crawling neglects. The only way to initiate the roll to elbow is by pressing into the giant globe beneath us. This pressing into the ground is what generates the needed stability to move into a vertical position.

The point of this? Everyone who has read Simple and Sinister or has the initials SFG behind their name have the tools to apply the greatest (until someone can emphatically disprove it) neurological movement ever. Can you crawl? By all means, go for it. But my question to you is just like my question about Apple - are you crawling to get better or are you crawling because you have been convinced you can't get stronger without it? The benefits of mastering the get up have been swallowed up by the recent craze in popularity of crawling and other movement based systems. If it is good enough to balance out the swings in the Simple and Sinister program, there is probably a good reason why.

Appendix 2

Red / Yellow / Green Charts

The thought process behind the R/Y/G classification of exercise based off of the FMS scores is the process of addition by subtraction - remove those drills that will only make things worse. Loading (in any way that volume can be increased) as well as velocity added to any of the problematic patterns will only make the asymmetrical or 1/1 scores get worse. In this approach, anything that does not strengthen the identified patterns is removed. This information can be used in determining training groups, identifying home work drills or home exercises, and for intervention selection - how it is applied is based heavily on the situation.

Abbreviations:

1/2	Half
1/2K	Half Kneeling
S-Leg	Single Leg
TGU	Turkish Get up
TK	Tall Kneeling
OH	Overhead
DL	Deadlift
KB	Kettlebell
1/2S	Half Standing

ASLR (1/1, 1/2, 1/3)

	Kettlebell	Barbell	Bodyweight	Other
Red	Swing(2arm, 1 arm)	Back Squats	Sprinting	Pitching
	Clean	Clean	Squats	
	Snatch	Snatch		
	S- Leg Deadlift			
	Windmill			
	Overhead swing			
	Squats			
Yellow	Front Squats	Good Morning	Running	Throwing
	TGU - high bridge	Hang clean	Asymmetrical Stance Drills	
	Deadlift	Hang Snatch	Rolling Drills	
		Deadlift	Seated Drills	
Green	Tall Kneeling (TK) press	Elevated Deadlift	Skipping	Chops
	TK Press		Galloping	Lifts
	1/2 Kneeling press		Supine Drills	
	1/2K Windmill			
	TGU to elbow			
	Elevated Deadlift			

SM (1/1, 1/2, 1/3)

	Kettlebell	Barbell	Bodyweight	Other
Red	Press	Military Press	Pull up	Pitching
	Snatch	OH squat	Hand stand press	
	TGU - beyond post			
	Overhead Swing			
	Windmill			
	Push press			
	Jerk			
Yellow	1/2 TGU	Bench press	Crawling	Throwing
	OH walks		Chin ups	
	Low Windmill		Quadruped	
	Single Arm Deadlift		Brachiation	
Green	Swing		Prone drills	chops
	Clean		Supine Drills	lifts
	TGU to elbow		Seated Drills	
	Arm Bar			
	Farmers Carry			

RS (1/1, 1/2, 1/3)

	Kettlebell	Barbell	Bodyweight	Other
Red	Snatch	Bent Press	Sprinting	Asymmetric loaded drills
	TGU past elbow		Crawling	
	Clean		Rolling Drills	
	Windmill		ALL Single leg strength work	
	Bent press			
Yellow	Front Squat		Running	Throwing
	1 Arm Swing		Skipping	Half standing drills
	Suitcase DL		Galloping	
	1 Arm Press			
	1 Arm DL			
	S-Leg DL			
Green	Arm Bar	Squats	Supine Drills	Chops
	TGU to elbow	Pressing	Prone Drills	Lifts
	2 Arm Swing	Deadlifts	Quadruped drills	Half kneeling drills

TSPU (1/1, 1/2, 1/3)

	Kettlebell	Barbell	Bodyweight	Other
Red	TGU past 1/2 kneeling	Back Squat	1 Arm Push up	
	2 KB Press	Snatch	Hand stand push ups	
	2 KB push press	Military Press		
	2 KB Jerk			
	2 KB Snatch			
Yellow	1 KB Snatch	Front Squat	Crawling	Plyometrics
	1 KB Press	Zercher Squat	Push up progression	
	1KB Push Press	Deadlift	Pull ups	
	Swing	Bench Press	Chin ups	
	Clean			
	1 KB Jerk			
	Goblet Squat			
Green	1/2 TGU		Supine Drills	Half kneeling drills
	S-Leg Deadlift		Prone Drills	Chops.
			Quadruped Drills	Lifts

ILL (1/1, 1/2, 1/3)

	Kettlebell	Barbell	Bodyweight	Other
Red	TGU past bridge	Traveling Lunges	Lunges	Pitching
	Windmill		Deceleration drills	
	Bent Press		Cutting drills	
Yellow	Swing	Split squat variations	Jogging	1/2 Standing Drills
	Clean		Running	
	Front Squat		Split squats	
	Snatch		Bulgarian split squats	
	Deadlift		S-Leg strength work	
	Press		Skipping	
			Galloping	
Green	1/2 TGU			1/2K Drills
	1/2K Press			chops
	Suitcase DL			lifts
				halos

HS (1/1, 1/2, 1/3)

	Kettlebell	Barbell	Bodyweight	Other
Red	TGU past the 1/2K	Step ups	Sprinting	
	Single leg drills		Single leg strength work	
			Step ups	
			Single leg drills	
Yellow	Swing	Snatch	Running	Throwing
	Clean	Clean	Split squats	
	Windmill	Split squats	Rolling drills	
	Snatch	Squats	Sitting drills	
	Front Squat		Crawling	
	S-Leg Deadlift		Skipping	
Green	TGU to 1/2K		1/2k drills	1/2 S Chops
	Suitcase DL		1/2 standing drills	1/2S Lifts
	1/2k drills		Supine drills	
			Prone Drills	
			Galloping	

DS (1)

	Kettlebell	Barbell	Bodyweight	Other
Red	Squats	Back Squats	Pistols	Jumping Drills
	Clean	Military Press	Hand Stand pressing	Plyometrics
	Snatch	Snatch	Squats	
	Press	Clean		
Yellow	Swing	Hang Snatch	Split Squat variations	
	TGU passed 1/2K	Hang Clean	Single leg strength work	
	Split squat	Pin Squats	Pull ups	
	Tactical Lunge	Zercher Squats	Chin ups	
		Front Squats		
Green	TGU to 1/2 K	Deadlifts	Supine drills	TK Chops
	Deadlift	Bench press	Prone Drills	TK Lifts
	1/2K drills		Quadruped Drills	
			Kneeling Drills	
			Push ups	

Appendix 3
"This only works because of the patient population you work with - it doesn't apply to mine."

We will officially call out two groups of individuals that have consistently stated that this model will not work with the individuals they work with - PT's and Athletic Trainers in a Collegiate Setting. The PT's claim that this model will not work with their patients because of age and mobility problems. The AT's claim this is not applicable because in the collegiate setting they have limited one-on-one time with their patients. The real problem in both these instances are in the individual(s) applying the model. Each will be addressed individually.

For those who say that following this model cannot work because of the limitations (age, injuries, age related problems, etc) of their patients, these patients are the ones who need this model the most. Movement is universal - everyone regardless of age should possess the same minimal movement competencies. One of the most important is the ability to get up from the ground. In the older population, the ground is feared. They fear falling and getting injured or falling and not being able to get back up. Look at how this problem is typically addressed in the elderly - walking aids (canes, walkers, scooters), special orthopedic shoes, Falls Prevention Programs. All do very little to address the actual problems and are geared at teaching this group to live with the problems. This Falls Prevention Program actually is looking to address the problems that lead to falls in the elderly in a manner that is attacking it head on (www.youtube.com/watch?v=KlaNVnFssmg).

We have applied this model successfully to individuals recovering from total hip replacements, total knee replacements, and almost every other type of surgical procedure that is routinely done (NOTE - this is applied by licensed Athletic Trainers and licensed Physical Therapists in a rehab clinic). All of those completing the program returned to levels of function that they had thought was out of reach.

One current individual that is being trained is a former Army Ranger that made a career of jumping out of airplanes. His list of injuries is quite lengthy. In the past 5 years he has had a total hip replacement, a shoulder reconstruction, and several other orthopedic conditions that have led to his movement in general being uncomfortable. His goal is to move better, feel better, and drop some weight. He has many restrictions, but getting him on the ground and going through the NDS postures and patterns have him back to working out (in a completely new manner) without hurting. The NDS sequence is being followed but clinical discretion is allowing for the appropriate modifications to be made so that the benefits of the postures/patterns are being gained without any negative effects. The FMS was also performed at the onset of his training - he scored a 7 (1's on everything). Many professionals think the FMS is not applicable to certain individuals, but in fact it is very applicable in anyone -regardless of age- where movement quality is be addressed. This score of 7 gives us an objective measure to gauge our progress. As long as our training does not cause any 1's to turn into 0's and we are working towards 2's, then we are on the right path.

In those instances when one-on-one training is not possible, this program still can serve a greater purpose. Having a movement quality base line (the FMS) is the key. This can then generate individualized daily "homework" for each athlete to work on in an effort to reduce the likelihood of injury (by addressing and removing asymmetries). The first domain of Athletic Training is injury prevention- this goes above and beyond taping ankles, and the standard pre-participation physical. Having the FMS (which is a screen - just like blood pressure and the eye test) can allow the AT in a collegiate setting to know which athletes need to have a more thorough orthopedic exam. Anyone that scores a 1 or a 0 on any FMS test automatically go into a group that gets a more complete assessment in an effort to identify the causative factors - which the FMS cannot find. The real benefit of this model is in preventing issues from turning into problems.

The Movement Restoration model has been and can be applied to any individual in any type of setting - the key is in the person applying the model. Even if the best application is in the ordering of exercises being performed (like was modeled in the North Carolina Drill), the benefits will be seen.

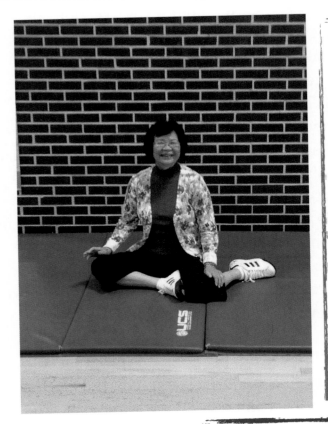

This is Takeko. She is a ripe, young, 75 years old. Born and raised in Okinawa she moved to the US after World War II. She continues to be very active and her movement patterns reflect this. This is a typical posture for her to be seated in while reading. Attached is a link to a video of Takeko going through the FMS and also a video of her going through some of her basic everyday movements.

Video Links:

Takeko's Movements- http://youtu.be/i5HfCO6wv5U
Takeko's FMS - http://youtu.be/aQUfbyzGp1M

Acknowledgements

This project began when my son was born, almost 5 years ago. We have had several individuals who have helped us and provided feedback, insight, and reality along the way. Without the help of these individuals, this project would have fizzled away a long time ago. There is no order to this list, so the first was just as valuable as the last:

Gary Herman
Jeff O'Connor
Dr. Mark Cheng
Clay Holman - Model #1
Eric Pohl - Model #1
Pavel Tsatsouline
Nikki Shlosser
Mark Toomey
Lee Burton
Gray Cook
Laree Draper
Tona Hetzler
Derek Miller
Jeff Stratton
Kalen

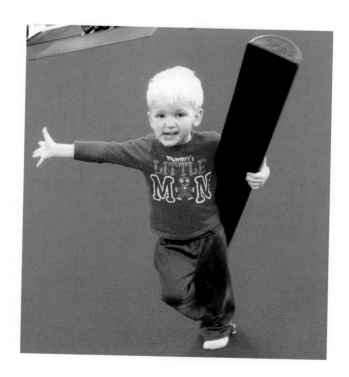

Thank you all.

Until next time.........

Bibliography

Bertoti, D. (2004). Functional Neurorehabilitation through the life span. Philadelphia, PA, F.A. Davis Co.

Blakeslee, S., Blakeslee, M. (2008). The Body Has a Mind of Its Own. New York NY, Random House Paperbacks.

Bolton, A. and P. Tsatsouline (2012). Deadlift Dynamite. Little Canada, MN, Dragon Door Publications, Inc.

Cech, D., Martin, S. (2012). Functional Movement Development Across the Life Span. St. Louis MO, Elsevier Saunders Inc.

Cook, G. (2010). Movement. Santa Cruz, CA, On Target Publications.

Cook, R., G. Bird, C. Catmur, C. Press and C. Heyes (2014). "Mirror neurons: from origin to function." Behav Brain Sci 37(2): 177-192.

Delforge, G. (2002). Musculoskeletal trauma : implications for sports injury management. Champaign, IL, Human Kinetics.

Dodds, R., H. J. Denison, G. Ntani, R. Cooper, C. Cooper, A. A. Sayer and J. Baird (2012). "Birth weight and muscle strength: a systematic review and meta-analysis." J Nutr Health Aging 16(7): 609-615.

Doidge, N. (2007). The brain that changes itself : stories of personal triumph from the frontiers of brain science. New York, Viking.

Feldenkrais, M. and E. Beringer (2010). Embodied wisdom : the collected papers of Moshé Freldenkrais. San Diego, Calif.

Grindstaff, T. L., R. R. Hammill, A. E. Tuzson and J. Hertel (2006). "Neuromuscular control training programs and non-contact anterior cruciate ligament injury rates in female athletes: a numbers-needed-to-treat analysis." J Athl Train 41(4): 450-456.

Hannaford, C. (1995). Smart moves : why learning is not all in your head. Arlington, Va., Great Ocean Publishers.

Key, J. (2010). Back pain : a movement problem : a clinical approach incorporating relevant research and practice. Edinburgh ; New York, Churchill Livingstone/ Elsevier.

Loudon, J. K., A. J. Parkerson-Mitchell, L. D. Hildebrand and C. Teague (2014). "Functional movement screen scores in a group of running athletes." J Strength Cond Res 28(4): 909-913.

McGill, S. (2004). Ultimate Back Fitness and Performance. Ontario, Canada, Wabuno Publishers; Waterloo.

Melillo, R. (2009). Disconnected kids : the groundbreaking brain balance program for children with autism, ADHD, dyslexia, and other neurological disorders. New York, Perigee Book.

Merriam-Webster Inc. (2005). The Merriam-Webster dictionary. Springfield, Mass., Merriam-Webster.

Myer, G. D., A. M. Kushner, A. D. Faigenbaum, A. Kiefer, S. Kashikar-Zuck and J. F. Clark (2013). "Training the developing brain, part I: cognitive developmental considerations for training youth." Curr Sports Med Rep 12(5): 304-310.

Myers, T. W. (2009). <u>Anatomy trains : myofascial meridians for manual and movement therapists</u>. Edinburgh ; New York, Elsevier.

Myers, T. W. (2014). <u>Anatomy trains : myofascial meridians for manual and movement therapists</u>. Edinburgh, Elsevier.

Ramachandran, V. S. (2011). <u>The tell-tale brain : a neuroscientist's quest for what makes us human</u>. New York, W.W. Norton.

Roshanravan, B., C. Robinson-Cohen, K. V. Patel, E. Ayers, A. J. Littman, I. H. de Boer, T. A. Ikizler, J. Himmelfarb, L. I. Katzel, B. Kestenbaum and S. Seliger (2013). "Association between physical performance and all-cause mortality in CKD." <u>J Am Soc Nephrol</u> 24(5): 822-830.

Simons, D. G., J. G. Travell, L. S. Simons and J. G. Travell (1999). <u>Travell & Simons' myofascial pain and dysfunction : the trigger point manual</u>. Baltimore, Williams & Wilkins.

Sonnon, S. (2012). <u>Primal Stress</u>. Atlanta GA, RMAX International.

Spanu, C. E. and M. S. Hefzy (2003). "Biomechanics of the knee joint in deep flexion: a prelude to a total knee replacement that allows for maximum flexion." <u>Technol Health Care</u> 11(3): 161-181.

Starrett, K. and G. Cordoza (2013). <u>Becoming a supple leopard : the ultimate guide to resolving pain, preventing injury, and optimizing athletic performance</u>. Las Vegas, NV

Stewart, K., Hetzler, T., Mitchell, D., Hetzler, B. (2014). <u>Crawling Pattern Movement Effects on Fine Motor Skills Among Children With Autism Spectrum Disorder</u>. Masters of Science, Athletic Training, Missouri State University.

Trokey, T., Hetzler, T., Mitchell, D., Hetzler, B. (2014). <u>Effects of SubOccipital Release Soft Tissue Technique on Toe Touch Measurement</u>. Masters of Science, Athletic Training, Missouri State University.

<u>Tsatsouline, P. (2004). The Naked Warrior. Little Canada MN, Dragon Door Publications, Inc.</u>

Tsatsouline, P. (2013). <u>Kettlebell Simple and Sinister</u>. Reno, NV, StrongFirst, Inc.

Tsatsouline, P., John, D. (2011). <u>Easy Strength</u>. St. Paul, MN, Dragon Door Publications, Inc.

Varier, S., M. Kaiser and R. Forsyth (2011). "Establishing, versus maintaining, brain function: a neuro-computational model of cortical reorganization after injury to the immature brain." <u>J Int Neuropsychol Soc</u> 17(6): 1030-1038.

Voight, M. L., B. J. Hoogenboom and W. E. Prentice (2007). <u>Musculoskeletal interventions : techniques for therapeutic exercise</u>. New York, McGraw-Hill, Medical Pub. Division.

Wyckoff, S. L. (2010). <u>Infant Gross Motor Variability within an Ecological Niche: A Study of Infant Development and Care Giving in Rural Papua New Guinea</u>. Doctor of Philosophy, University of Washington.

Printed in Great Britain
by Amazon.co.uk, Ltd.,
Marston Gate.

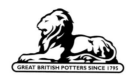

Churchill China

Great British Potters since 1795

Broadhurst – Bridgwood – Myott Meakin
Crown Clarence – Queen's Fine Bone China

Staffordshire Heritage Series

General Editor
J. H. Y. Briggs, M.A., F.S.A., F.R.Hist.S.

In print
1. PIT BOY TO PRIME MINISTER
The Story of the Right Hon. Joseph Cook
Graham Bebbington

2. AGENTS OF REVOLUTION
John and Thomas Gilbert – Entrepreneurs
Peter Lead

3. THE WATER MILLS OF THE BOROUGH OF
NEWCASTLE-UNDER-LYME
George Riley

4. THE MINERS OF STAFFORDSHIRE 1840–1914
John Benson

5. CHURCHILL CHINA
Great British Potters since 1795
Rodney Hampson

———

Also by Rodney Hampson
LONGTON POTTERS 1700–1865

Susie Cooper Bryn Youds.
pub. Thames & Hudson 1996 Large pb. $24.95 now £5.95

Churchill China Rodney Hampson.
pub. Keele University 1994 Large pb.   £19.95 now £9.95

The Water Mills of the Borough of Newcastle
George Riley. pub. Keele University 1991 pb.   £4.95 now £2.45

The Miners of Staffordshire 1840 - 1914
Ed. John Benson. pub. Keele University 1993 pb.   £5.00 now £2.50

Agents of Revolution (Staffs. Canal Entrepreneurs)
Peter Lead. pub. Keele University 1989 pb.   £8.95 now £4.45

Short Circular Walks from Local Churches Vol. 3
P & G. Shufflebotham. pub. Gladwyn 1996 pb.   £2.99 now £1.49

The Trent & Mersey Canal Peter Lead.
pub. Moorland Publishing 1993 pb.   £9.99 now £4.99

From Inferno to Flowers (Etruria) Bryan / Fisher.
pub. By the authors 1986 pb.   £2.50 now £1.25

The Little Gold-Mine (Burslem Novel)
Arthur Berry. pub. Bullfinch 1991 pb.   £5.99 now £2.99

A Staffordshire Quiz Book John Godwin.
pub. S.B. Publications 1994 pb.   £4.50 now £2.25

Wedgwood And His Times (In Rhyme)
Anon. pub. Rose Bank Publishing. 1999 thin pb.   £1.75 now 85p

Lest We Forget (North Staffs. Mining)
Fred Leigh. pub. Rose Bank 1994 pb.   £6.99 now £3.49

Whom God Hath Joined Arnold Bennett.
pub. Alan Sutton 1994 pb.   £4.99 now £2.49

Tales of the Five Towns Arnold Bennett.
pub. Alan Sutton 1990 pb.   £3.95 now £1.95

A Vision of Splendour (Gothic Revival Architecture in Staffordshire)
Michael Fisher. pub. By the Author 1995 pb.   £9.99 now £4.99

**If you would like to order any of the local history books, please tick against the
relevant titles and fill in the section below then return to the address overleaf.
N.B. Post and Packaging extra, at cost.**

NAME..

ADDRESS...

POSTCODE.. **TEL. NO**...

ABACUS GALLERY / THE VILLAGE BOOKSHOP
56/58 Millrise Rd, Milton, Stoke on Trent. ST2 7BW
Props: Dave & Margaret Mycock.   Est. 1980.
Tel: (01782) 543005

A SELECTION OF NEW LOCAL HISTORY BOOKS
AT HALF THE PUBLISHED PRICE

Capital Crimes (Staffordshire Hanging Offences)
Ros Prince. pub. Churnet Valley 1994 pb.   £8.95 now £4.45

Stoke on Trent A Pictorial History Alan Taylor
pub. Phillimore 1995 hb   £12.95 now £6.95

The Potteries - A Photographic Record Donald Morris.
 pub. Sigma 1998 pb   £9.95 now £4.95

Stoke on Trent in Old Photographs
Corum & Lawley. pub. Budding Books 1998 pb.   £7.99 now £3.99

A - Z of Stoke City (Football Club) Tony Matthews.
pub. Breedon Books 1997 Large hb.   £15.99 now £7.99

Whitchurch to Market Drayton in Old Photographs
Marianne Morris. pub. Alan Sutton 1994 pb.   £7.99 now £3.99

Crewe. A Portrait in Old Picture Postcards Vol.1
pub. S.B. Publications 1991 pb.   £4.95 now £2.45

Crewe. A Portrait in Old Picture Postcards Vol. 2
pub. S.B. Publications 1992 pb.   £5.95 now £2.95

The Dane Valley A Portrait in Old Picture Postcards
pub S.B. Publications 1991 pb.   £5.95 now £2.95

Stafford & District Postcards from the Past
Roy Lewis. pub. Sigma 1998 pb.   £6.95 now £3.45

Kidsgrove, Talke & Mow Cop Postcards from the Past
Roger Simmons. pub. Sigma 1998 pb.   £6.95 now £3.45

Newcastle under Lyme & District Postcards from the Past
pub. Sigma 1998 pb.   £6.95 now £3.45

Staffordshire Place-Names Anthony Poulton Smith.
pub. Countryside Books 1995 pb.   £6.95 now £3.45

Staffordshire - A Century in Photographs Staffordshire W.I.
pub. Countryside Books 1997 pb.   £6.95 now £3.45

Staffordshire Privies Anthony Poulton-Smith.
pub. Countryside Books 1998 pb.   £6.95 now £3.45

Derbyshire Privies David Bell.
pub. Countryside Books 1998 pb.   £6.95 now £3.45 P.T.o

Churchill China
Great British Potters since 1795

Broadhurst – Bridgwood – Myott Meakin
Crown Clarence – Queen's Fine Bone China

by
Rodney S. Hampson, M.A.

Staffordshire Heritage Series Volume 5

Editor: J. H. Y. Briggs, M.A., F.S.A., F.R.Hist.S.

The Centre for Local History, Department of History
University of Keele, 1994

First published in 1994 by
The Centre for Local History
Department of History
University of Keele
Staffordshire
© 1994 The Centre for Local History
Department of History, University of Keele

Rodney S. Hampson has asserted his right to
be identified as the author of this work.

British Library Cataloguing in Publication Data
A catalogue record for this book
is available from the British Library

ISBN 0 9513713 5 5 *(paperback)*
ISBN 0 9513713 4 7 *(hardback)*

Composed and originated by
Keele University Press Services
Printed by The Amadeus Press Ltd
Huddersfield, England

CONTENTS

This book is dedicated to the late
Reginald Haggar who showed me the way
and to my wife Eileen in appreciation
of her unfailing support

FOREWORD

By the middle of 1994 Churchill was Britain's largest family-owned ceramic manufacturer producing over 1.5 million pieces of pottery every week. The two main divisions of Hotelware and Tableware employ around 1,300 people at five sites throughout Stoke-on-Trent.

In addition Churchill has now formed a bone china division by the acquisition of the Crownford company in Longton, manufacturers of bone china giftware and tableware under the Queen's trademark. The Group sees an opportunity for expansion in this section of the market through quality products and independent distribution.

I am also pleased to announce that Churchill intends to seek a listing on the London Stock Exchange in October 1994. We at Churchill are proud of our products and place great value on our customers, our workforce and our suppliers. I hope you enjoy Rodney Hampson's splendid book.

E. Stephen Roper
Group Chief Executive

PREFACE

The university is always seeking ways of entering into partnership with local industry and, therefore, I am delighted to welcome this volume which arises out of fruitful collaboration between Keele's History Department and Churchill China. Expert at its task, the department has found fifty more years of history for Churchill than the company thought it possessed. This explains why the company is celebrating its 200th anniversary rather precipitously on the heels of its 150th.

The record here spelt out is a highly instructive one, indicating that the pottery industry has far more history than simply that of the prestige tableware companies that are household names. Not that Broadhursts and Bridgwoods, who are the forerunners of Churchill, were in any sense ordinary companies. Their very durability over so long a period of time would argue against that. As yet, however, too little has been written about such companies, which are of great significance both in terms of the number of workers employed and the quantity of pottery produced.

Both companies exhibit in their histories a willingness to experiment with new techniques, for example Broadhursts' development of transfer printing by roller in the 1870s and Bridgwoods a little later by pioneering the installation of gas-fired kilns and new techniques in lithography. At the same time you will find in this story a down-to-earth recognition of the importance of exploiting the tried and the tested. Innovation was often more instructive for other companies than profitable for the innovators, who paid the price of experimentation in their balance sheets.

Never far from the technologies, markets and accounts, however, are people – risk-taking entrepreneurs and a skilled labour force. This story of family businesses has been associated now with the Roper family for four generations, and they, like their Bridgwood and Broadhurst predecessors, have brought to the manufacturing of pottery very special qualities of vision and implementation.

Both Broadhursts and Bridgwoods, and more recently Churchill, have sought at several junctures in their histories to pioneer the layouts of model factories, believing that good working conditions were essential to quality production. It is this which has guaranteed this group success in exporting to worldwide markets from the beginning, with very early penetration of, for example, the Asian and Latin American markets.

CHURCHILL CHINA

I welcome the telling of this story of long traditions, the constant updating of manufacturing and management processes to meet changing demands, and of a company where the skills of potters and management have enabled the company not simply to survive but to move to new strengths of industrial achievement.

This is a good story and I am glad Keele has had a part in telling it.

Professor B. E. F. Fender
Vice-Chancellor
University of Keele

ACKNOWLEDGEMENTS

The generous assistance of the following people in the compilation of this history is gratefully acknowledged:

Mr. K. E. Allerton, Mr. J. M. Aynsley, Miss D. Baker, Mrs. K. Barker, Simon Bell, Mr. H. Blakey, His Excellency the Brazilian Ambassador in London, and colleagues in Brazil; Mrs. T. Brookfield, Mr. B. Burns, Mr. D. H. Chitty, Mr. B. Clarke, Mr. R. Colclough, Dr. E. Collard, Mr. P. Day, Mr. A. Dobraszczyc, Mr. G. W. Elliott, Dee Frankish, Gladstone Pottery Museum staff, Dr. G. A. Godden, Mr. I. Griffiths, Mrs. E. M. Hampson, Dr. C. J. Harrison, Professor M. Harrison, Dennis Heywood, Mr. R. J. C. Hildyard, Horace Barks Reference Library staff, *Instituto Historic e Geografico Brasileiro* staff; Mr. W. H. T. John, Mrs. G. Johnson, Dr. M. Johnson, Candida Kelsall, Mr. T. A. Lockett, Mr. J. C. Lloyd, Mr. K. T. Mason, Mr. J. W. Michener, Alan Miles, Mr. P. Millington, Wendy Morton, Mr. W. Morgan, Mr. C. Morris, Mr. D. Morris, Newcastle-under-Lyme Reference Library staff, Mrs. K. Niblett, Mr. P. O'Reilly, Mr. E. E. Orme, Mr. M. J. Phillips, Sue Platt, Mr. J. Potter, Mr. R. Pomfret, Public Record Office staff, Miss A. Roberts, Mr. M. Rogers, Mr. Andrew D. Roper, the late Mr. E. Peter Roper, Mr. E. Stephen Roper, Mr. Michael J. Roper, Mrs. W. S. Rowley, Royal Doulton Tableware Ltd., Mrs. A. Seaton, 'Signalman', Mr. J. Smith, Staffordshire Record Office staff, Stoke-on-Trent City Museum and Art Gallery staff, Mr. W. N. Suckling, Mr. G. R. Tams, Mrs. V. Timms, Mr. S. R. Twigg, Mr. C. Tyzack, Mr. H. B. Walker, Mrs. N. Whitehouse and Mrs. P. Woodhouse. Apologies are sincerely offered to anyone involved whose name has been omitted.

Every effort has been made to trace the copyright owners of illustrations used. The following are thanked for granting permission to reproduce material in their copyright, custody or possession: the Ordnance Survey for figures 1, 2, 9, 22, 23, 24, 25 and 40; *Tableware International* (formerly *The Pottery Gazette*) for figures 14, 16, 17, 18, 19, 20, 21, 27, 31, 33, 34, 37 and 41, and colour plates 7 and 8; the Public Record Office for figures 5, 6, 7, 10, 11 and 30; the Controller of Her Majesty's Stationery Office for figures 29, 35 and 36; the Gladstone Pottery Museum for colour plate 25; the Trustees of the Wedgwood Museum for archive material; and the Warrillow Collection, University of Keele for figure 38 and the cover illustration.

LIST OF COLOUR PLATES

INTRODUCTION

Churchill has always been too busy looking forward, to bother looking back, and so it turned to its local University for help when it did become curious about its distant past. It was a tempting challenge to uncover what turned out to be two hundred years of continuous history – the recent past from personal recollections and the forethought of a few individuals, the rest from an amazing variety of locations, evident from the long list of acknowledgments and even longer list of sources.

The business of 1994 is made up of many strands – the oldest, Bridgwoods, now Churchill Hotelware, reaching back two hundred years to the time of George Washington, first President of the United States, and the French Revolution. Broadhursts, the heart of Churchill Tableware, began fifty years later, before the Great Exhibition of 1851 – the firms to be united by the Roper family in 1965. Another strand is Myotts, itself almost a hundred years old, now part of Churchill Tableware.

These are not the famous names, Wedgwood, Minton, Spode, but more modest firms, the backbone of the Staffordshire pottery industry. They are essentially family firms, though not always bearing the family name. Edward Roper took over Broadhursts in the 1920s, but the Broadhurst name was retained until 1984, and likewise, the Aynsley family took charge of Bridgwoods in 1891 without changing the name. Churchill was adopted as an easily recognisable name for the entire group in 1984.

The histories of the constituent firms are typical of family businesses. Both Bridgwoods and Broadhursts came successfully through difficult times – Sampson Bridgwood's 'noble struggles against adversity' in 1823–25, and Peter Roper's resurrection of Broadhurst after enforced closure during the Second World War – both instances where family support gave continuity. It can only be this personal 'will to win', backed by dedicated staff, that has brought the enterprise through two hundred years to today's proud position as the largest family-owned ceramic company in the UK.

Both Bridgwoods and Broadhursts started in Longton, most southerly of the six towns and innumerable villages which make up the Staffordshire Potteries. In medieval times, individual potters had made domestic pots wherever there was clay, fuel and a market. North Staffordshire was unusual in being a poor upland farming area, with both coal and clay, surrounded by the richer lands of Cheshire and South Staffordshire. The poor moorland farmers supplemented their farming income by making pots for the adjoining lowlands.

One requirement was earthenware butter pots, in which the lowland farmers packed butter for market, a steady demand which encouraged specialisation. From the beginning of the eighteenth century, finer ware was developed, exemplified by Josiah Wedgwood's cream-coloured earthenware and jasper. John Turner of Longton (then called Lane End) was Wedgwood's contemporary and equal, and set standards of potting in Longton which encouraged emulation.

When Bridgwoods started potting two hundred years ago, Longton was a 'small but populous village' of four thousand inhabitants, with a church, chapels, market hall, collieries and twenty or so master potters. It lay on the great road from Derby to Chester, well-placed to serve the travelling pot-sellers who bought for 'ready-money', a tradition that kept Longton prosperous sixty years later, when other pottery towns lost business in the American Civil War.

A high tariff on imported Chinese porcelain in the 1790s encouraged British production, and Spode perfected bone china about 1800. Longton potters, already expert in earthenware, took up his reliable formula, and developed a new trade in simple, cheap china teaware. Bridgwoods changed to the new material, and prospered.

Earthenware production continued. James Broadhurst grew up in the same town, and rose from being a working potter to a sizeable manufacturer of earthenware. By the time he was in business in 1847, Longton had trebled in population, and almost a third of its inhabitants were employed in its forty potworks.

Both Bridgwoods and Broadhurst moved to new factories – Bridgwoods to the present Hotelware site in 1853, and Broadhursts to nearby Fenton in 1870, a site abandoned in 1981 for lack of space to expand. The other five towns of the Staffordshire Potteries experienced similar growth, and other factories developed which were eventually to become part of the Churchill Group – Clarence Works in Longton, Alexander Works at Cobridge, and Marlborough Works at Tunstall, the most northerly town.

North Staffordshire's specialisation in pottery manufacture for three hundred years has developed a unique combination of inherited skills and technical expertise, supported by a power-base of materials and machinery suppliers. The history of the Churchill Group is a microcosm of the development of the North Staffordshire pottery industry.

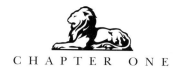

BROADHURSTS IN LONGTON
1847–1870

Peter Hampson, James Broadhurst I and William Broadhurst started in partnership at the Green Dock Works, on the south-west side of New Street (present-day Cooke Street), Longton in 1847. They leased a four-oven works (Figure 1) valued for rates at £111 from William Batkin, a works previously occupied by Job Broadhurst and earlier owned by Richard Newbold, of Mayer and Newbold.[1]

Peter Hampson seems to have been a member of a Longton family who were carriers, beer retailers, painters, modellers and designers.[2] William Broadhurst may have been the twenty-one-year-old son of Job Broadhurst, who had just vacated the works.[3] William Broadhurst left the partnership in 1849[4] and joined Josiah Perry in a new partnership at Fenton, which failed in 1852.[5] Perhaps James Broadhurst was his uncle, brought into the business to provide practical experience, but no family relationship with Job or William Broadhurst has been found.

James Broadhurst was termed a 'Potter Journeyman' in the 1841 census, when he was aged about forty, living in Paradise Street.[6] He had married Drusilla, daughter of a working potter, John Lockett, at Stoke on 5 April 1824.[7] They had six children: Thomas born 24 August 1824, Ellen born 26 October 1827, Ann born 27 September 1830, James II born 14 May 1832 and Samuel born 26 June 1835, (all baptised at Longton New Connexion Methodist Church); and John, born about 1839.[8]

The partnership made earthenware.[9] There are records of printed patterns with the mark 'H & B', but these could also have been made by Heath and Blackhurst of Burslem.[10] Hampson and Broadhurst treated their workpeople at the annual hiring at Martinmas 1851:[11]

> On the evening of Friday, the 14th instant, about 150 of the workpeople of Messrs. Hampson and Broadhurst, with a few invited friends, sat down to a substantial supper in the new warehouse of their manufactory, Providence Bank, Green Dock, Longton. After the repast Mr. James Miller was called to the chair; Mr. P. Hampson senior officiated as vice-chairman.

The usual loyal toasts having been given, the chairman gave 'Success to the Firm of Hampson and Broadhurst' which was drunk with three times three [cheers], and one cheer more for the Providence Bank. Mr. J. Broadhurst, in responding to the toast, made a suitable reply. Other toasts followed, which elicited remarks showing the proper and kindly feeling subsisting between the employers and the employed. The social character of the meeting was kept up to a late hour, and all separated to their homes well satisfied with the evening's proceedings.

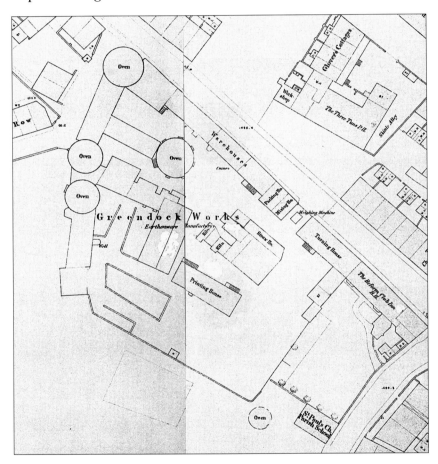

Figure 1 Green Dock Works, New Street (now Cooke Street), Longton, occupied by Hampson and Broadhurst 1847–54. Reproduced from Ordnance Survey 1/500 Plan OST (20) Longton, 1856

The mention of the new warehouse shows that some new building had been done. There had been a works on this site since about 1800, and the 1856 Ordnance map shows an irregular works layout behind a straight roadside facade, perhaps the 'new warehouse'.

James Broadhurst I lived in Orchard Place in 1851, alongside three other Longton manufacturers: James Colclough, William Green and William Hopwood.[12] Three sons were working potters: Thomas, a presser, aged 26; James aged 18, a thrower; and the youngest, Samuel, a warehouseman. By 1853, James Broadhurst I had found other partners, and on 20 February 1854 his partnership with Peter Hampson was dissolved by mutual consent. Peter Hampson continued at the Green Dock Works.[13]

In 1851, John Goodwin, who had been an earthenware manufacturer in Longton for thirty years, took the unusual step of moving to a new purpose-built works at Seacombe, near Birkenhead, Cheshire.[14] He left vacant the Crown Works, at the corner of Flint Street (now The Strand) and Commerce Street. Goodwin had been innovative at Longton: his sale of utensils included a Fourdrinier's Patent Sifting Apparatus, which replaced silk lawns by metal plates and sieves.[15] The owner of the Crown Works, Ralph Steele, a Longton wine merchant, leased the works for seven years from 11 November 1851 to James Bradbury, for a yearly rent of £236.[16] James Bradbury had lived in Longton, but was now farming at Mobberley, Cheshire. From 1852, the partnership at the Crown Works was Bradbury, Mason and Bradbury. Richard Mason had been a pottery manager, and the second Bradbury is assumed to be a son of James.[17]

Although there had been a potworks on the 'Crown' site since the 1790s, the factory taken over by Bradbury was a regular two-courtyard arrangement with two large biscuit and three smaller glost ovens (Figure 2), much of it still standing today as the John Tams Group Crown Works. In 1853, it was valued at £3,400.[18] James Broadhurst joined Bradbury and Mason there about 1853, and formally left his partnership with Peter Hampson at the Green Dock Works on 20 February 1854.[19] James Bradbury died about that time, and the partnership between his executors and Richard Mason and James Broadhurst was dissolved on 28 August of the same year.[20]

James Broadhurst I had been in partnerships from 1847 (which justified the firm's claim of being established in that year) but in 1854 he was his own master. By 1856 he had taken some or all of his sons into the business, and the firm was known as James Broadhurst and Sons:[21] Thomas would be 32, James II 24 and Samuel 21. A directory records them as making both china and earthenware. A Willow pattern plate is on record in America, marked 'James Broadhurst / Crown Pottery / Longton', which would have been made between 1854 and 1870.[22] James Broadhurst I died 23 February 1858 aged 59, leaving personal estate of 'under £4,000'.[23]

Drusilla Broadhurst, widow of James I, continued the family business at the Crown Works, probably under the active management of her eldest son, Thomas, as her younger sons, James II and Samuel, had separate ventures in an earthenware works in Gold Street, Longton in 1860, and in Commerce Street in 1861.[24] At the 1861 census, Drusilla Broadhurst lived in Peel Street, Dresden, and was described as a widow of 62 who was a 'retired earthenware manufacturer'. Thomas, aged 36, lived at the old family address of Orchard Place, as did Samuel, then aged 25, who claimed to employ 185. James Broadhurst II lived at Peel Street, aged 28, with his wife Emma (from Derbyshire), his two-year old son Samuel, seven-months old daughter Gertrude and a thirteen-year-old girl servant.

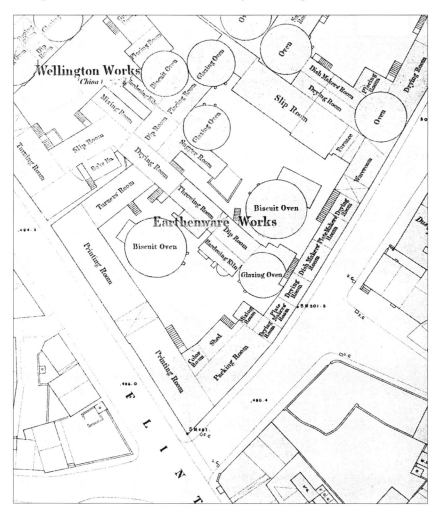

Figure 2 Crown Works, Flint Street (now The Strand), Longton, occupied by James Broadhurst (and Sons) 1853–70. Reproduced from Ordnance Survey 1/500 Plan OST (20) Longton, 1856

The death of Mrs. Drusilla Broadhurst on 5 October 1861, aged 62,[25] precipitated further changes in the business. An advertisement dated 6 September 1862 offered an unidentified earthenware business for sale, with all the details pointing to

Broadhursts' Crown Works. The reason for selling was given as 'declining business on account of the death of the senior partner'. The property possessed frontages of 100 yards to two principal streets in Longton, and had two biscuit and three glost ovens, and two hardening and enamelling kilns. The business had been established for forty years, trading with Turkish, Australian and East Indian markets. The premises were to be leased, with offers to be made to local solicitors.[26] No satisfactory bids must have been forthcoming, and a further advertisement in December offered the business for auction on 23 January 1863.[27] Inquiries were to be made to James and Samuel Broadhurst, Crown Pottery; and it looks as if the Broadhurst brothers contemplated selling the family business after the death of their mother. 'Established forty years' must have referred to John Goodwin's start in business in the same factory in 1822.[28]

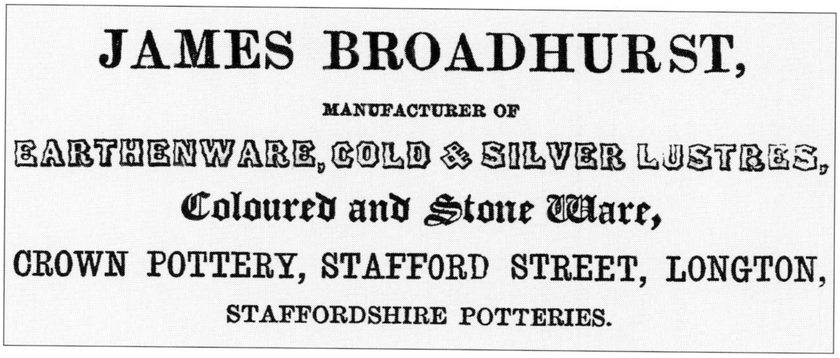

JAMES BROADHURST,

MANUFACTURER OF

EARTHENWARE, GOLD & SILVER LUSTRES,

Coloured and Stone Ware,

CROWN POTTERY, STAFFORD STREET, LONGTON,

STAFFORDSHIRE POTTERIES.

Figure 3
Advertisement for James Broadhurst in *Jones's Mercantile Directory of the Pottery District of Staffordshire 1864* (London, February 1864), 277

It seems however that no sale took place: on 24 April 1863, James Broadhurst and Samuel Broadhurst, manufacturers of china and earthenware, trading as James Broadhurst & Sons, dissolved partnership.[29] Samuel Broadhurst continued the separate business at Gold Street, and again a James Broadhurst was his own master at the Crown Works. An advertisement in a directory published in 1864 (Figure 3) lists his wares: earthenware, gold and silver lustres, coloured and stoneware.[30] Like Bridgwoods, James Broadhurst received his encomium from Lidstone in 1866 (Figure 4), with mentions of trade with Stamboul and the Golden Horn (Turkey), South America and Austerlands (Australia) in earthenware, gold and silver lustres, and coloured stoneware.[31] The destinations agree fairly well with the 1862 sale advertisement naming trade with Turkey, Australia and the East Indies. Overseas trade was obviously well-established: Keates & Ford's Directory for 1865–6 listed nine china and earthenware merchants in Longton, including James Broadhurst's brother, Samuel.

JAMES BROADHURST,

Manufacturer of Earthenware, Gold and Silver Lustres, Coloured and Stone Ware, Crown Pottery, Stafford Street, Longton, Staffordshire Potteries.

LIKE a renaissance morn upon me burst,
The art-achieved miracles of James Broadhurst,
And all in keeping, all with action rife,
Or for Mussulmen nought of breathing life.
Yet who shall say their Hist'ry is a waste
Of mental worth, for we can trace their taste.
Long years, thro' the Moorish palaces of Spain,
Thence as from th' Arabs we *that* style obtain.
Specimens that now my cabinet adorn,
Once graced Stamboul by the Golden Horn,
First had existence, yea, they flourish'd erst
In the establishment of James Broadhurst.
Thro' South Americ', too, his goods are sent,
Ay to ev'ry market on either continent.
O'er undisputed empire doth he reign,
In Auster-lands, beyond the roaring main,
And for that far meredional clime
He hath well worked for some length of time.
Hail! Manufacturer of Earthenware,
Art's laurels are thine own, and none the wreath
    may share.
'Round Minerva's monument thy glory clusters,
Ages trump thy fame for Gold and Silver Lustres,
Beside, in coloured stoneware none have durst
Compete with our enlightened James Broadhurst.

Figure 4 Poem in praise of James Broadhurst, in J. T. S. Lidstone, *The Thirteenth Londoniad ... giving a Full Description of the Principal Establishments in the Potteries etc.* (The Potteries, 1866), 31

James Broadhurst started to register his own designs: in 1866, an Oriental scene engraved for decorating jugs (Figure 5), and in 1870 a flag and crest, and an intertwined garland plate border (Figures 6 and 7).[32] The flag and crest are of the then Empire of Brazil. A plate with the flag design is in the collection of the *Instituto Historico e Geografico Brasileiro*, supplied by James Broadhurst for the Rio de Janeiro Police Force; and a saucer lined in pink with the same Broadhurst design is in the Brazilian National History Museum.[33] Another Longton manufacturer, Thomas Waterhouse Barlow, said in evidence to a Parliamentary Inquiry about a new railway in 1862, that business with South America had developed in the past six to eight years. He had shipped 2,500 crates there in the past year, and neighbouring manufacturers did the same: one Longton potter had established a place of business at Rio (de Janeiro) and sent his son as resident agent.[34] Registered designs were exceptional: 'open stock' patterns common to many firms (Willow, Asiatic Pheasants) were much more frequently used.

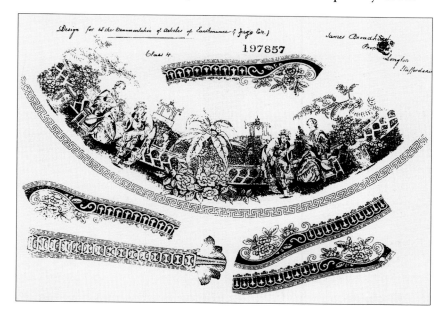

Figure 5 Design no. 197857, Oriental scene for body, neck and handle of jug, registered by James Broadhurst 4 June 1866. PRO: BT 43/68

James Broadhurst II took an interest in affairs outside his factory. When there was concern about the employment of children, James Broadhurst was one of the eight public-spirited Longton manufacturers who signed a memorial to the Home Secretary in 1862, asking for an inquiry and legislation, as 'a portion only of the employers could be brought to consent to [a voluntary] agreement'.[35] An inquiry was launched, and James Broadhurst gave evidence. He said it was good that children should not work after six; he would not take an order that put pressure on them; but he thought half-time working was impracticable, as there were not enough lads. In Broadhurst's plate shops, Samuel Key, aged 13, said he had worked there five years, running moulds and wedging clay. He came in at six, sometimes five-thirty, and went at six or seven, sometimes seven-thirty or eight. Keys was a fair example of the problem: running moulds into and out of hot stove rooms, and wedging heavy blocks of clay were considered to be two of the most harmful occupations in pottery making for young children. Legislation came in 1864, resulting in the employment of more girls and women (to replace the boys who had to attend school half-time) and the gradual introduction of machinery.

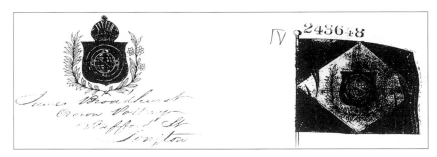

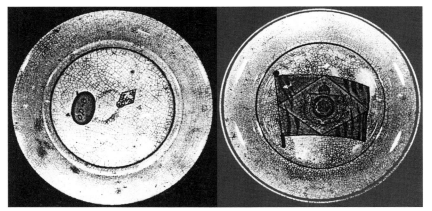

Figure 6 Design no. 243648, flag of the Brazilian Empire, registered by James Broadhurst 4 August 1870. PRO: BT43/68; and a plate supplied by James Broadhurst between 1870 and 1889 (when the Empire ceased) for the Rio de Janeiro Police Force. *Collection of the Instituto Historico e Geografico Brasileiro*, Rio de Janeiro, Brazil, OP-8

As a proprietor, James Broadhurst was bound by the economic pattern of boom and slump. He joined his Longton fellow-manufacturers in a notice to operative potters in 1864,[36] stating that there could be no price (wage) changes during the current year (for which they were hired); that there should be an agreed revision of prices in August for the coming year; and reminding employees that they were bound to their employer for the year. James Broadhurst maintained firm workshop discipline within his own works. He prosecuted a new employee who stole lead in 1863;[37] and two printers and a thrower for neglect of work whilst absent, drinking, in 1865.[38]

In 1867, James Broadhurst II lived at 16 Trentham Road,[39] but he had returned to Orchard Place by 1869,[40] and was still there in 1871, aged 38, with his wife Emma aged 35, and six children: Samuel, 12; Gertrude, 10; James, 7; Harry, 5; Drusilla, 2 and Laura of nine months. Mrs Broadhurst had her 16-year-old niece, Elizabeth Blewit from Derbyshire, and a Welsh girl servant to help her.[41]

Hampson Brothers of Green Dock Works, successors to Hampson and Broadhurst, with whom James Broadhurst II said he had served his apprenticeship,[42] became insolvent in 1869. Their assignees were John Aynsley of Longton, china manufacturer, and Oliver Lodge (senior) of Hanley, commission agent. In July 1869, Aynsley and Lodge invited tenders for

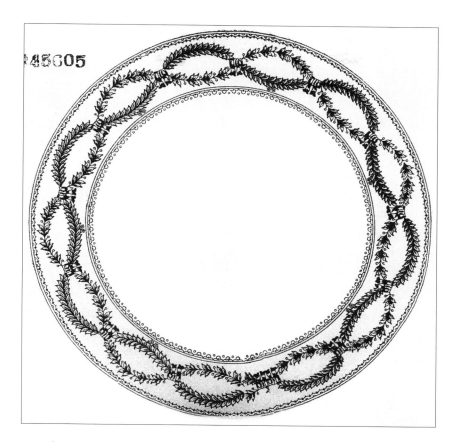

Figure 7 Design no. 245605, border of intertwined garlands, possibly of coffee and tobacco, which form part of the national emblems of Brazil, for a plate border, registered by James Broadhurst 6 October 1870. PRO: BT 43/68

one lot of finished and unfinished earthenware lying at Green Dock Works.[43] James Broadhurst was the successful tenderer, with an inspired offer of £605, over-topping a rival bid by only £5.[44] That transaction, if nothing else, brought him into contact with John Aynsley, who at that time was proposing to build a new works at Fenton.

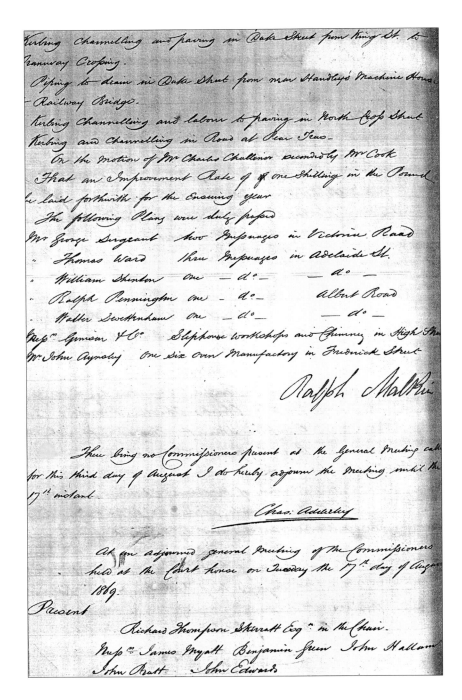

Figure 8 Extract from Fenton Improvement commissioners' Minutes, 1865–73, 6 July 1869, showing that plans were passed for 'Mr. John Aynsley One Six Oven Manufactory in Frederick Street'. Hanley Reference Library: SA-LG-60

BROADHURSTS IN FENTON
— 1871–1922 —

When the Fenton Improvement Commissioners met on 6 July 1869, they passed plans for 'Mr. John Aynsley One Six Oven Manufactory in Frederick Street'. The Commissioners had been set up in 1839 as an elementary form of local government, and their Minute Book survives (Figure 8).[1] About 1840 a road had been made from 'the Albion Inn at Shelton' (present-day Hanley) to 'Masons' manufactory at Fenton',[2] the present-day Victoria Road. There was a national movement to set up building societies, and the Fenton Freehold Land Society was founded 30 January 1864.[3] It bought twenty-four acres of land at Fenton Low, straddling Victoria Road, for £6,700, in the auction of parts of the Whieldon Estate on 12 October 1865.[4] A layout was planned by Mr. Chapman of Newcastle,[5] and John Aynsley of Longton bought Lots 388 to 408, 4161 square yards, for £420 on 1 December 1869.[6]

John Aynsley had been Samuel Bridgwood's partner in a works adjoining Longton's Lower Market from 1857 until it was demolished in 1861, when they built a new china factory in Sutherland Road, Longton, the Portland Works. Their partnership ended in 1863.[7] John Aynsley carried on alone, so successfully that he was able to launch this new venture at Fenton six years later, funding it by borrowing £3,000 at 4½% on 21 December 1869.[8] The mortgage recited 'whereas the said John Aynsley has erected certain buildings of considerable value ... intended to be used as a china manufactory'[9] suggesting that work was well advanced, six months after the plans had been passed. When the Chief Bailiff of Fenton retired in June 1870, he said that 'within the two years 150 or 160 new houses had been erected, a large earthenware manufactory had been built.'[10] Again, when the Fenton Freehold Land Society was wound up in 1874, it took pride in 'a large manufactory, a foundry and hotel, and over 200 houses' having been built.[11]

The 1875 Ordnance Map shows the factory as built, between Frederick Street and Brunswick Street (present-day Beville Street), an elongated courtyard with a central arched entrance in Frederick Street, two ovens and two kilns in the yard, and a row of four ovens along the western side (Figure 9), a layout substantially unchanged until after the 1939–45 war. The works did not then extend to Victoria Road, and there were no houses immediately opposite in Frederick Street. John Aynsley and Samuel Bridgwood had called their Longton factory 'Portland Works', probably because of the local interest in the 1859 centenary of Josiah Wedgwood's start in independent business, and in his most famous creation, the copies of the Portland Vase. (Both the Wedgwood Statue at Stoke Station and the Wedgwood Institute at Burslem date from this centenary.) When John Aynsley built another factory at Fenton, no doubt to his own design, he called it Portland Pottery, and included a replica of the Portland Vase on the pediment.[12]

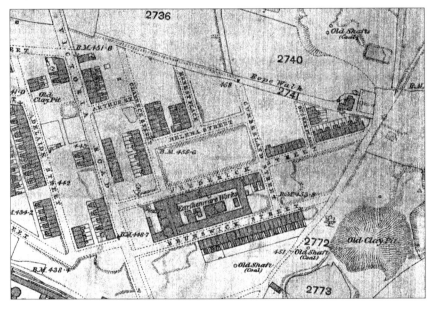

Figure 9 Reproduced from Ordnance Survey 1/2500 Map XVIII No. 6 Fenton, 1875, showing Broadhursts' Portland Pottery as 'Earthenware Works' between Frederick Street and Brunswick Street (now Beville Street), Fenton

On 12 November 1870 the *Staffordshire Sentinel* stated 'Mr. Aynsley's new earthenware works at Fenton are now almost completed, and some hundred hands, will, it is believed, be busy engaged there before the close of the present month'.[13] On 12 January 1871 the Crown Works at Longton was offered for auction 'lately occupied by Mr. James Broadhurst' where 'a successful business has been carried on ... for many years past'.[14] In a directory dated September 1872,[15] James Broadhurst is listed at Fenton as an earthenware manufacturer at Portland Pottery, and when the Crown Works was sold 22 March 1872,[16] it was stated to be occupied by Frederick Jones and 'recently by James Broadhurst the younger'. Clearly it was James Broadhurst II who had rented the new Portland Pottery from John Aynsley and commenced business there in November 1870. Here John

Aynsley forms a link between his erstwhile senior partner, Bridgwood, and his new tenant, Broadhurst, a link which became a bond, ninety-five years later.

The Crown Works had no steam power or machinery. When it failed to sell at auction, it was offered to be let, and the owner was willing to adapt the premises for the introduction of machinery.[17] Probably, James Broadhurst was attracted to a brand new works with a steam engine. When he died in 1897, it was said that he was a pioneer of the newer style of manufacture. Trade had been depressed in the 1860s, but recovered in the early 1870s.[18] John Aynsley and James Broadhurst must have been either far-sighted or fortunate to build and occupy a new steam-operated works at the beginning of a prosperous period.

James Broadhurst was able to buy the manufactory and premises from John Aynsley 10 April 1876 for £8,300, leaving £3,000 on mortgage to him, and raising another (prior) mortgage of £5,000 from the Tunstall £50 Permanent Building Society to do so.[19] Two years later, James Broadhurst bought the land between his works and Victoria Road for £200.[20] By 1883, he had paid off £2,000 of Aynsley's advance, and settled both Aynsley's remaining £1,000 and the Tunstall Society's £5,000 mortgages by a new £6,000 5% mortgage to Percy Frederick Meakin of Hanley.[21] This mortgage mentions for the first time 'steam engines, boilers, millgear fixed and moveable' but it is reasonable to expect that a factory designed in 1869 would include steam power and machinery from the start. The factory is termed a china works and James Broadhurst is called a china manufacturer in the title deeds at several dates, but the 1870 retiring Chief Bailiff, the local newspaper of November 1870 and directories[22] all refer to 'earthenware'. It is reasonable to accept that only earthenware was made at the Portland Pottery.

The new houses surrounding the works were obvious accommodation for Broadhursts' workers, and the 1881 census shows many pottery workers resident, though no preponderance of people born in Longton which would have suggested that James Broadhurst brought workers with him. Elizabeth Broadhurst, a widow, kept a shop at 5 Frederick Street. As she had a daughter named Drusilla it seems likely that her husband had been a descendant of James Broadhurst I and his wife Drusilla. A carter, John Broadhurst, lived at 54 Frederick Street, aged 27, born at Longton, surely another relative; and a James Broadhurst, a common thrower aged 21, lived with his mother-in-law at 10 Ernest Place. James Tams, a potters' fireman, lived at 97 Victoria Road. He was born in Longton; his three sons were respectively an engraver's apprentice, a presser and a mould-runner, and his eldest daughter was a burnisher, but his two younger daughters had been born in Ohio, U.S.A., in 1874 and 1876, so that family had been to America in the meantime. Herbert Deakin, potters' manager, aged 47, another Longtonian, lived at 7 Adelaide Street.

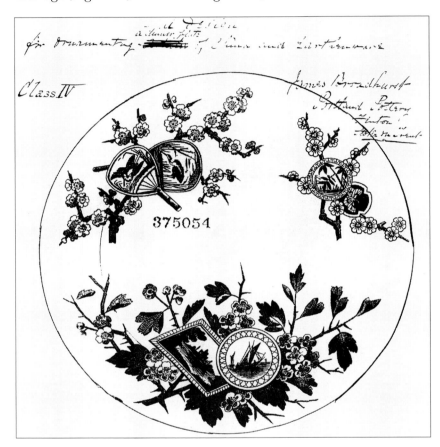

Figure 10 Design no. 375054, hawthorn blossom, fans etc. for a plate, registered by James Broadhurst 24 December 1881. PRO: BT 43/73

Beyond the directory entries for earthenware, little is known about the products of the factory at the time. 'Mocha' is said to have been made: earthenware mugs, jugs and chamberpots, banded with coloured slip and decorated with drops of colour which ramified into tree-like forms.[23] A few designs were registered in the 1880s: an 'aesthetic' print for dinner plates, engraved with hawthorn blossom and fans (Figure 10), in 1881.[24] Shown without a border, this design may have been for a coupe shape. Another plate print was registered in 1883, with camels and a chevron border (Figure 11).[25] Between 1892 and 1895, John Aynsley, himself a china manufacturer at Longton, made quarterly payments averaging £65 to Broadhursts, his former tenants, presumably for earthenware required for Aynsley's customers.[26]

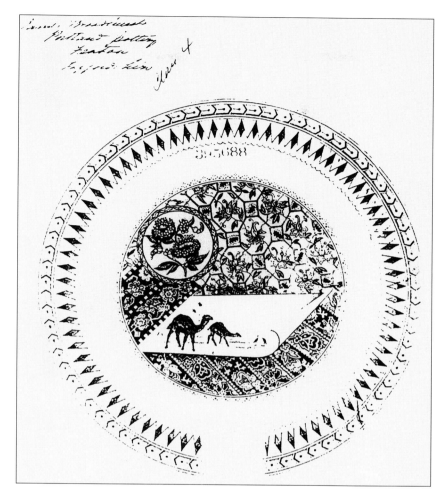

Figure 11 Design no. 395688, camels and a chevron border for a plate, registered by James Broadhurst, 16 March 1883. PRO: BT 43/74

A surviving invoice dated October 1896 (Figure 12) is to a customer, Hering and Jabes in Philadelphia, for 'Toy Teas Sponged Asstd' – children's ware, decorated with cut-sponge patterns.[27] Five-inch plates were eightpence a dozen. The particular cask was marked H & J / J B / 105, suggesting that 104 casks had previously been sent to this one customer. This 1896 bill-head is from 'James Broadhurst & Sons', showing that another generation of Broadhursts had joined the family firm. It includes a magnificent if somewhat exaggerated view of the factory from Frederick Street, with a three-storey facade and eight ovens.

Business was not good in 1885: a report indicated that, since the palmy days of the early seventies, trade had been either normal or below, and that from the end of 1883 depression was increasingly acute, caused by foreign competition and resulting in reduced production and much lower prices.[28] In early 1891, Broadhursts were busy: a court case, where an apprentice placer sued Broadhursts for 15 shillings wages stopped, revealed that they were short of ware and James Broadhurst insisted that wet ware should be placed and fired, despite the foreman placer's objection. The ware came out 'stewed' and the apprentice placer's wages were stopped. He won his case.[29] The 1890s were a period of renewed concern about the health of pottery workers. Legislation led to special rules for cleanliness, overalls and eating facilities, followed later by the control of the use of raw lead.[30]

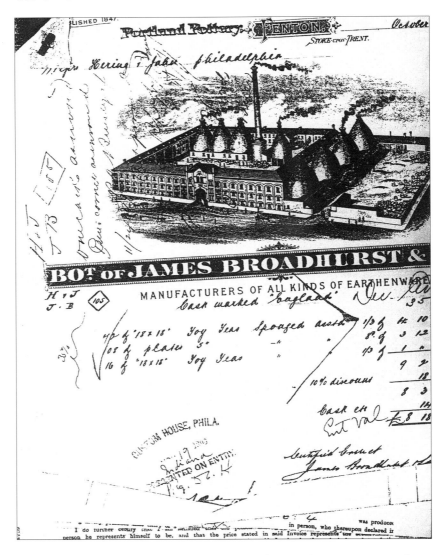

Figure 12 Bill head from James Broadhurst and Sons, October 1896, to Hering and Jabes, Philadelphia, for a cask of 'Toy Teas Sponged asstd.' and plates, showing an 'aerial' view of Portland Pottery from the north-west. Courtesy of Mr. J. Smith

James Broadhurst II was about 38, living in Longton, when he took over his new works. By 1873 he had moved to Pentonville House, Stoke Road, Shelton,[31] and two further daughters were born there: Frances in 1873 and Minnie in

1874. By 1876 he had moved again, to Blythe Villa, Blythe Marsh, and he remained there until his death in 1897.[32] In 1881 he was a widower, with seven children: he and his sons Samuel, 22, and James, 17, all calling themselves earthenware manufacturers.[33] Harry, then fifteen, was perhaps away at school. The 1896 billhead referred to James Broadhurst *and Sons*, and in 1894, James Broadhurst II conveyed the land, manufactory and premises at Fenton to James Broadhurst III and his brother Harry Broadhurst, with £5,000 still owing on the property.[34] Nothing further has been found about the eldest son, Samuel.

James Broadhurst II had put his affairs in order in 1894, by transferring his business to his sons.[35] Whilst on a visit to Southport in 1897, he was 'seized with paralysis' and died on 20 July, aged 65.[36] His obituary recorded that he was 'one of the pioneers of the newer style of manufacture' and spoke of his 'model works'. James Broadhurst II had served his apprenticeship with 'Hampson & Co., Longton', presumably starting his apprenticeship aged fourteen, about 1847, when his father joined the business. Like his 'potter journeyman' father, James Broadhurst II had learnt practical skills: he was described as a thrower at the 1851 census. He had begun business himself about forty years ago at the Crown Pottery 'now occupied by Mr. Tams'. He left personal estate of £2,747.[37]

Despite the death of James Broadhurst II, the firm continued under the style of 'James Broadhurst and Sons' until it became a limited company in 1922.[38] In 1898 the mortgage of £5,000 owed to Percy Meakin was transferred to Arthur G. Prince, a Longton chemist.[39] Mr. Prince died 17 February 1904, and the debt was paid off by instalments, completely by 29 January 1918.[40] Harry Broadhurst continued to live at Blythe Bridge, probably at the family home with his unmarried sisters.[41] He is remembered as a lively character, visiting the works in a wheel chair, having had his legs amputated due to thrombosis.[42] James Broadhurst III was married and lived first in Blythe Bridge, then at Claremont House, Regent Street, Stoke in 1900, and between 1904 and 1916 at Sidmouth Avenue, Newcastle.[43] It was stated in 1922[44] that Broadhursts had a long and unbroken record of activity in the production of a strictly competitive type of earthenware that aimed to satisfy the requirements of the 'ordinary classes' (a mass market), making neither china nor sidelines. They made cheap printed dinner sets, printed and under-glaze shaded toilet sets, half tea-sets with printed or lithographed borders and loose stock lines in printed plates and dishes, dipped bowls, pudding bowls, sets of jugs and white and gold teaware, for export and home markets. Business was obtained quietly, without either advertising or exhibiting, not even as locally as at the King's Hall Exhibition of 1913 at Stoke, nor at the British Industries Fair in 1919, after the end of the Great War.[45]

Broadhursts was one of the first firms in the Potteries to institute roller transfer printing,[46] superseding traditional printing from flat copper plates. Although this had been pioneered in the Potteries in the 1830s by Machin & Potts, and revived by Albert Wenger in 1878, it did not become popular until George Hassall of Hanley patented changeable rollers and cheaper machines in 1898.[47] Mr. Morgan, decorating manager at the Portland Works after 1945, recalled that his first floor office had formerly been used for the printing machine, the transfers passing through a slit in the floor to the transferrers below.

The 1922 report[48] spoke of the factory being wonderfully well equipped. One of the managers during this period was Mr. Asaph Leese, who had been a founder member of the new technical association, the North Staffordshire Ceramic Society, in 1901, and who spoke regularly at its meetings.[49] His first contribution was in 1902, jointly with H. W. Edwards, on work they had done at the Sutherland Institute, Longton on 'The Influence of Grog in Saggar Marls'; and later contributions were on loss in saggars, speck in the biscuit oven, and discolouration in biscuit earthenware.[50] When he was President of the Society in 1916–17, his presidential address[51] was on 'Unestimated Losses in Pottery Manufacture', and it was full of practical instances: neglectful enginemen; heat losses through boiler scale which caused slow running throughout the factory; and slovenly slip-making. The moisture content in materials and slipshod flat-making also called his attention, and his entire lecture was permeated with his experience of day-to-day work at Broadhursts. Later he spoke on tensile strength, cylinder and pan grinding, drying of cast ware, the effects of calcination of flints, black and grey flints, drying stoves, boiler feed water, and discolouration of clays, all of which revealed him to be a master of practical detail. When he died in 1934, aged seventy, the Ceramic Society stood in silence at its 9 April meeting as a mark of respect.[52]

Although he had able management, James Broadhurst III had no sons to succeed him, and he was in failing health.[53] He had paid off the mortgage on the property in 1918, and in 1922, when he was in his late fifties, he sought outside help to continue the business for the benefit of himself, his wife and his sisters. He found it in Edward Roper, then in partnership with a Mr. Meredith at Longton.

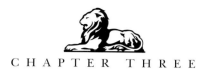

BROADHURSTS UNDER EDWARD ROPER
———— 1922–1941 ————

James Broadhurst's arrangement to secure the future of the family business was to take a partner: formally, in a private limited liability company. James Broadhurst and Sons Ltd. was registered (No. 184,289) in 1922, with a capital of £12,000, to take over the business of earthenware manufacture at Portland Pottery, Fenton.[1] James Broadhurst of New Lodge, Oakhill, Stoke-on-Trent and Edward R. Roper of Windhaven, Weston Road, Meir were the first directors. Official records of the formation of the company no longer exist, but Roper family tradition has it that Edward Roper took a half share and replaced the disabled Harry Broadhurst as managing director.[2]

Edward Robert Roper (Figure 13) was born about 1880 at Belgrave Road, Dresden, Longton, second son of Isaac and Mary Ann Roper.[3] His first job was as a junior clerk for James Kent, earthenware manufacturers,[4] at the Old Foley Pottery, King Street, now Hadida Fine Bone China Ltd. after many changes in control. James Kent succeeded Moore & Co. in 1897,[5] who themselves had followed the younger Samuel Bridgwood in 1876. Edward Roper married Ida Constance Allerton, daughter of William Allerton of the old-established Longton firm of manufacturers, in March 1908; their daughter Joan was born in 1909 and their son Edward Peter Roper in 1911.[6] In 1912 Edward Roper was a cashier, living with his wife and young family at 363 Uttoxeter Road, Longton.[7]

A Longton earthenware manufacturer, Albert E. Jones & Co., of the small Garfield Pottery, High Street, took over the larger Palissy Pottery in Commerce Street in 1907, and re-equipped it.[8] In 1912 Jones's concentrated their production at their larger works.[9] Edward Roper formed a partnership in 1913 with a fellow Freemason, Llewellyn Meredith of Gordon Villa, Blythe Bridge, to manufacture earthenware at the vacant Garfield Works.[10] Despite his Welsh-sounding name, Meredith described himself in 1924 as 'the only Irish-born pottery manufacturer in the district'. The partnership of Roper and Meredith at the Garfield Works lasted through the 1914–18 war and until 1922.[11]

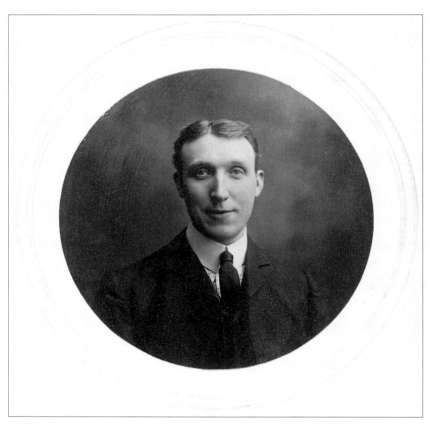

Figure 13 Edward Robert Roper (1880–1941), Managing Director of Broadhursts from 1922 to 1929, Chairman from 1930 to 1941

The Garfield Works was an old three-oven works,[12] presumably re-named in 1881 to commemorate the American President, James Garfield, who was assassinated in that year. Roper and Meredith made 'Earthenware and Semi-Porcelain for all Markets'.[13] In 1924, Mr. Meredith said that they produced tea, dinner and toilet ware at moderate prices, for many years specialising in the cheap Crown Derby type of ware and decoration, and with their Hawthorne, Willow and Chatsworth patterns deservedly popular.[14] The factory mark was R & M in a circle under a crown.[15] The partnership between Edward Roper and Llewellyn Meredith was dissolved 30 June 1922,[16] but Mr. Meredith continued the business as Roper and Meredith for two or three years afterwards. He opened a London Showroom in 1923[17] and introduced crested china (so-called 'Goss' ware), with the 'R & M' mark.[18] Mr. Meredith later migrated to Australia, and by 1928 the Garfield Works was operated by Alfred Clough.[19]

Broadhursts' new limited company sought publicity: an illustrated article in the *Pottery Gazette* for December 1922 (Figure 14) remarked that 'Mr. Edward R. Roper, who is well known in the popular earthenware trade as a manufacturer,

James Broadhurst & Sons, Ltd., Portland Pottery, Fenton, Stoke-on-Trent, are a firm of earthenware manufacturers who can claim to have had a long and unbroken record of activity in one special direction, viz., the production of a strictly competitive type of earthenware that aims at satisfying the requirements of ordinary classes. Unlike many of the older factories, they have not mixed both china and earthenware; nor have they embarked from time to time on a thousand-and-one sidelines in

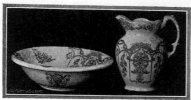

[Photo. by the West End Studios, Stoke.
JAMES BROADHURST & SONS, LTD.

order to keep up their turnover. They have increased their output from year to year with an essentially practical line of useful earthenware, such as most retailers of pottery require to provide them with a turnover in good and bad times alike. Their specialities are cheap printed dinner sets, printed and very effective under-glaze shaded toilet sets, half tea sets with printed or lithographed borders, loose stock lines in printed plates and dishes, dipped bowls, pudding bowls, sets of jugs, white and gold teaware, and similar useful everyday wares. For the export markets they have always catered most successfully, and for the home market they are in quite as good a position to meet the wholesaler's or retailer's needs, and we can quite believe that there are hundreds of our readers who would do well to get into touch with the line. It will, no doubt, be read with interest that Mr. Edward R. Roper, who is well known in the popular earthenware trade as a

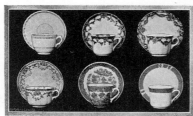

[Photo. by the West End Studios, Stoke.
JAMES BROADHURST & SONS, LTD.

manufacturer, and who has been associated with the production of earthenware all his life, has recently become associated with James Broadhurst & Sons, Ltd., and it is by the kindness of this gentleman that we are now able to give our readers for the first time some particulars as to the firm's staple productions. The writer, who was permitted by Mr. Roper to make an inspection of the workshops and warehouses, was much impressed by the general layout of the factory and the sound and solid

classes of productions upon which it is engaged. It seems almost inconceivable that a seven-oven factory, turning out such an impressive range of goods for the cheaper and middle-class trade, has not been heard of to a far greater extent in the home market, for the works are wonderfully well equipped and handle the very types of goods that are now in favour. The body of the ware is very strong, and a good colour, the patterns are pleasing and sensible, and the glaze is smooth and hard. The printed patterns, which, in the dinner ware, are mostly of the rim-width type, are done economically by means of machine printing, and, if we remember rightly the firm under notice was one of the very first in the Potteries to institute roller printing with a view to lowering the costs of production. And it is this which enables them to handle a bulk business in loose dinner ware or tea ware, and to offer to the trade solid crates of useful lines at prices which are bound to make for quick repeats. Canton, pink, peacock, and cobalt blue prints can be had from this house in a large variety of patterns. They have a very good "Blue Willow" pattern and hosts of border designs, and in every case fairly quick deliveries can be guaranteed. Likewise, they have many very saleable toilets, from plain white upwards. In teaware, they offer

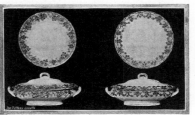

[Photo. by the West End Studios, Stoke.
JAMES BROADHURST & SONS, LTD.

a good line in a new fluted shape, and they have also some interesting treatments in simple underglaze painted and sponged patterns, which are suitable either for cottage use in this country or for a number of the export markets. Their dipped bowls, which are made in all sizes from 48's up to 3's, are well finished, and should appeal to a very wide market. We have pleasure in illustrating a few lines which are typical of the firm's productions in general, and in doing so we feel sure that many of our readers will be glad to have this information and to get into touch with such a useful source of supply.

The Alexandra Pottery Co., Dudley-st., Maindee, Newport, Mon., is one of those numerous small potteries that one encounters from time to time in the course of one's journeys up and down the country, which cater for a more or less local trade in redware for the kitchen and pantry. In dealing with these coarser types of household pottery one of the most important factors to consider is naturally the price. It is clear that the moderate prices at which the ware has to be sold will not admit of heavy transit costs, and consequently a radius of forty or fifty miles or so is very often considered to be the limit of the permissible working area. This seems to be the case with the pottery under notice, which the writer happened to stumble across in taking a journey to South Wales quite recently. The following particulars may not, therefore, be of any real use to quite a large proportion of our readers, but they may, at all events, be of interest to

Figure 14 Publicity for James Broadhurst and Sons Ltd. in *The Pottery Gazette and Glass Trade Review* 1 December 1922, 1819

and who has been associated with the production of earthenware all his life' had joined Broadhursts. Printed border patterns in Canton, pink, peacock and cobalt blue were offered, and a very good 'Blue Willow' pattern, as well as fluted teaware, sponged and under-glaze painted patterns and dipped bowls in all sizes.[20] An accompanying advertisement named their Canadian agent: William Smith of Toronto, an agent they shared with Sampson Bridgwood. At that time, the manufacturers' home trade scale for a 21 piece five inch earthenware tea set started at six shillings.[21] Advertisements continued in 1923.[22]

Mr. Leese continued as a manager: in 1923 he was commenting to the Ceramic Society on dunting problems caused at his firm when grey flints were used instead of black;[23] and the need for improved drying stoves, since those existing were mostly jerry-built and placed too near the workpeople, so that heat was wasted and working conditions were uncomfortably hot. In 1926 he recalled problems of twenty years earlier, when 'they' (Broadhursts) had trouble with flat ware discoloured in the centre, a problem overcome then and since by 'seasoning' the oven. 'Seasoning' was to open the firemouth doors for about three hours, after forty hours' firing, to allow the heat to permeate right through the ware.[24] Mr. Leese, who died aged 70 in 1934, was remembered for his 'sideline' in making ceramic tubes to fit over iron placing 'pillars'.[25]

James Broadhurst's wife, Constance Amelia, died 24 May 1923 at their home, New Lodge, Oakhill.[26] When J. G. Aynsley, head of Sampson Bridgwoods, died in 1924, Mr. and Misses Broadhurst sent a wreath 'in kindest remembrance of an old friend', evidence of amicable contact at a personal level between two firms which were to be united forty years later.[27] James Broadhurst himself died on 13 October 1929, aged 65.[28] He left £35,321, and probate was granted to his unmarried sister Frances Louisa (Fanny) Broadhurst, and a schoolmaster, Charles Edward Averill of Forsbrook.[29] They sold James Broadhurst's share of the business to Edward and Peter Roper; and the freehold of the factory was bought by the limited company on 7 April 1933 for £6,000.[30] James Broadhurst's three unmarried sisters had lived at Blythe Bridge,[31] but Frances Louisa Broadhurst died 3 August 1934 at Leamington Spa,[32] and another sister, Drusilla Elizabeth, died 20 December 1940, also at Leamington Spa.[33] Laura lived on to 1953.

Edward Roper's son, Edward Peter Roper, joined the firm in September 1928, aged 17.[34] After attending Denstone College, he underwent technical education at the North Staffordshire Technical College. At the time he started, business was very difficult: the world was in full recession and the firm was fighting for survival. One hundred and twenty staff were employed, and all the equipment was driven by rope and pulley, powered by a single steam engine. There were two large biscuit intermittent ovens, four glost ovens and two enamel kilns. Making was by jiggering flatware, jolleying hollow-ware, and casting.

The ware made (tableware, toilet ware, jug sets) was decorated with under-glaze transfers, banding, aerographing or on-glaze lithographs. Peter Roper had a large input into designs, some of which were bought in. Trade was done with Eatons in Canada, and with Australia, but sales were mainly in the home market.[35] Shards found on the factory are probably representative of the ware made then: under-glaze painted and printed ware, sponged ware and banded ware.[36] When Peter Roper was twenty-one, he began sales trips, covering Britain by car, from London to Inverness.[37] Broadhursts exhibited at Olympia in 1939.[38]

Mrs. Nellie Whitehouse recalled working in the biscuit banding shop at Broadhursts from 1931 to 1936, between the ages of sixteen and twenty-one, with her school-friend, Gertie Stanier. It was very dusty, hot in summer and cold in winter, with brick floors and a little stove. She did green band-and-line, using water and gum arabic. Mr. Tams was the lodge man, and Mr. James Fenton was decorating manager. She remembered Mr. Edward Roper as a tall man, a concerned employer, who made sure she received unemployment pay when she was pregnant and unable to continue working.[39]

The company was re-formed in 1939 as James Broadhurst and Sons (1939) Ltd., registered number 352,895.[40] The *Pottery Gazette* reported that the new company had share capital of £10,000 in £1 shares, and was formed to carry on the business of manufacturers of china, earthenware, pottery, stone and glass ware and tiles. Mr. E. R. Roper and Mrs. Ida C. Roper of Windycote, Blythe Bridge were life directors, and Mr. F. Harding was company secretary. A letter of 14 June 1939 from George E. Harding, formal liquidator of the old company, has been kept.[41] It enclosed a schedule of the assets acquired by the new company:

	£. s. d.
Cash in hand and at Bank	3,600. 0. 0
Freehold Works and buildings adjoining known as Portland Pottery, Fenton, Stoke-on-Trent	5,000. 0. 0
Sundry Debtors	1,450. 0. 0
Motor Cars	300. 0. 0
Stocks	650. 0. 0
Tenants Fixtures Plant and Machinery	370. 0. 0
Value of unexpired insurance	130. 0. 0
	11,500. 0. 0
Less Creditors of James Broadhurst & Sons Limited to be discharged by James Broadhurst & Sons (1939) Limited.	1,500. 0. 0
Net Assets to be acquired by James Broadhurst & Sons (1939) Limited.	£10,000. 0. 0

During the 'twenties and 'thirties there had been increasing dissatisfaction in the Potteries with the economics of coal-fired intermittent ovens,[42] and by 1939 there were 66 town gas kilns and 24 electric kilns in use in the area.[43] Of the electric kilns, 23 were enamel kilns and one was glost, and a second electric glost kiln was anticipated at Wedgwoods' new Barlaston factory. There were eight new gas-fired earthenware ovens in 1939, and Broadhursts themselves contemplated installing a gas-fired glost tunnel kiln.

The gas-fired kiln was ordered in 1941, but the second World War had started in September 1939 and the kiln was not installed until after the end of the war.[44] The war brought increasing restrictions on trade, and in 1941 a 'Concentration Scheme' was enforced by the government on the pottery industry.[45] Seventy-seven businesses were to be closed or 'concentrated' on seventy-eight 'nucleus' firms. James Broadhursts, together with Barkers & Kent at the Foley, and Rigby & Stevenson of Hanley, were to be concentrated on W. H. Grindley & Co., Ltd., Woodland Pottery, Tunstall. The intention was that Broadhursts should continue to trade from Fenton, supplied with ware by Grindleys for Broadhursts' existing home trade customers as far as their quota allowed. Broadhursts' factory was to be 'liberated' for other use.

The factory was used for storing hemp for a tyre company at Etruria. The secretary, Mr. Harding, and three labourers operated the store on behalf of the government and also sold a small amount of Grindleys' ware.[46] Mr. Peter Roper joined the Royal Air Force in 1941, and Mr. Edward Roper died on 3 September of the same year, after some months' illness.[47] He was aged 61, and apart from being Churchwarden at Meir Parish Church and a member of the Etruscan Lodge of Free-masons, had 'steeped himself in his work'. He left a widow, Mrs. Ida Roper, living at Brackenlea, Weston Road, Meir; one son, Peter, and one daughter, Mrs. Flower.

After seventy years in production, the Portland Pottery was all but closed down, as a contribution to the war effort.

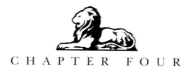

BROADHURSTS UNDER PETER ROPER
—————— 1941–1964 ——————

During the 1939–45 war, production had ceased at Portland Pottery. Mr. Edward Roper died in 1941; Mr. Peter Roper was away in the Royal Air Force; and Mrs. Ida Roper acted as chairman of the company. Mr. Harding, company secretary, and three labourers dealt with the modest amounts of ware provided by Grindleys for Broadhursts' customers, and stored hemp for a tyre company. The pre-war staff was dispersed to war work or military service.[1]

Peter Roper (Figure 15) returned from war service in 1945 to re-start the works, with only £5,000 in the bank.[2] Some of the pre-war staff lived in the houses surrounding the works and returned to their former jobs;[3] others had to be recruited in competition with other pottery firms, anxious to begin or increase production to meet the pent-up demand after the war. By October 1945 production for export only had begun.[4] An announcement in the *Pottery Gazette* of April 1946 stated that Broadhursts had received a licence to re-start manufacture of earthenware for home and export. Production had started, but the company was not in a position to accept any further home trade orders since its total allocation was booked for months ahead. The firm was concentrating on teaware with much of the output diverted to export. That was representative of the time: despite enormous demand, home supply was strictly limited by government order, so that much-needed foreign currency could be earned by exports. For seven years, until 1952, only undecorated ware (and decorated seconds) could be sold at home: even unhandled cups were readily saleable.

Peter Roper's experience was principally in sales, but he determined that as his father had 'made a go of it' before the war, so should he. His aim was to increase both output and sales by modern mass-production techniques.[5] Peter Roper's initial experiences were daunting. His biscuit fireman died after the first firing of the biscuit oven, and he and the warehouseman had to finish firing their first glost oven when the glost fireman became incapable through drinking.[6] Mr. Fred Starkey was clay manager: he appointed a fitter and established a workshop in

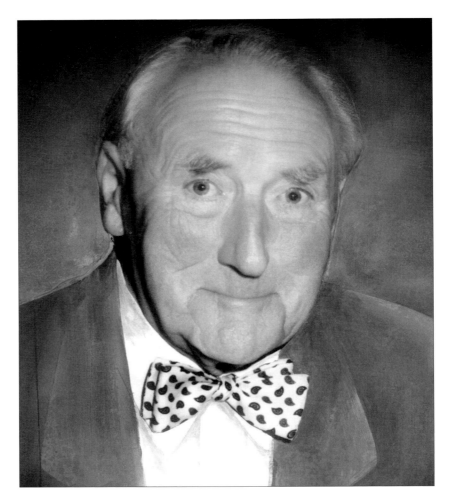

Figure 15 Edward Peter Roper (1911–1991), Managing Director of Broadhursts from 1945 to 1959, Chairman from 1959 to 1984, Chairman of the Churchill Group from 1984 to 1989, President from 1989 to 1991

the erstwhile Jenkinson's undertaker's business which stood in one corner of the yard adjoining Victoria Road,[7] an indication of the increasing mechanisation of the industry. Formerly, the engineman had done all mechanical repairs.

Mr. Wilfred Morgan joined Broadhursts on 5 May 1947 as decorating manager. Before the war he had worked for Doultons, Woods and then Susie Cooper;[8] and during the war at the ordnance factory at Swynnerton. In 1947, the firm had a total staff of about seventy, and was firing two large and one small biscuit ovens a fortnight. A few semi-automatic making machines had been installed, but everything was driven by the single steam engine. Decoration then was under-glaze painting and lining, and rubber stamping by hand, since transfer printing had not been resumed (Colour Plate 21). There were about six people hand-stamping and between twenty and thirty paintresses. The decorators worked hard and could earn good money at Broadhursts: as much as five pounds a week in the late 1940s.[9] The new Gibbons gas-fired tunnel glost kiln was in use when Mr. Morgan arrived, taking 6,000 dozen pieces of ware per week. Ordered in 1941, it was not to be installed until after the war, assuming that funds were then available.[10]

In the rush to resume production, poor working practices developed and the workforce had to be trained into new ways. Glost ware drawn from the new kiln had merely been stacked randomly against a wall, an impossible situation for getting up orders; and the biscuit warehouse was over-staffed.[11] Many of the workers lived nearby, and women would go to their homes to make their children's meals. Extended families worked together in departments: for example, Mr. and Mrs. Charlie Shaw ran the glost warehouse. A 'works outing' to New Brighton about 1948 resulted in a domestic tiff in the making shop! The Broadhurst family name, found in the 1881 census, still survived amongst employees: Jim Broadhurst, the glost kiln man; Bill Broadhurst, the head mould maker; and John Broadhurst, the 'oddman'.[12] Their sisters, Freda Yates, Winnie Ford and Gertie Jones, were also employed at the works. In 1947 there were still stables in the yard, and a descendant of the carter, another Jim Broadhurst, did Broadhursts' haulage.[13]

Mimosa, designed by a Mr. Shelley, was an early export pattern.[14] Advertising of the late 1940s shows the types of ware made then: moulded shapes with small floral patterns such as Clyde (Figure 16),[15] Crocus,[16] Tyne,[17] and unnamed designs such as No. 1146, a small stylised flower centre in maroon.[18] In the early 1950s came Saxon, a lined design, with handles in solid blue or pink,[19] Tudor[20] and Maytime. The advertisements listed overseas agents: W. E. Bird in Australia and Andrew Hawley in New Zealand. Other foreign markets were covered by agents in England: Sasha in Manchester, and Hales, Hancock & Goodwin in London. Coronation mugs and plates were, of course, made for 1953. By 1950 production was up to 10,000 dozen a week. Broadhursts were one of the first firms to have a Ryckman gold edge lining machine from Malkins, about 1950, and eventually had three.[21]

A link with the past was broken when Mr. Harding retired from the office about 1950, to be succeeded by Mr. R. J. Heyes before 1952.[22] Laura, last of James Broadhurst's sisters, died in 1953, aged about 82.[23] Mr. Starkey, clay manager, left about 1952, to be replaced by Joe Bentley and an assistant, Ray Colclough.[24] In the early days after the war, Mr. Roper had kept his close interest in sales,[25] but by 1954 British Pottery Ltd. covered sales in London and the South of England, whilst Lt. Col. E. Broughton Eyre was the firm's Sales Manager for the Midlands, Northern England and Scotland.[26]

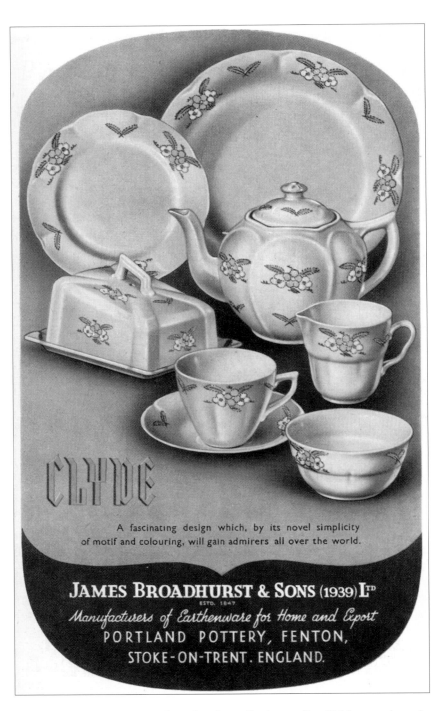

Figure 16
Advertisement for
James Broadhurst &
Sons (1939) Ltd. Clyde
pattern, in *Pottery
Gazette Reference Book
1949*, 57

On the production side, the installation of a Webcot electric decorating kiln about 1950 improved the facility to do on-glaze decoration, replacing the old coal-fired enamel kilns.[27] Saggars were bought from Diamond Clay or Hewitts, and glaze mixtures from Kents, until an over-flinted delivery caused faulty ware, a claim for compensation from Kents for £5,000, and a change of supplier to Harrisons. When Ray Colclough came to Broadhursts in 1952 he found an office staff of four: Mr. Heyes, Mr. Heath and two girls, only two telephones, and no adding machine. Only Mr. Roper and Mr. Morgan ran cars. A new building had been erected on the Victoria Road side, but they were chronically short of space. Three biscuit bottle ovens were still in use for production of about 12,000 dozen pieces a week. Decoration was by hand-stamping and hand-painting. Clay was tipped in Frederick Street, at first weathered and wet, but when it was later delivered dry, it caused dust problems with neighbours. The clay was shovelled manually into the cellar, moved by trucks and a mangle hoist to the blunger at ground level, then carried by hand to the first floor makers. The steam engine was replaced first by a large electric motor, then by motors to individual machines.

In the early 1950s, Broadhursts were thoroughly back in business, with renewed management and some new equipment. Shortly before he died, Peter Roper commented that he was surprised how successful the business became during the late '40s and early '50s, and he had the foresight to invest much of the profit of the post-war boom years in re-equipping. In sole charge, Peter Roper found a good friend in Tony Hayek. Mr. A. G. Hayek came to the Potteries after the war as a technical officer with the Board of Trade's Production Efficiency Service,[28] an outcome of the 1946 Working Party Report which featured Bridgwoods' modernisation plans. Broadhursts became one of his clients, and when the Production Efficiency Service closed down in 1950, Tony Hayek stayed in the Potteries, formed his own consultancy, and continued to advise Broadhursts. A. G. Hayek and Partners were deeply involved in formulating Broadhursts' 1955 large-scale modernisation plans[29] and as he had no fellow-directors, Mr. Roper found Tony Hayek 'a good listener and a very useful person to have to discuss and talk through various ideas and problems'.

Broadhursts launched a programme of thorough modernisation in early 1955,[30] to increase production by a third (an extra 5,000 dozen per week), involving demolition of the existing bottle biscuit and glost ovens and their replacement by continuous kilns, the reorganisation of the biscuit warehouse and the enlargement of the glost warehouse. The completed operation was well described and illustrated in an article in the *Pottery Gazette* of November 1956. All the coal-fired bottle ovens and enamel kilns had gone, and the central courtyard was filled in with a large building in which the work was organised round a number of conveyors. A dozen semi-automatic making machines and a Gibbons electrically fired Gottignies biscuit kiln were installed and working by September 1955. The Gottignies type of kiln was described in 1953 as:[31]

> long used on the continent, particularly for firing tiles, is now being tried in this country ... consists of a number of passages, 24 being typical, heated by gas or electric ... ware is pushed through on bats ... and it is claimed that fuel consumption is comparatively low in relation to the volume of ware fired.

Broadhursts' Gottignies kiln, 44′ 6″ long, was featured in the supplier's 1959 *Pottery Gazette* advertisement (Figure 17). It had 24 passages and operated on a contra-flow system with one man at each end, placing on and taking off. There were three others in the Potteries, at Empire Porcelain, Biltons and James Kent, and Broadhursts' lasted longest.[32] It required a harder glaze and produced harder ware, an improvement in quality.[33]

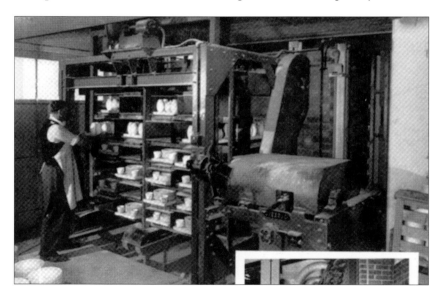

Figure 17 Gibbons-Gottignies electrically heated Multi-Passage Kiln, 44′ 6″ long, for the biscuit firing of general earthenware at James Broadhurst & Sons (1939) Ltd. *Pottery Gazette Reference Book 1959*, 431

About 200 staff were employed in 1956, only about a quarter of them on decorating, because of the high proportion of under-glaze work done.[34] With an output of 16,000 dozen per week by the end of 1956, new designs were brought out: Alton, Star and Bouquet;[35] Hawaii in 1957,[36] and Revel in 1958[37] amongst them. Peter Roper recalled 'Revel' (Colour Plate 22) as a major advance in quality of decorating, and one of their most successful designs, together with 'Rushstone' of the 1960s.[38] Exports were made to Australia (Coles), New Zealand and South Africa; and good home customers such as Littlewoods were acquired.[39] The trade fairs (Earls' Court, Olympia and later Blackpool) were regularly and successfully attended. The firm earned a reputation for efficiency. Mr. Morgan took pride that they never stopped work and had a reputation for high productivity and quick reliable delivery.

All was not plain sailing: a rail strike in 1955 led to clay being brought in by lorries previously used for iron ore. The iron contaminated the clay and 10,000 eighteen-piece tea sets sent to Australia were found to be be so badly stained that the customer was given a full refund.[40] Purchase tax was imposed on pottery in the same year, a deterrent to home sales but a stimulus to production efficiency.[41] A new showroom at first floor level was initiated at the beginning of 1957 (Figure 18),[42] and 'boxed sets' were introduced.[43]

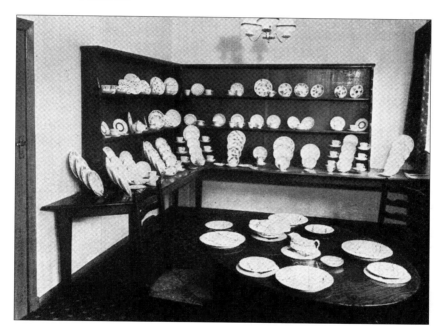

Figure 18 The new first-floor showroom at James Broadhursts' Portland Pottery, Fenton, 1957. *Pottery Gazette and Glass Trade Review* February 1957, 272

Despite its 'limited company' status, Broadhursts continued to be a family firm. In 1957 Peter Roper's eldest son, Michael, joined the business at the age of 17 (Figure 19).[44] His interest was in production, and like his father he furthered his technical education at the College of Ceramics. On 6 May 1959, a new company with the pre-1939 name of James Broadhurst & Sons Ltd. was formed, registered no. 628267, the '(1939)' being dropped from the title.[45] The new firm had a nominal capital of £75,000 in £1 shares, with Edward Peter Roper and Mrs. Muriel Elizabeth Roper as the first directors. Mrs. Joan Flower, sister of Mr. Roper, held a nominal ten shares. The new company took over the assets of the old company for £32,539.

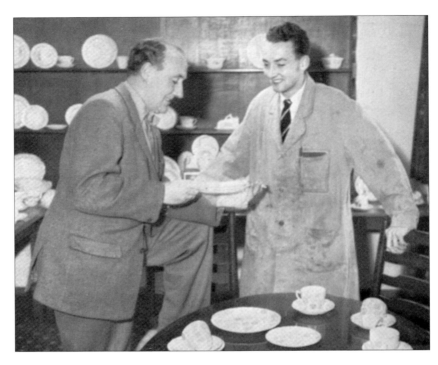

Figure 19 Mr. Peter Roper and Mr. Michael Roper in the showroom, Portland Pottery, October 1958. *Pottery Gazette and Glass Trade Review* November 1958, 1370

Stephen Roper, the second son, joined the firm in 1960 and took an interest in sales.[46] Mr. Heyes continued as company secretary and Mr. John Pedder was appointed sales manager for the Midlands, North of England and Scotland.[47] In the works, Mr. P. Clarke, engine maintenance man, retired after 56 years' service, and warehouse workers Mr. and Mrs. Charles Shaw, each with sixty years' service, took lighter duties (Figure 20).[48] Like Mr. Shah at Bridgwoods in 1916, q.v., Saltani Hirji, a member of a Calcutta pottery and glass distribution firm, spent time at Broadhursts as part of his 1956–59 course at the College of Ceramics.[49]

The range of decorative finishes was extended. In 1956 the emphasis had still been on simple under-glaze decoration,[50] but gradually more on-glaze decoration was done; first one and eventually three gilding machines were installed.[51] An engobing process was developed 'in-house', and a small 3-tier 3-passage gas glost kiln was adapted for once-fired wares, egg-cups and cheap mugs. The standard body colour was made whiter, in response to customers' demands.[52] Broadhursts pioneered boxed sets, introduced to attract mail-order business, and also exported, first to Canada.[53]

Japanese competition was felt in Australia:[54] Mr. Peter Roper made a sales trip there in 1962 and Stephen Roper went again in 1964 (Figure 21).[55] A large order for Italy was unprofitable because of the many shapes required.[56] The Blackpool Trade

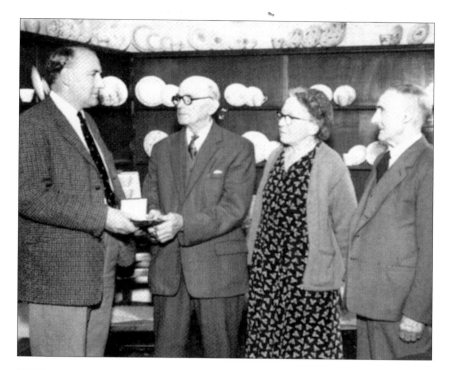

Figure 20
Presentation to three long-serving employees of James Broadhurst & Sons Ltd. From left, Mr. Peter Roper, Managing Director; Mr. P. Clarke, engine maintenance man; and Mr. and Mrs. Charles Shaw of the warehouse staff, Portland Pottery. *Pottery Gazette and Glass Trade Review* November 1961, 1335

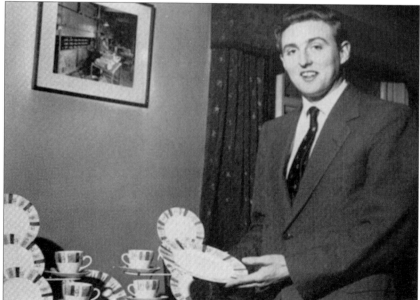

Figure 21 Stephen Roper pictured prior to a sales trip to Australia in 1964. *Pottery Gazette and Glass Trade Review* February 1964, 246

Fairs continued to be regularly attended, and Mr. Armstrong became repre-sentative for the north-east when Mr. Pedder moved to Beswicks. Broadhursts initiated selling direct to super-markets in presentation packs.[57] All the well-known mail order houses were supplied: Littlewoods, Great Universal Stores, Grattan Warehouses; business which has continued to the present time. Shapes and designs of the early 1960s included on-glaze Matador and Shanghai, at Blackpool in 1961;[58] Mayfield, carton-packed in 1962;[59] and Tahiti, Apollo in a candy-stripe gift pack and Calypso in an 18-piece carry-home pack in 1963.[60]

After the expansion programme of 1955–6, the Portland Pottery site was completely built over and clearly allowed little scope for further expansion of production. Purchase of other factories was considered,[61] including Bovey Potteries in South Devon, owned by Pountneys of Bristol, (in the market in 1957)[62] and later Clokies of Castleford, Yorkshire. When in 1964 a suitable factory for purchase was found, it was much nearer home: an old-established hotelware firm, Sampson Bridgwood & Son Ltd., of the Anchor Works in nearby Longton.

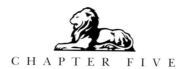

BRIDGWOODS IN LONGTON
—— 1795–1853 ——

A Sampson Bridgwood paid tax on one hearth at Aston near Stone in 1666,[1] and Bridgwoods were in the Longton area in the early eighteenth century. Thomas Bridgwood, a collier of Mear Heath, was buried at Stoke 9 March 1735/36, and left £21.16s.0d.,[2] and John Bridgwood paid three shillings rates in 1740.[3] The pottery industry in Longton developed from the early eighteenth century, with initially 'cottage potters' such as the six potters, including Samuel and Thomas Johnson, who were fined for making 'Claypitts for getting of Clay' at the Manor Court in 1733.[4] Thomas Bridgwood's coal would be in demand for firing their pots.

Samuel Bridgwood I, born 1762,[5] had married Kitty Johnson by 1785, when their first child was born.[6] Between 1783 and 1799, they rented the White Lion Inn at Lane End from Kitty's father, Richard Johnson I, himself an inn-keeper and cooper. Lane End and Longton were originally separate communities, Longton concentrated round Longton Hall and (Meir) Lane End a settlement where lanes (roads) met at the crossing of the Longton Brook (now Times Square). Lane End became officially known as Longton in 1848, and will be referred to throughout as Longton, except in direct quotations. Samuel Bridgwood also rented a property from the executors of the late William Edwards, from 1790 to 1794.[7] Edwards had been a master potter at Longton from c.1784 to his death c.1789,[8] and it may be that Samuel Bridgwood continued William Edwards' potting business, but there is no supporting evidence. It is not known what types of ware were made by Edwards at this period, but other potters in Longton were making cream-coloured, china glazed, and 'blue' (painted) earthenware, and 'Egyptian Black' and 'Red China' stoneware in the 1780s.[9]

Samuel Bridgwood I and his brother-in-law, Richard Johnson, went into partnership as Johnson & Bridgwood, manufacturers of earthenware or 'Staffordshire ware' in Longton about 1795, and were listed in directories of 1796 and 1797.[10] Both Bridgwood and Johnson were trustees of Lane End Chapel (later St. John's Church) in 1792.[11] When Richard

Johnson died in 1842, aged 85, he was described as the last link with the early (pottery) trade.[12]

Johnson & Bridgwood made earthenware: probably the standard cream-colour, made from ball-clay and flint, and the newer white body, containing china clay recently available from Cornwall. Their works seems to have been at the junction of the present Market Street and Transport Lane, where the National Westminster Bank branch stands.[13] The partnership ended 11 November 1799, after which they continued in separate businesses. Advertisements later in the century claimed that the firm of Sampson Bridgwood & Son was 'Founded 1800', but this was a continuation from the 1795 partnership.[14]

Samuel Bridgwood I took a factory across the road, about where Wood Street and Caroline Street join the Lower Market Place (Times Square)[15] and paid 4s.2d. rates on it in 1802.[16] The local historian, Simeon Shaw, wrote in 1829:[17]

> Roger Wood, Esq. of the Ash … in 1756, erected the manufactory (now occupied by Mr. Sampson Bridgwood, an excellent manufacturer of Porcelain,) on the side of the Brook at the lower Market-Place, Lane End. Here a person named Ford, for some years made common stone earthenware, and brown ware. There were not more than one hundred houses in Lane End at that time, and very few indeed in Longton liberty. We are told that at this factory the first cream colour was made on that side of the district.

Samuel Bridgwood I died 8 September 1805 at Golden Hill, Fenton,[18] and his widow, Kitty Bridgwood, continued his earthenware business. They had nine children, including Sampson who was born c.1792.[19] Mrs. Bridgwood inherited the White Horse alehouse, on the site of the present Crown Hotel, and it continued in family ownership until at least 1878.[20] She offered her potworks for sale in 1813, at a time of national depression because of the wars with Napoleon and the United States, but the factory was not sold:[21]

> Lot 1, A very convenient set of Potworks, advantageously situated in Lane End, and a constant supply of excellent water, late the property of Mr. Sam. Bridgwood deceased, and since occupied by Mrs. Bridgwood.

Presumably the 'Brook' provided the excellent water supply!

Richard Johnson, Samuel Bridgwood I's former partner, was bankrupt in 1810,[22] and his property was offered for sale repeatedly, until his sister-in-law, Kitty Bridgwood, bought his 'larger works' in 1814.[23] The advertisement described that works as:

> in the centre of Lane End, within a few yards of the New Market Hall now erecting ... a squeezing house, dipping house, saggar house, and chamber over, a very large and newly erected slip kiln (esteemed the best throughout the Potteries) a gloss hovel, greenhouse and pump, and a commodious warehouse bank, with a throwing and squeezing house.

Sampson Bridgwood was aged 22 in 1814 and no doubt well-trained to take an active part in the management of the two factories which his mother occupied until 1821.[24] Sampson Bridgwood's only son, Samuel Bridgwood II, was born c.1820.[25] Sampson and his wife Martha also had five daughters: Martha, Mary born 1827, Catherine baptised 1828, Maria baptised 1833 and Ann Maria baptised 1836.[26] In 1818, the business was 'Kitty Bridgwood & Son', making earthenware.[27] Fragments of two 10 inch diameter earthenware plates with under-glaze blue printed 'Willow' pattern, impressed 'BRIDGWOOD', have been excavated at the Gladstone Pottery Museum in Longton, probably examples of their production at this period.[28] 'Blue Willow' is still made by Churchill today, at Longton and Tunstall (Colour Plates 25 and 26).

It seems likely that Sampson Bridgwood had a mill in this period: in 1820, a boy left in charge of a small steam engine used for grinding potters' materials at Sampson Bridgwood's fell asleep, became entangled in the machinery and was killed. His drunken father had not relieved him that evening. Subsequently a young man in charge of the same engine had his foot nearly taken off by getting entangled in the wheels. The reporter suggested that these useful machines should be better guarded.[29]

The boom after the end of the Napoleonic war was followed by a slump. In 1822, John Lockett had taken over Kitty Bridgwood's 'Johnson' works.[30] Sampson Bridgwood, who had begun manufacturing china,[31] was insolvent that year, and briefly in Stafford Gaol as an insolvent debtor.[32] His creditors appointed an assignee to sort out his affairs, and Edward Royle operated 'Wood Street' works for him.[33] In 1824, the assignee offered for sale Sampson Bridgwood's expectations on the death of his mother, then aged about 64 and living at the Crown and Anchor Inn.[34]

Sampson Bridgwood was in business in his mother's 'Wood Street' works in 1825,[35] and in 1829 Simeon Shaw referred to him as 'an excellent manufacturer of Porcelain'.[36] Some fifty years later, another ceramic historian, Llewellynn Jewitt, wrote of the works: 'It was here that the late Mr. Sampson Bridgwood made his first start, and after noble struggles against adversity laid the foundation of his ultimate splendid success'.[37]

Directories from 1822 to 1853 specify that Sampson Bridgwood made only china.[38] In 1833, part of his china works was on fire due to a heated flue setting fire to a floor; and next year a fire at his High Street china works caused £70 to £80 of damage.[39] In 1836, Sampson Bridgwood paid a levy to the local Chamber of Commerce on six ovens, suggesting that he was in a large way of business.[40] Evidence was given to an inquiry into the employment of children in 1841 that Sampson Bridgwood had three china factories.[41] William Turner, aged 33, who was foreman of all three factories, said that they had no machinery further than hand-turned jiggers. The workers started at six in the morning and finished at nine at night four nights in the week, paying respect to 'St. Monday' by observing a long weekend:

> they never do much work on Saturday afternoons or Mondays; they can't buckle to, and idle their time on those days; the consequence of this is that they work over hours at other times to make up for it. It is distressing to see children do extra work in this way; sometimes I see the sweat running down from them in coming from the hot houses, which must weaken and make old men of them very soon … if we could oblige the men to come at proper hours to work, there would be no necessity for the children to come over-hours, and they could then go to evening-schools, which they cannot do now.

He said that they had no apprentice girls under 13, or not more than two or three, who worked by themselves, or with the women painters. The jiggers referred to required a boy to turn a handle to rotate the mould for the plate or dish maker. William Arnitt, aged 11, said that he 'turned jigger' for his brother. Two other brothers and his father worked at Bridgwoods also. The foreman said that Arnitt's father was improvident: between them, however, the five Arnitts earned at least 39 shillings (£1.95) a week for the year through, and yet he couldn't find clothes for his son to attend Sunday-school.

There was great concern at this time about the employment of young children in potteries, especially mould-runners, going into and out of the 'hot-houses' (drying stoves) as described by Turner. Nothing was done to prevent this happening, however, until manufacturers, including Sampson Bridgwood & Son (and James Broadhurst), memorialised the Home Secretary in 1862.

The rate book records show Sampson Bridgwood occupying two works in 1832 and three in 1837.[42] Probably one would be his original works at Wood Street, his second works would adjoin his house in High Street, and the third would be on Stafford Street (later to be the 'Strand' side of the present Market Hall). This works had been occupied by George Forrester from 1799 to 1830.[43] Writing in 1829, Simeon Shaw described it as being 'the *first* [in Longton] in which a regular plan for the arrangements of the separate places for the distinct processes was adopted', a purpose-built works along the lines of Josiah Wedgwood's 1769 Etruria Works.[44] It had three ovens in 1856.

From 1822 Bridgwood had made only china: although the bone china formula was known by 1800, it only gradually became popular. Out of some forty-five firms in Longton in 1822, thirty-one made earthenware, eight made earthenware and china, and six, including Bridgwoods, made china only.[45] There is no direct evidence of the type of china produced by Bridgwood. In an account of the development of the pottery industry in Longton, written in 1863, it is suggested that the town's distance from the canal (at Stoke) and its position on the highway from Derby led to its trade being with 'carts and waggons from the eastern and northern counties'; a business which brought in ready money and which called for articles more useful than ornamental, where 'price was of greater consequence than quality'.[46]

Bridgwood certainly employed 'women painters' for decorating, and in the mid-century he sold china 'in the white' to former artists of the Rockingham Works in Yorkshire: Isaac and Alfred Baguley at Swinton and Haigh Hurstwood at York, both in one of those northern counties already mentioned for Longton trade.[47] There is an old record of a porcelain cup stamped 'Bridgwood & Son' and dated 1853.[48] A writer of 1900 placed Bridgwoods equal with Samuel Alcock and Sons in the production of artistic china at the mid-century, inferior only to Ridgway, Minton and Copeland.[49] Sampson Bridgwood had some interest in the technicalities of his trade: he subscribed for a copy of Simeon Shaw's *Chemistry of Pottery* in 1837.[50]

In 1834 and 1841, Sampson Bridgwood was living in High Street, Longton (now Uttoxeter Road, probably on the site of the offices of Youngs, solicitors), with his wife Martha, son Samuel II (born 1820) and several daughters, and with a china manufactory adjoining.[51] In 1833 Sampson Bridgwood was High Constable of Longton, at a time when there was agitation

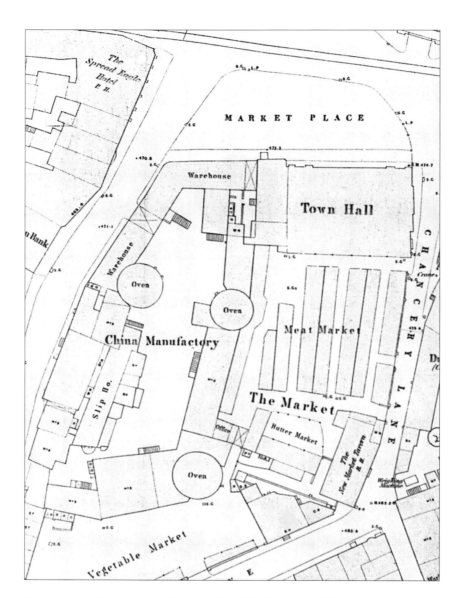

Figure 22 Plan of China Manufactory in Stafford Street (now the Strand), Longton, occupied by Sampson Bridgwood between c.1837 and 1857, and by John Aynsley and Samuel Bridgwood until demolition in 1861. Reproduced from Ordnance Survey 1/500 Plan OST (20) Longton, 1856

for the parliamentary borough of Stoke-upon-Trent to be incorporated.[52] When Town Commissioners were appointed for Longton in 1839, Sampson Bridgwood was the first Chief Bailiff.[53] Spratslade water mill, for flint and potters' materials, which he occupied, was offered to be let in 1843.[54]

In Sampson Bridgwood's life so far, Longton had grown from a 'small but populous village' of 4,000 inhabitants and about twelve potworks in 1800[55] to a 'thriving market town' of 12,400 inhabitants and forty-five factories in 1841,[56] with the attendant problems of uncontrolled growth. An 1839 description spoke of the 'odd jumble of houses, gardens, yards, heaps of cinders and scoria from the [iron] works, clay-pits, clay-heaps, roads made of broken pots',[57] reason enough for establishment of some form of local government. There had been a riot at Longton against the new police in 1839;[58] vigorous electioneering in 1841;[59] and Longton had its share of the Chartist riots which rampaged through the Potteries in 1842.[60] On the credit side, a fire engine was provided in the town in 1840 for the use of the new police,[61] and Zion Chapel was rebuilt in 1841.[62]

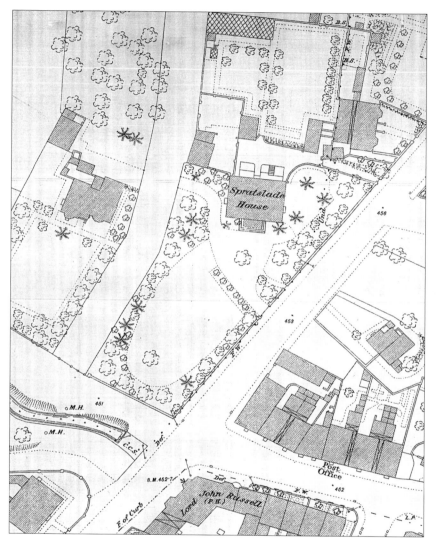

Figure 23 Plan of Spratslade House, (Belgrave Avenue, Longton, 1994) occupied by Sampson Bridgwood c. 1846–1857. Reproduced from Ordnance Survey 1/500 Longton Sheet XVIII.10.20 (1878), surveyed 1875

From 1841 to 1854, Bridgwood's factory address was Stafford Street,[63] and by 1847 he was only operating the Stafford Street Works (Figure 22), owned by the Proprietors of the Market Hall and valued for rates at £130.[64] At that date, Sampson Bridgwood owned a china-works himself in either High Street or Market Street, rated at £42 and occupied by his son, Samuel Bridgwood

II, and John Burgess,[65] perhaps where he formerly lived himself, one of his three potworks of the late 1830s. The Bridgwood and Burgess partnership in manufacturing china seems to have only lasted from 1845 to 1847,[66] but they were also earthenware dealers in Birkenhead in 1843 and 1845, and in Liverpool in 1845.[67] Burgess went to America in 1847 with Robert Dale in a partnership with John Hackett Goddard as American merchants, Longton and New York.[68] Goddard had been a potter, and continued as an 'American merchant' until his death in 1885. Samuel Bridgwood must have also continued to trade with America: he was lampooned as 'The Yankee' in 1862.[69]

Sampson Bridgwood and his son, Samuel, occupied two mills at Gom's Mill, Longton, between 1847 and 1851,[70] and in 1846 Sampson Bridgwood was also a partner with John Goodwin and John Hawley in Mossfield Colliery,[71] then a shrewd investment which was later to be disastrous for the family interest in pottery manufacturing. It can be seen that, besides manufacturing china, at this time he also controlled his fuel supply and ground his own raw materials. With his son as an American merchant the chain was complete from raw clay to retailer.

By 1846, Sampson Bridgwood lived at Spratslade Mansion (now a residential home in Belgrave Avenue, Longton) (Figure 23),[72] and in 1851 he was recorded as a china manufacturer employing 155 workers (64 men, 42 women, 24 boys and 25 girls).[73] With him lived his son Samuel, 31, his daughters Mary, 24, and Anne Maria, 15, a governess, two maids and a coachman. Sampson Bridgwood left Spratslade Mansion in 1857 and moved into Lightwood House.[74]

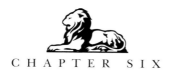

BRIDGWOODS AT ANCHOR WORKS
1853–1876

Sampson Bridgwood was aged 61 in 1853. He had been a china manufacturer for thirty years, and was currently employing about 150 workers in a three-oven manufactory in Stafford Street, Longton.[1] A partner in Mossfield Colliery, he also tenanted a flint mill.[2] Samuel Bridgwood, his only son, aged 33, had been in a short-lived china manufacturing partnership between 1845 and 1847;[3] he was an 'American merchant';[4] and he shared the flint-mill tenancy with his father.[5] A new partnership of 'Sampson Bridgwood and Son' had been formed by 1853.[6]

The building of a new works commenced about 1852. The Ordnance Map of 1856 (Figure 24) showed the new factory as a courtyard works with two biscuit ovens, two glost ovens and a granite oven, on the north-east side of the new railway between Stoke and Derby. The coal tramway from Mossfield Colliery, part-owned by Bridgwoods, passed the front of the factory *en route* to the coal depot in Wharf Street. The original factory formed the northern of the two courtyards of the complete works and much of its structure remains today. Although the works is named 'Anchor Works (China)' on the 1856 map, the presence of a 'granite oven' shows that Bridgwoods now intended to produce the new hard earthenware body for the growing American market, as well as their traditional china. The work had been started as early as 1852, because an 80 yard chimney built in August 1852 for 500 guineas blew down in the storm of January 1853.[7] A date stone (now lost) over the archway, dated the works 1853,[8] but building continued in 1854, when Mr. Bridgwood broke his leg, as he stepped on an arch at his new flint mill, which gave way.[9]

The new partnership seems to have been for the new works, although for a short time it ran both old and new factories. In 1857 Samuel Bridgwood and John Aynsley II formed a partnership, Bridgwood being the '& Co.' of 'John Aynsley & Co.', which produced china at the Stafford Street works until 1861, when the factory was demolished to make way for a new Town Hall and Market Hall.[10] John Aynsley II, born 1823, had already had a colourful career, working in the pottery industry from the age of nine, first as a presser and then as a thrower, for several Longton firms, then for Mintons at Stoke between 1841 and 1848. Next he tramped the country, looking for work, before returning to Longton to work for Bridgwoods and other firms. In 1854 John Aynsley joined a small partnership with Thomas Cooper and Samuel Cope, making china and 'toys' on the present-day Lloyds Bank site until 1857, when Samuel Bridgwood took him into partnership.[11] As will be seen, John Aynsley took over the stricken Bridgwood concern, thirty-three years later.

It is said that John Aynsley designed the Anchor Works for Bridgwoods: certainly he had a wide experience of different factories. Samuel Bridgwood bought land on Sutherland Road in 1857, and when the Stafford Street works had to be demolished in 1861, Samuel Bridgwood and John Aynsley built a model works there, the Portland Works. It can safely be assumed that John Aynsley designed that works. By 1863, Aynsley was able to buy the site for £1,500, end his partnership with Samuel Bridgwood and continue alone.[12]

Building continued at the Anchor Works. A preserved datestone for 1859 from the southern courtyard archway indicates that the factory had been doubled in size by then, and celebratory dinners were held at Martinmas 1860.[13] The report in the local weekly newspaper, *The Staffordshire Sentinel* for 17 November 1860, is worthy of reproduction in full:

FESTIVITIES AT THE ANCHOR POTTERY. LONGTON.

One of the most extensive and successful treats ever given in Longton by employers to those in their service was on Tuesday and Wednesday last by Messrs. Sampson Bridgwood and Son, of the Anchor Pottery to their numerous work-people. Some portions of the works have been in use for several years, but it is only lately the entire manufactory has been completed, and the spirited proprietors determined to celebrate the finish and opening by a sumptuous treat to every person in their employ. The new workhouse [query warehouse], a noble room 150 feet in length, was decorated for the occasion in a most profuse and tasteful manner with flowers, evergreens, &c. At the upper end of the room was a beautifully executed motto "God save the Queen," surmounted by a Staffordshire Knot; at the lower end was another motto in large letters "Success to our Employers," surmounted by a most elegant device, worked in leaves, consisting of a knot in the middle and an anchor on each side, the whole device being symbolical of the name of the works. We also observed the following appropriate mottoes, "Live and let Live," "Life is not all Sunshine," "Onward," "Work and Win," "God bless our own Country," "We are United," &c., &c. A large number of good pictures were also hung upon the walls and, with the mottoes, and evergreens, devices, &c., gave the room a most joyous and festive appearance. The decorations were under the superintendence of Mr. George Mountford, the manager at the works, who was assisted by several others. We also observed in the room a most admirable and life-like bust of Mr. Sampson Bridgwood, executed by J. Mc Bride, Esq., of London.

At four o'clock, on Tuesday afternoon about 200 of the adults sat down to a most sumptuous dinner, the bill of fare comprising an extensive list of creature comforts, with many choice delicacies, to which we hardly need say ample justice was done by the company. The chair was occupied by Mr. Samuel Bridgwood, (his father being unavoidably prevented from being present through indisposition), and the vice-chair by Mr. Mountford. The chairs of both these gentlemen, besides being decorated with flowers and evergreens, were literally covered with grapes, apples, oranges and other fruits, which were afterwards given away among the guest [sic]. After dinner the cloth was withdrawn and abundance of rum punch was served up, with a rich dessert, and the usual loyal, patriotic, and other toasts were proposed and drunk with customary honours.

After these came the toast of the evening, "Success to our employers," which was proposed by the VICE-CHAIRMAN in a brief but pithy address. He then read and presented to the Chairman the following address from the workmen.

"Respected Sirs, – At this customary festive season of the year, when the employers and the employed enter into a new and a mutual engagement for a definite period, the workpeople connected with your establishment, individually and collectively, embrace the opportunity of expressing their feelings and sentiments entertained towards you as their employers, dictated by kindness of heart and purity of motive. Amid the multitudinous changes which have occurred, and are occurring in this densely populated manufacturing district, your firm has ever maintained a high position for commercial enterprise, uprightness of character, and honesty of purpose, but above all for a dignified deportment, blended with urbanity of manners towards those in your employ; excellencies and characteristics which could not fail, and have not failed to make an enduring impression on the minds of all who are capable of appreciating exalted worth. And in confirmation of this fact we remark, with pride and satisfaction, because we think it alike honourable to both parties that no magisterial interference has ever been required to adjust any difference that may have arisen between master and servant, as we have at all times found you of easy access, and both willing and prompt in removing any well-founded grievance that existed. This line of conduct is eminently worthy of imitation, and we sincerely regret that it is not invariably pursued. It would prevent many unseemly exhibitions in courts of justice, and allay irritation and discontent between the employers and employed, whereby the interest and comfort of both parties would be promoted. We trust, however, that our social relations are improving in this respect. We think there are indications that, as intelligence increases, masters are much more inclined to listen to complaints and the men much less unreasonable in their demands. Should this be the case, the result cannot fail being beneficial and satisfactory. We hail the present occasion with delight. It is a gathering of an interesting and gratifying character, the virtual opening of the new manufactory, which takes a commanding position in the locality. We hope the fabric manufactured may be entitled to the same pre-eminence that has been accorded to the porcelain department, and that the same good-feeling and success may accompany the undertaking. And, in conclusion, respected sirs, we, your workpeople, beg your acceptance of this address, with our ardent and sincere wishes for your health, prosperity, and happiness."

Mr. BRIDGWOOD replied to the address in a few feeling remarks, his emotions being evidently too powerful to enable him to do so at any great length. He spoke, however, of the great pleasure it gave him to meet them that evening, thanked them for their expressions of good-feeling towards himself and father, and hoped those feelings would ever subsist between them.

The toast was drunk and most rapturously honoured, the entire company rising and giving several hearty rounds of deafening cheers followed by the Pottery fire [sic]. – A number of other toasts were given, including "Our Employed," proposed by the CHAIRMAN, and responded to by Mr. ISAAC TUNNICLIFFE, an old servant of 20 years standing. "The Town and Trade of Longton," and "The health of the Vice-Chairman" were given and suitably responded to, after which the company enjoyed themselves with dancing, singing, &c., till a late hour.

At two o'clock on Wednesday, the whole of the boys and girls were treated to an excellent dinner, and spent the afternoon in a variety of amusements until six o'clock when they were sent home. At seven o'clock about 140 of the adults again sat down to a good dinner, served up as on the previous evening, and some pleasant hours were again spent in dancing, songs, recitations, &c. The band of the Longton Volunteer Rifle Corps was present each evening in uniform and supplied excellent music. Mr. Samuel Bridgwood was present the whole of each evening, and by his free and generous deportment and unwearied attentions to even the humblest person, greatly enhanced their enjoyment.

We do not remember ever attending any similar treat in which there was more real enjoyment and good-feeling among all parties than on this occasion. The firm have earned and secured for themselves the deepest respect and sincerest attachment of all in their service, and it is pleasing to know that the anxious solicitude of the proprietors for the welfare of those dependent upon them is permanent, and has developed itself in a manner no less creditable to them than beneficial to the people. In the arrangement of the new workshop the convenience and health of the workpeople have been studied to the fullest extent. Instead of the small, low, dark, dusty, and ill-ventilated workshops, so common in the Potteries, Messrs. Bridgwood have provided for their employes [sic] such workshops that, for light, pure air, and plenty of space, are not to be surpassed, if equalled, in the district. We can only say in conclusion that we most sincerely hope the good-feeling existing between Messrs. Bridgwood and their operatives will continue to grow, and ever characterise the establishment.

Clearly, the completion of the works provided for production of a new 'fabric'; almost certainly granite earthenware, for which there had been a single oven in 1856, and for which Bridgwoods became well-known in the coming years. Some 340 adults were employed, compared with 106 adults in 1851, a measure of the firm's progress. The 1878 Ordnance Plan (Figure 25) shows the additional southerly courtyard with four more ovens, nine in all, and the complete mill at the rear, a main-line railway siding, and tramways within the mill area.

A year later, November 1861, the American Civil War (1861–5) was being felt severely by the North Staffordshire

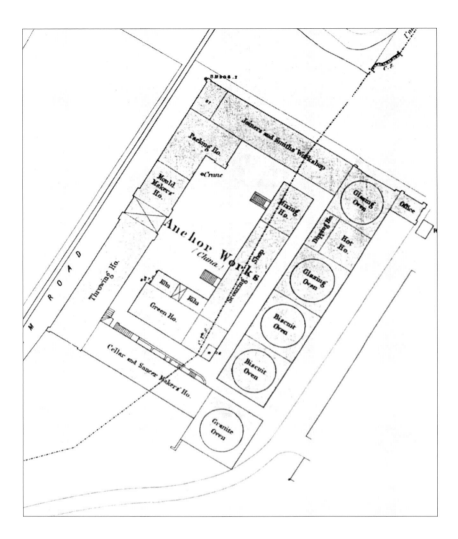

Figure 24 Anchor Works, Bridgewood (*sic*) Street, Longton, in 1856, as built by Sampson Bridgwood and Son in 1853. Reproduced from Ordnance Survey 1/500 Plan, Longton OST (20) 1856. See Figures 25 and 35

pottery industry, and over forty manufactories were said to be closed. Longton was least affected, dependent as it was on a large number of small dealers.[14]

There are a few known examples of Bridgwoods' products at this period. Fine china with gold 'vermicelli' or laid-ground borders and hand-painted centres is known from marked services (Colour Plates 1 and 2), showing the high quality of work done at this time,[15] and the same shape is known with a blue printed Chinese pattern.[16] A sycophantic poem of 1866 (Figure 26) claims Sampson Bridgwood and Son as the largest exporters of china in the Potteries, and mentions their imitation 'Capo-Di-Monte' ware.[17] (A contemporary work describes Capo di Monte ware as known at that date as 'perhaps the most beautiful description of porcelain which has ever been manufactured in Europe'.)[18] The verse goes on to enumerate their

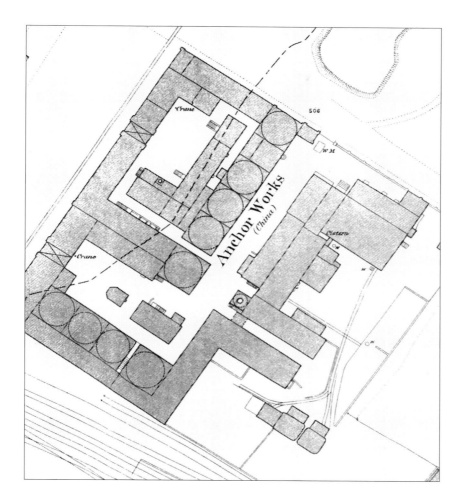

Figure 25 Anchor Works in 1878, as extended by Sampson Bridgwood and Son in 1860. Reproduced from Ordnance Survey 1/500 Plan, Longton Sheet XVIII.11.1, 1878. See Figures 24 and 35

products: first jugs, plates, desserts, dinners and teas; medicine and pickle spoons, mugs and breakfast cups, toilet trinkets, dejeuner and luncheon sets; and then their Porcelaine Opaque (a fine hard earthenware, see Colour Plate 6) including a Stilton cheese cover and a Bread Tray ornamented with Ceres, and dinner-ware in Etruscan shapes; ending with the bold claim that Bridgwoods' mill was the largest in the Potteries.

An 1870 directory describes Samuel Bridgwood and Son as manufacturers of china and earthenware for home and foreign markets and grinders of all kinds of potters materials.[19] A sober assessment of their production was given in 1878 by Llewellynn Jewitt: china tea, breakfast and dessert services partly for the home but principally for the North American markets. White granite was made for home, United States, Canadian and Australian markets, including 'Parisian Granite', stamped 'Limoges'.[20] In 1870, the earthenware manufacturers for the United States and British North America (Canada) met at

Figure 26 Poem in praise of Sampson Bridgwood and Son, 1866, in J. T. S. Lidstone, *The Thirteenth Londoniad ... giving a Full Description of the Principal Establishments in the Potteries etc.* (The Potteries, 1866), 42–3

42   THE LONDONIAD.

To them high rank each British Isle allots
For superior toilets and Drab Teapots.
From Trent to Mediterraneum Mare
Goes their Torquoise, their Black Egyptian Ware.
When Minerva, patroness, shall muster
Her Immortal Legions, she shall bless their Lustre.
Thus they march, ye living age, untrammelled—
They've plenty of the Willow and Ware Enamelled.

    P.S. There is a legend connected with "a dish to match," received from Messrs. Tams & Lowe. At the Railway Office in Longton, where I was in the habit of leaving, every day, articles of greater or lesser value, the principal officer said, " we cannot possibly take in this dish, Sir, nor can we allow it to remain here for a single moment during your absence, this is no common dish, and a very expensive one, and if it should become broken I am sure the Company—" the rest of the official's remarks, as the newspapers said regarding part of Mr. George Melley's speech during the late election, "would not look *the thing* in print." This was the first and last article I had to remove on account of its *extraordinary value!*

SAMPSON BRIDGWOOD AND SON,

Manufacturers of China and Earthenware, Longton, Staffordshire.

Th' largest exporters of China in the Potteries,
And the pioneers of ev'ry good the Art-Minstrel sees,
As in Homer's Iliad, rises Samothrace's ridge-wood,
So o'er Longton towers the eminent house of Bridgewood.
I hailed an air of substantiality in their
China, seldom seen in the district elsewhere ;
And their imitation Capo Di Monte Ware,
So called from that place in Naples ; who has not heard
That on this famous Ware personally work'd Charles the Third.

THE LONDONIAD.   43

Jugs, Plates, Desserts, Dinners and Teas in all their full renown,
Thro' most of th' civilized nations o' th' world are known.
Medicine Spoons, Pickle ditto, are here I ween,
Mugs, and, too, the best Breakfast-cups I've seen.
Of lovely contour, lo, their Toilet trinkets,
Beside their rare Déjeuner and Luncheon sets.
Toilet Stand, here heights of Arts they have attained,
Oft' with the sight of too much gold I have been pain'd,
But here 'tis properly adapted and Art maintain'd.
Their Porcelain Opaque must bear the palm away,
Their Stilton Cheese Cover, and glorious Bread Tray,
Appeared with Ceres, radial of a classic day.
Dinner Ware, Etruscan shapes, I too, salute,
And Toilet Ware, Tea ditto, the market to suit.
And here that which doth an entire district fill
With echoes, long the largest, and the largest still,
In the Potteries, is their Grinding Mill.
The world under obligations they have laid,
For all the improvements that our firm hath made.
Here I saw ye CIPPI, as from Partheonic era sent,
Art's spirit enshrining itself in sepulchral monument.
As erst 'midst Garamantian Sands I see Ammonian Jove,
Just ent'ring into brutal form from shining courts above,
Miracle of Art on Earth ! with Life Celestial strove,
So intelligent *that* look ! I felt the great I AM
Was looking still upon me though in the form of Ram ;
And the Solar Sphinx was watching amid her rival spheres.
Out-looking, over the Desert Sands and wider waste of years.
Kindly deeds perform'd by the honored Sire,
Seem the whole British Nation to inspire,
While in the Noble Son and Captain, we
See revived th' Wondrous age of Chivalry.

Burslem and decided on the extreme measure of only working half time for three months, in view of the depressed state of trade.[21] Subscriptions to Longton Cottage Hospital in that year by Bridgwoods' china workers (£13.7s.2d.) and granite workers (£4.13s.8d.) might be regarded as an indication of the proportion of each body produced, or of the comparative generosity of the workers in each branch.[22]

The 1860s saw changes in pottery employment. Lord Shaftesbury initiated another inquiry into the employment of children in 1861, and twenty-six pottery manufacturers memorialised the Home Secretary for legislation to prevent children from being employed at too early an age. Sampson Bridgwood and Son (and James Broadhurst) were amongst the eight Longton manufacturers who signed, urging that voluntary agreement could not be obtained amongst pottery employers.[23] As in 1841, an Assistant Commissioner visited the Potteries, and took evidence. One of the problems in controlling the hours of work of children was that they did not work directly for the master. Sampson Bridgwood, like most manufacturers, preferred the saucer-makers to employ their own lads as jigger-turners and mould-runners. A saucer-maker took work at a price and employed one, two or three lads. If the employer found the lads, they might not suit, and they would have to be paid for doing nothing when the men were away.[24]

The upshot of the inquiry was that pottery work was included in the *Factory Acts Extension Act* of 1864: children under eight were not to be employed, whilst those between eight and twelve had to attend part-time school daily, and older children up to seventeen had to produce a medical certificate confirming their age before being employed. Neither women nor children were to work between six at night and six in the morning. The master-potters were dissatisfied with the half-time arrangements: they were unable to find the extra children to work two shifts. Gradually, extra women and girls were employed to make up for boys attending school half-time and those boys who went into the better-paid iron trade. Drying stoves were improved, and steam-driven machinery, used for twenty years in the 'out-potteries' of Glasgow, Yorkshire and the North-east, began to be introduced. Seeking to abolish the system of workers allowing their employers so much in the shilling off their wages for various expenses, the Holloware Pressers' Union wrote to Sampson Bridgwood in 1864, and received a 'satisfactory report'.[25]

Bridgwoods were prosecuted in 1868 for four offences under the Factory Act, and the reports of the Court proceedings give valuable insights into their factory arrangements.[26] Bridgwoods were referred to as 'the extensive manufacturing firm' and 'the important firm', and many other manufacturers attended the hearings. The charges concerned employing children without current proof of school attendance and failure to keep a register of children employed. Bridgwoods were represented by a barrister (instructed by Mr. E. Young of Longton, presumably the founder of Churchill Tableware's solicitors, Young & Co.), who argued at length that the children were actually employed by independent workmen and not by the masters. He emphasised that 'no manufacturers [had] done more for the advancement and benefit of the persons in their employ than Messrs. Bridgwood' and that 'Mr. Bridgwood senior had been a manufacturer at least fifty years and had, seeing that the act was calculated to benefit the workpeople in the district, taken an active part in getting it introduced into the Potteries'. Notices were displayed all round the works, instructing workmen who employed young people to register them at the office; and Mr. Bridgwood junior went round the works four or five times a week and went into some workshops as often as twice a day to see that the act was observed. Mr. Bridgwood senior had said that he would dismiss the first person he found infringing the act. The factory inspector said his opinion was that it was the personal wish of Messrs. Bridgwood that the act be strictly observed, but when he had pointed out irregularities at the works some months ago, they had not been rectified. Bridgwoods were fined 20 shillings (£1) and costs for employing one boy without a school attendance certificate; and a work-man, Charles Birks, was fined 40 shillings and costs for a similar offence. Two charges were dismissed.

A visitor to Longton in 1860 wrote:[27]

I alight still early in the forenoon at Longton, under clouds of smoke that darken the air, and amid heaps of broken crockery that bestrew the ground, as we shall see, for miles around. The town looks busy enough, has indeed the aspect of a hardworking town, with furnaces – huge cones peering here and there above the houses, and is dingy and dusty even in its best parts; and because that the furnaces are low, the smoke sweeps and eddies through the streets before rising up to the murky cumulus. That it lives by brittle ware is manifest; crockery and china-shops and workshops not a few, and exhibitions of moulds and earthenware at upper windows, mark the staple; and men and boys, and women and girls, aproned and labour-stained, whose appearance harmonises with their habitation, out-number all other folk on the foot-ways. Though the booksellers' shops display indications of a taste for reading, Longton, which dislikes being identified with its ugly consort Lane End, is the scapegoat for the whole district. Censure the consequences of neglect, note an eye-sore, blame manners and habits wherever you may happen to be in the Potteries, you will be told in reply that your observations are true as regards Longton, but not the other places. Find no fault with Stoke, Hanley, Burslem or Tunstall; but abuse Longton as much as you will.

This was the Longton in which Sampson Bridgwood became an old man. At the 1861 Census he was aged 68, living with his son and partner, Samuel aged 40, a cook, housemaid and groom, at Lightwood House, a little out of the smoke. Samuel was the man of affairs: elected to Longton's first Borough Council in 1865, he was quickly an Alderman and was made second Mayor, in November 1866.[28] Together with other Longton Liberals, he was savagely lampooned in a 'Catalogue of Waxwork Figures', an election squib of 1862.[29] Under the pseudonym of 'Sam Tidgerud the Yankee', he was accused of selling his partner's (John Aynsley's) patterns to his father's customers, of penny-pinching, promising everything and doing nothing, and staying the night at beerhouses kept by widows and single ladies. His effigy was alleged to be seven feet high, two-faced and with special provision for patrons to kick him for an extra charge.

Samuel Bridgwood was Captain of the Longton Volunteers, and allowed his grounds to be used for rifle practice. He was a County Magistrate, and both Samuel and his father were appointed to the first bench of Borough Magistrates in 1867.[30] He was described as a merchant at the 1871 census, and in 1875 he had an independent earthenware business at Old Foley Pottery, later Moore & Co. In that year Samuel was a member of the East Vale Board of Health, the local authority for the area of Bridgwoods' Anchor Works.[31]

Sampson Bridgwood died 2 June 1876 at Lightwood Lodge, Longton, at the age of 84.[32] His obituary described him as 'an old townsman … a gentleman much esteemed'. His place in public affairs had long been taken by his son, Samuel, who died aged 56 less than five months later, on 23 October.[33] Samuel merited a much more fulsome obituary, noting his mayoralty and aldermanship, his captaincy of the Longton Rifle Corps from 1861 to 1868, and his membership of the county magistracy. Mention was made of his protracted illness. Flags were flown at half-mast at the Town Hall and Courthouse, and many blinds were drawn. The note concluded 'we understand that the important manufactory of which he was the head will in all probability be carried on by his executors', and this was to be so.

Samuel Bridgwood was the sole executor of his father's will, and so his own executors proved both wills. Sampson Bridgwood left 'under £20,000' and Samuel Bridgwood left 'under £45,000', both handsome sums in nineteenth-century terms, and to these sums the value of property owned had to be added. Of course, Samuel's fortune included his inheritance from Sampson. The executors were Sampson Bridgwood's two sons-in-law, George Webster Napier of Alderley Edge, Cheshire and the Revd. James Harold Walker of Dilhorn, Staffs., and his nephew, Arthur Sampson Napier, a student of Exeter College, Oxford.[34]

Sampson Bridgwood had first partnered his mother in his father's earthenware business, then taken up the newer china manufacture for thirty years; built a model works and added granite ware. He lived to be 84 and left a thriving business, including coal mining and flint milling as well as china and earthenware.

December 1, 1883.

white and ivory) is clean and soundly fired. Their decorated patterns, both under-glaze and enamelled, are artistically coloured, and show a good taste. We particularly noticed a variety of patterns in the old "Crown Derby" style of decoration, which for colouring and effective decoration always looks well. A new pattern which they are just now bringing out in printed and also decorated is called "Kenilworth," which is very effective—a dado style of decoration, covering half the plate obliquely, with a lighter style of finish for the other half. It is very novel in style, and both pleasing and artistic. It is capable of finish in several styles of decoration. In toilet ware the "Lorne" is the last new plain shape which they have just got out, and it is well designed, both for elegance and usefulness. The patterns made to the different shapes are well adapted and are effective; the printed patterns are good, and the decorated patterns show care in the disposition of the different colours. The Crown Derby styles are well represented in this line of goods. To go through the different patterns would require more space than we can give here. We would, however, particularly notice their embossed shaped "Derby." As will be seen from the

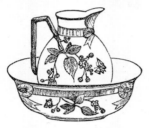

above illustration, a blackberry spray on the side of the ewer forms a bramble handle, with a ribbon, tied in a bow round the neck of the ewer, and outside the basin. The *tout ensemble* is very pretty. It is finished in a variety of ways, from a medium style of decoration to a very elaborate and expensive style, but in each case there is the appearance of elegance and chasteness. Majolica occupies a good part of their attention. This firm have lately opened show-rooms in London, at 21, Charterhouse - street, Holborn - circus (Mr. Briggs, agent), where a nice assortment of patterns can be seen.

Messrs. Sampson Bridgwood and Sons, of the Anchor Pottery, Longton, have recently brought out a new dinner service in china. It will be seen from the following illustrations of it, that it is quite a departure

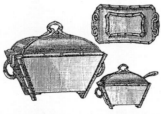

from many of the shapes now in vogue. The soup tureen is made very deep, with square ends, and the sauces are made to match.

December 1, 1883.

The following illustrates the cover-dish, salad, and baker. The jug is after their "Diamond" tea-ware.

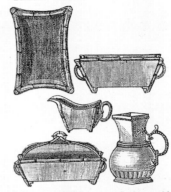

The dishes and plates are made square, with the corners turned over to represent ears.

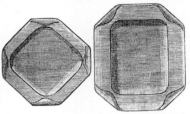

We have simply shown it in plain white china, but the shape is one that will bear any amount of decoration, the square sides or panels giving scope to the artist to display his talent to meet the requirements of individual purchasers or markets. It is not often that firms produce dinner services in china, and Messrs. Bridgwood are justly celebrated for the clear transparency of their china bodies. The following represents the high compote of a new dinner service which

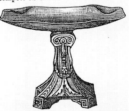

will be out during the month. The stand is very elaborate, it being of a clear sharp embossed pattern. They also have it made with the dish having an open worked pattern round the edge, after the style of Sevres china. As this has to be cut out by hand it is a very delicate process and requires careful manipulation.

At the sale of Mr. Hudden's plant, this firm bought several of the copper plates, and will consequently be able to furnish the trade with many of the patterns supplied by Mr. Hudden before his failure.

Figure 27 Publicity for Sampson Bridgwood and Son's new dinner service in china, also showing the 'Diamond' shape jug. *Pottery Gazette*, December 1, 1883, 1152–53

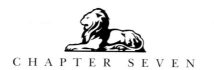

CHAPTER SEVEN

BRIDGWOODS AT ANCHOR WORKS
1876–1890

At the death of both Sampson Bridgwood and Samuel Bridgwood in 1876, the business was left to Sampson Bridgwood's daughters, Martha and Mary, wives of two of the executors.[1] Martha had married George Webster Napier, a cotton spinner; and Mary married the Reverend James Harold Walker, an Irishman, who was curate at St. John's Church, Longton, between 1858 and 1860. He became curate at Dilhorn in 1862 and succeeded the Revd. C. F. Dawes as vicar there in 1863.[2] Mr. Napier managed the business for his wife, Martha, and sister-in-law, Mary, who were partners as Sampson Bridgwood & Son, china, earthenware and granite manufacturers and millers.[3] The partnership was dissolved 1 January 1879 and Mary Walker carried on alone.[4] She also owned the factory and adjoining mill, and continued the family interest in the Mossfield Colliery Company.

Mr. Gaskell, a Liverpool cotton broker, managed the business for Mrs. Walker from 1879 until 1884.[5] He was probably her cousin, as Sampson Bridgwood's sister, Catharine, had married a John Gaskell at Stoke on 22 April 1817.[6] Mrs. Walker's son, George Edward Walker, came into the business in 1880 at the age of twenty-two, and became his mother's partner in 1882. Unlike his forebears, brought up 'in the clay', G. E. Walker had been educated as the son of a well-to-do country clergyman. Another son, Harold Bridgwood Walker, born 26 April 1862, became a Lieutenant General; his son was an Admiral, and his grandson, Harold Berners Walker, was British Ambassador to Iraq in 1990.[7] A daughter, Miss M. B. O. Walker, married Douglas Brownfield of William Brownfield and Sons, potters at Cobridge, in 1883.[8] Mr. Gaskell left in 1884.[9]

It seems that the factory was 'ticking over' under Mr. Napier's supervision between 1876 and 1879, though there is a general 1878 reference to the granite trade with America improving, and orders coming in, 'notably in the case of Bridgwoods'.[10] From the time that Mrs. Walker took full control and Mr. Gaskell became manager, there were many innovations.

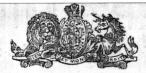

IMPORTANT TO POTTERS, BRICKMAKERS,
AND OTHERS.

CLEMENT ROBEY'S
UNRIVALLED
PATENT OVEN

*(Working most satisfactorily on the Continent, and in
various parts of England and Scotland),*

POSSESSES THE FOLLOWING ADVANTAGES :

1.—Saves One-third to One-half in the Cost of Fuel,
thoroughly disseminates the heat and insures uniform firing, lessens
the wear and tear of brickwork more than one half, greatly reduces
the loss in saggars, and is easy to manage by any Fireman.

2.—Is perfectly simple in construction, and being flat-bottomed,
facilitates the placing, prevents reeling, and holds more ware ; fires
and cools in less time, thus giving the opportunity of drawing extra
Ovens, without additional erections.

3.—*Existing Ovens* requiring a new bottom, can be altered for less
than *Five Pounds* additional cost, as neither foundations nor outward
structure have to be interfered with. As a Smoke Consumer its
general adoption will be a public benefit.

Testimonials and a Model of the Oven can be seen, and the Terms
known, on application to the Patentee, Sylvan Cottage, Basford
Park, near Etruria, Staffordshire (five minutes' walk from the
Station) on the Main and Loop Lines.

C. R. sells Liquid French Gold, requiring no burnishing.

All kinds of Insurances, Patents, and Registration of Designs,
effected as usual.

Figure 28 1879
advertisement for
Robey's Patent Oven;
as installed by
Sampson Bridgwood
and Son in 1880.
*Keates's Directory of the
Potteries and Newcastle
1879*, 13

Some of the 'Granite' (earthenware) ovens were converted in
1880 to 'Robey's Patent' (Figure 28). This was a system whereby
existing ovens were converted from up-draught to down-
draught, with the floor flues discharging into a separate
chimney stack.[11] Such a chimney was built at the 'Granite
Works' in late 1880.[12] At this time there was a great deal of
interest in improving the performance of pottery ovens:
Wilkinson and Minton patent oven designs were also available,
and the Robey design had been on the market since 1873.[13]

Its merits were claimed to be a saving of from 35 to 50% in fuel costs, uniformity in ware, reduction in saggar loss and a flat floor to the oven.[14] In 1890, however, it was stated that the alterations to the ovens 'were decidedly a failure'. Bridgwoods proposed to build a new works on the opposite side of Wharf Street (now Bridgewood (*sic*) Street) in 1882, but this does not seem to have materialised.[15]

Another attempted improvement to the firing was the introduction in 1886 of gas as the fuel for ovens. Gas, in fact, had been used as early as 1873 for firing porcelain at Charlottenburg, Germany.[16] At Bridgwoods, an un-named Scottish firm installed a 'costly gas manufacturing plant' and converted two china biscuit ovens to gas firing, but the trials were reported as being very expensive and not concluded.[17] In 1890, it was stated that six or eight kilns had been converted (perhaps including enamel kilns?) and very good china produced, but difficulties arose because the form and arrangement had been wrong. This had been a plucky trial from which the trade had benefited. In 1889 the installation of electric light was commenced, to save money, but this innovation was not completed.[18]

In production too, there were new ideas. In 1880, Bridgwoods were reported to be using rubber backstamps, which was three times as quick as using tranfer-printed marks.[19] More revolutionary was the announcement in 1885 that Bridgwoods were employing the process of photography on china, producing magnificent plaques which were copies of the work of celebrated painters.[20] On 9 November 1885, Mary Walker, George Edward Walker and Jean Baptiste Germeuil Bonnaud 'of Longton, photographer' registered a provisional patent for producing 'Copies for Lithography from Photographs or other Designs' (Figure 29).[21] In September 1886 the process was stated to be not so successful, and no surviving examples have been reported. A loss of £5,000 to £6,000 in 1885 was attributed to these experiments.[22] Bonnaud was one of a group of foreign artists and technologists who contributed to the development of ceramic production in North Staffordshire in the late nineteenth century. Bridgwoods' management was prepared to experiment at this period, as did Minton, Wedgwood and Brownfield.

More conventional ways of increasing business were also being pursued. Registration of new designs, which provided three years' protection against copying, had been available since 1843. Bridgwoods had never taken advantage of it until 1881, but in the next two years they registered some twenty-one designs, for both shapes and patterns.[23] Most were for unusual

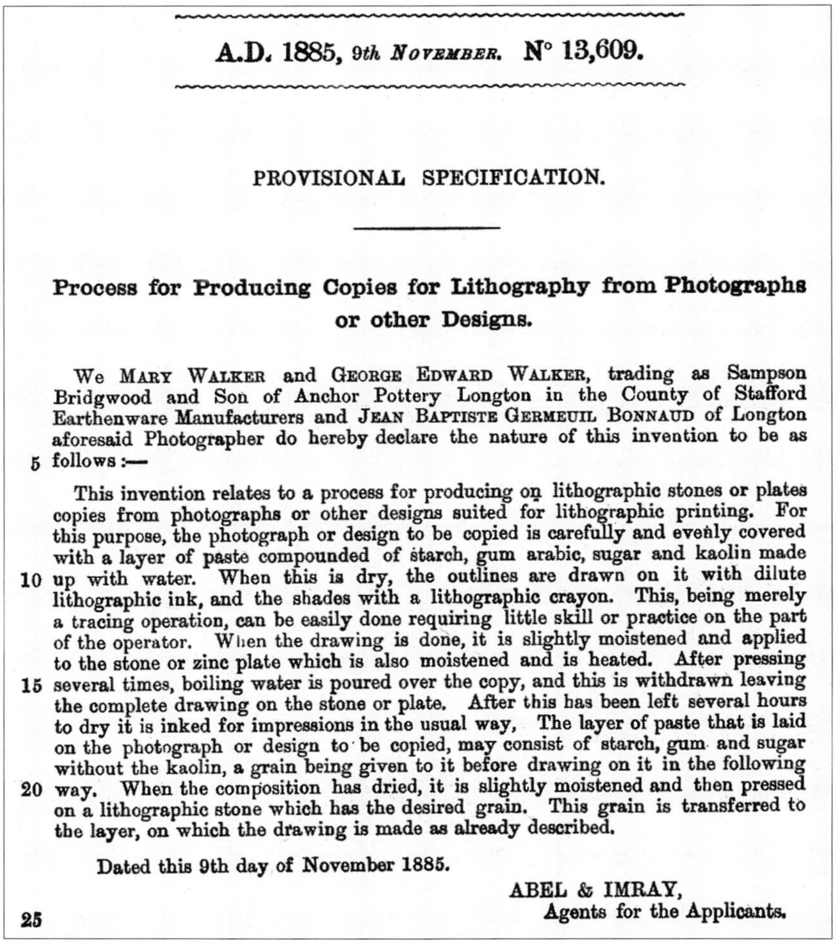

A.D. 1885, *9th November.* N° 13,609.

PROVISIONAL SPECIFICATION.

Process for Producing Copies for Lithography from Photographs or other Designs.

We MARY WALKER and GEORGE EDWARD WALKER, trading as Sampson Bridgwood and Son of Anchor Pottery Longton in the County of Stafford Earthenware Manufacturers and JEAN BAPTISTE GERMEUIL BONNAUD of Longton aforesaid Photographer do hereby declare the nature of this invention to be as
5 follows :—

This invention relates to a process for producing on lithographic stones or plates copies from photographs or other designs suited for lithographic printing. For this purpose, the photograph or design to be copied is carefully and evenly covered with a layer of paste compounded of starch, gum arabic, sugar and kaolin made
10 up with water. When this is dry, the outlines are drawn on it with dilute lithographic ink, and the shades with a lithographic crayon. This, being merely a tracing operation, can be easily done requiring little skill or practice on the part of the operator. When the drawing is done, it is slightly moistened and applied to the stone or zinc plate which is also moistened and is heated. After pressing
15 several times, boiling water is poured over the copy, and this is withdrawn leaving the complete drawing on the stone or plate. After this has been left several hours to dry it is inked for impressions in the usual way. The layer of paste that is laid on the photograph or design to be copied, may consist of starch, gum and sugar without the kaolin, a grain being given to it before drawing on it in the following
20 way. When the composition has dried, it is slightly moistened and then pressed on a lithographic stone which has the desired grain. This grain is transferred to the layer, on which the drawing is made as already described.

Dated this 9th day of November 1885.

ABEL & IMRAY,
Agents for the Applicants.
25

Figure 29 British Patent Provisional Specification 9 November 1885, No. 13,609, for Bridgwoods' process for producing lithographic copies from photographs

shapes: a tazza, a coffee-pot, an eight-sided plate and an oval one, and a helmet-shaped cup amongst them. The shapes were registered with small sepia photographs and are very indistinct. A single design for a transfer print, registered in November 1882, is much more attractive visually, with a crescent moon, mosques, a tiger, a palm tree and a yashmak-ed figure looking from a window, all over a scimitar blade (Figure 30). Though advertisements of the period invited export orders,[24] this pattern owed more to European or American ideas of oriental scenes, rather than to reality. Bridgwoods' London showroom was at 15 Charterhouse Street with Mr. J. W. Pulley as agent. China was exported successfully to both U.S.A. and Canada (Figure 31).

Bridgwood marked china of this period, decorated with a blue sprig, has been recorded in Canada, together with items of the 1883 china dinner service with 'folded corners', referred to below. Nine-inch plates in this design are known, incribed 'New

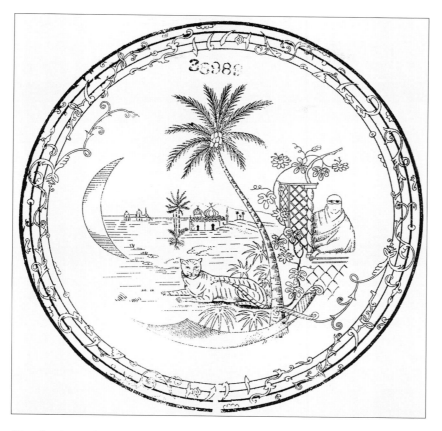

Figure 30 Design no. 389894, pattern for plate, registered by Sampson Bridgwood and Son, 13 November 1882. PRO: BT 43/73

Year's Greeting / 1885 / E. K. Barnsdale & Co.'. Barnsdale was a grocer in Stratford, west of Toronto. Bridgwood 'Parisian Granite', enamelled with three sprigs of apple blossom on a printed outline, has also been found in Canada.[25] Because of the frequency with which nineteenth-century Bridgwood marked ware has been discovered in Canada, items are included in the window of the 'crockery shop' of the Ontario street scene in the History Hall of the new Canadian Museum of Civilisation.

In the late nineteenth century, it was regarded as unusual to produce dinner services in china, but Bridgwoods did so in 1883, and the principal shapes were duly registered, rectangular shapes with 'bamboo' edges, the dishes and plates square with turned over corners (Colour Plate 9). Besides the design photographs, which included a pierced edge version for a comport, the shapes were featured in the *Pottery Gazette* (Figure 27).[26] Reference was made to the skill needed for the 'open worked pattern ... after the style of Sevres china'. At a more mundane level, dealers were informed that Bridgwoods had bought some of Mr. Hudden's copper plates at his failure, and would be able to furnish patterns. J. T. Hudden had built the

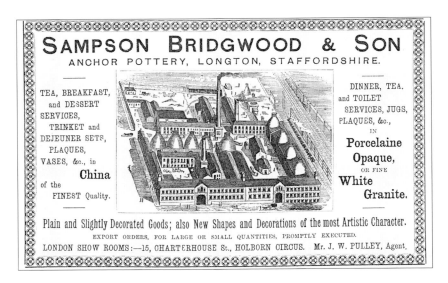

Figure 31 Sampson Bridgwood and Son's advertisement in 1883, showing an 'aerial' view of Anchor Pottery from the west. *Pottery Gazette*, 1 January 1883, 40

neighbouring British Anchor Works by 1875, but he failed in 1884. (Churchill China now owns this works, see Chapter 11.)

Further designs were registered in the 1884–86 period, and advertisements referred to a designer named H. J. Kane, employed by Bridgwoods, of whom nothing more is known.[27] Colour advertisements in the *Pottery Gazette* for April 1886 and January 1887[28] show Bridgwoods' capabilities in multi-colour decoration and gilding on both porcelain and 'Granite' earthenware. The 1886 picture shows seven shapes in china tea-cups: Bamboo, Glasgow, Salisbury, Strasburg, Sutherland, Trentham and Worcester, with floral pattern numbers between 1169 and 2317. The later advertisements are for china tea-ware with floral patterns, numbers between 2457 and 2722 (Colour Plate 7); and for Parisian Granite earthenware in a new 'Alpha' shape, showing a tureen and cover with a choice of four floral decorations and gilding (Colour Plate 8). Princess, Clarence and Rosslyn patterns, examples of Bridgwood china of this period, are shown in Colour Plates 3, 4 and 5.[29]

The Longton china manufacturers were in difficulty generally in the 1880s. In 1882 it was reported that bone and borax prices had practically doubled in four years, whilst the selling price of china had dropped. There was increasing foreign competition and selling prices were reduced still further in 1887 'to a non-paying point'.[30]

Despite the new shapes and expensive publicity, the business was having problems under its new and youthful management. In July 1887 it was announced that china production would cease, apart from a few plain shapes,[31] and in November of that year, all the fancy china shapes and associated copper plates were auctioned off:[32]

Charles Butters is under instruction from Messrs. Sampson Bridgwood & Son (who are declining the China business of the manufactory) to arrange for sale and sell by public auction on Wednesday, 30th November 1887 upon the above works, Warehouse No. 1 and 2, The whole of the valuable Copper Plates weighing over 1,000 lb., of most saleable patterns and designs, together with a large collection of Blocks and Cases with the working moulds.

Following cessation of china production, that part of the works was to be converted by the introduction of machinery to almost double the production of Bridgwoods' 'Porcelain Opaque', a high quality thinly-potted earthenware (Colour Plate 6). Prompt delivery, new patterns and shapes, and patterns previously done in cheap china were promised. Enamelling was continued, some granite ware was decorated with a moss rose pattern, and they commenced printing in 'still' colours.[33]

In order to make the changes, Bridgwoods gave all their employees a month's notice in February 1888, 'to allow of a readjustment of making prices'. Presumably the former china workers were to be paid lower prices. The points in dispute were both intricate and perplexing. Arbitration decided in favour of the employees, and Bridgwoods accepted the award, although it was said that 'the majority of the old hands had been removed in order to carry out their reduced rates of wages'.[34]

Business continued: Bridgwoods maintained their London Office, now at 22 Thavies Inn, Holborn Circus; and offered patterns to please American tastes, and special attention to badged ware. A patent well dish was made, with a bridge across to stop the meat sliding into the gravy and causing a splash![35] However, in June 1890, the *Pottery Gazette* reported that the event of the month was the 'not unexpected' failure of Sampson Bridgwood and Son, the collapse of what was one of the soundest and most respectable businesses in the Potteries. China production had been discontinued some time ago because it was difficult to get a good price for a really superior article.[36]

The causes of the failure were stated to be manufacturing at a loss, losses by experiments and loss in purchasing bone. A private meeting of creditors at the North Stafford Hotel on 2 May 1890 was told that that there was a deficiency of £11,536.[37] Mrs. Martha Napier (sister of Mrs. Walker) and Mr. C. Butters (auctioneer, Hanley) offered to pay ten shillings in the pound. This was rejected, although subsequently creditors agreed to accept seven shillings and sixpence in the pound from the same source, rather than force a bankruptcy.[38]

The partners knew that the business had been carried on at a loss for some years, but its assets had far exceeded liabilities until the recent tragic explosion at the Mossfield Colliery, in which Mrs. Walker had large interests.[39] Mr. Walker said that he and his mother were partners for ten years from 1882, when she had given him £2,000 of the £12,000 capital. In 1885, the works had been mortgaged for £8,000 to Thomas Crompton of Leek, of which £3,000 went into Turnhurst Colliery. £5,000 had been lost in 1885, attributed to the photography experiment and to gas-firing, but they threw aside the experiments, and worked more economically, reducing the loss to £2,000. The business, including the manufactory and the mill, was worth £30,000 and Mrs. Walker had given Mrs. Napier £15,000 for her half share in 1879. Mrs. Walker had since put in an additional £7,700 and had received nothing back other than rent for the works and mill.

In 1889 there had been an attempt by several manufacturers to form a ring in bone, and Mr. Walker became alarmed and bought bone at £9 a ton. The syndicate collapsed, and he had to sell bone at around £6 a ton, losing about £1,550. Mrs. Walker had £10,000 invested in Mossfield Colliery, but this had depreciated heavily because of the explosion in October 1889, in which sixty-four lives were lost, allegedly because of lack of supervision.[40] Mr. Walker had come into the business without experience in 1880, aged twenty-two, and had to contend with the consequences of the photography and oven experiments initiated by Mr. Gaskell. The County Court Judge approved the schemes of arrangement accepted by the creditors, saying that the conduct of the bankrupts was irreproachable, that they kept proper books and produced balance sheets regularly, and that there was nothing against their conduct. Both Mrs. Walker and Mr. G. E. Walker paid twenty shillings in the pound on their personal insolvencies, and the receiving orders against them were rescinded.[41]

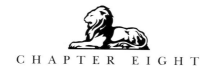

C H A P T E R   E I G H T

BRIDGWOODS UNDER
JOHN GERRARD AYNSLEY
—— 1890–1924 ——

The manufactory and mill were put up for auction by Butters on 30 July 1890 at the Crown and Anchor Hotel, Longton:[1]

Lot 1 | Earthenware manufactory and mill, 13,000 square yards, with private siding and electric light; sliphouse, 4 glost and 3 biscuit ovens and 2 hovels with old granite ovens; 5 x 6-mouth enamel kilns, accommodation for upwards of 20 printers, capacity 80-100 crates per week.

[The mill had 2 x 12 foot and 6 x 9 foot diameter pans for bone and stone; 2 x 9 foot and 7 x 7 foot diameter glaze pans; 7 drying pans; 12 arks, 2 washtubs; a 60 horse-power engine; 2 Galloway and one patent tubular boiler.]

Lots 2–10 | Areas of building land.

Lot 11 | Land and Mr. Lovatt's crateshops.

Lot 12 | Land, stables and coach-house.

Lot 13 | Tramway land [in front of manufactory].

Lot 14 | Mining and mineral rights.

The trade magazine commented that 'should it [Bridgwoods] fall into the hands of Longton capitalists it will probably not remain empty long' and such was the case. The local newspaper reported that 'Bidding [for Lot 1] opened at £10,000 and rose with spirited competition to £13,000 when the sale was declared open. Mr. F. Aynsley bought at £13,250.'[2] 'F.' Aynsley was perhaps a misprint for J. (John) Aynsley, who had been Samuel Bridgwood's partner from 1857 to 1863. Thirty years earlier, Bridgwoods had helped to set up John Aynsley in his new works at Sutherland Road: now he had bought Bridgwoods' works outright. In the meantime, he had built a new works for James Broadhurst. The Aynsley family was to own the works for the next fifty years, but the mill was in the hands of W. Lockett & Co. by 1896.[3] Aynsleys were not interested in this, since they had their own mill.

The contents of the works were next offered for sale, again by Butters, 20–24 November 1890: the implements, utensils, effects and goodwill:

> The valuable copper plates, which have commanded a most extensive sale; the whole of the Blocks and Cases, comprising the Firm's present-going-shapes, with the working moulds, printers' presses, about 3,000 workboards, Jiggers and Whirlers, wheels, stools, rests and baskets, kiln and oven bars, bats and props, large quantity of iron and wood shords, saggars, potters' stoves and piping, dynamo, valuable plaster and slate slabs &c; safes, office furniture and appointments, and a large quantity of loose and miscellaneous effects.

> Notice – The *Goodwill* and *Recipes*, *together* with the *right to use the name of* Sampson Bridgwood and Son, and the benefit of *current orders*, and use of the *Firm's books*, will be Sold by Auction on Monday, November 24th at three o'clock.

The only report of the sale was that the copper plates sold for from 3s. to 9s.3d. and other lots sold well.[4] It seems likely that Aynsleys purchased much of the contents of the works, and certainly they bought the right to use the name. Apart from possibly the jiggers (and the dynamo) there was no mention of the additional machinery proposed to be installed in 1887 when production of 'Opaque Porcelain' was to be practically doubled: perhaps it was never purchased. Apart from the mill engine, there was no motive power in the works. Following these sales, it was possible to pay dividends to the creditors, and the promised 7s.6d. had all been paid by April 1891.[5]

The *Pottery Gazette* stated in January 1892 that, after the failure, Sampson Bridgwood & Sons [*sic*] came into the hands of John Aynsley, who had decided to carry on the works and confine trade to high-class earthenware 'Considering the great reputation Messrs. Bridgwood and Sons gained for their ware not only in England but in the best markets of the world, it would have been a great pity' argued the *Gazette*, 'for such a well-known house to have passed into oblivion.'[6] The firm advertised its 'Porcelaine Opaque', and noted E. W. Jones, 24 Bartletts Buildings as its London agent.

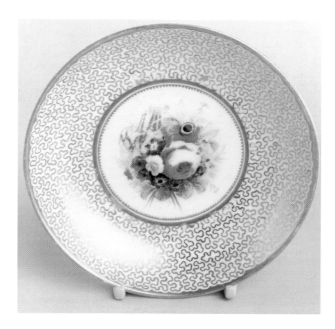

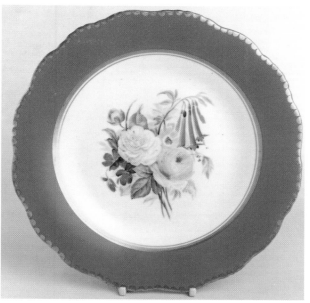

Colour Plate 1 Bone china saucer, hand-enamelled with a floral spray, surrounded by a gilded 'Vermicelli' border, representative of fine tea services made by Bridgwood and Son at their Anchor Works, Longton, in the 1860s. Diameter 5½ in., impressed mark Bridgwood / & / Son. See page 64. *Private Collection*

Colour Plate 2 Bone china dessert plate, decorated with a hand enamelled floral centre and a wide laid ground border and gilding, part of a rich dessert service made by Bridgwood and Son in the 1860s. Diameter 9 in., impressed mark Bridgwood / & / Son. See page 64. *Private Collection*

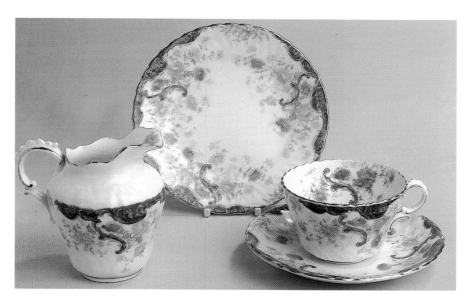

Colour Plate 3 Bone china cream jug, teacup, saucer and teaplate, part of a Princess pattern tea-set made by Bridgwood and Son in the 1880s. Outline printed in brown, it is typical of late-Victorian middle-class taste. 'Princess' probably refers to Princess Mary of Teck, who was to have married the Duke of Clarence. Plate 4 shows the same shape with the Clarence pattern. Plate diameter 6 in., printed mark Bridgwoods / China / Trade (Shield) Mark / Princess; pattern no. 5788 in gold. See page 76. *Churchill China Collection*

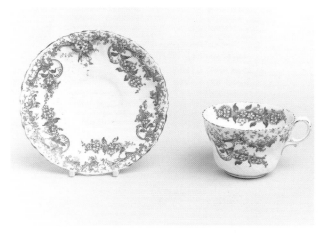

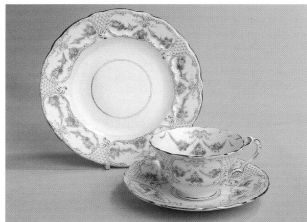

Colour Plate 4 Bone china teacup and saucer, Clarence pattern, transfer-printed in oxide red over the glaze with a rococo floral pattern and gilded, made by Bridgwoods in the 1880s. The shape is similar to that shown in Plate 3; the inside decoration is placed to face the (right-handed) user. 'Clarence' refers to the Duke of Clarence, eldest son of the Prince of Wales. He was to have married Princess Mary of Teck, but he died in 1892. Princess Mary (1867–1953) married his younger brother, and became Queen Mary. Saucer diameter 5½ in., printed mark Clarence / Bridgwoods / China / Trade (Shield) Mark. See page 76. *Private Collection*

Colour Plate 5 Teacup, saucer and dessert plate, bone china, transfer printed over the glaze in brown, and enamelled, Rosslyn pattern on an ornate rococo shape, made by Bridgwoods about 1885. The trellis border with reserves is better seen in Plate 6. 'Rosslyn' was the family name of Millicent, who married the heir to the Duke of Sutherland in 1884, 'the wedding of the year'. The Sutherlands' million and a half acres of land included large parts of Longton. Plate diameter 7 in., printed mark Bridgwoods / China / Trade (Shield) mark / Rosslyn. See page 76. *Private Collection*. A 'Sutherland' pattern is produced by Churchill Hotelware at the Bridgwood factory today

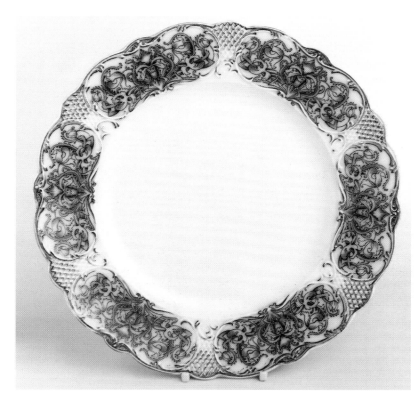

Colour Plate 6 Dinner-plate, in a high quality thinly potted earthenware, c.1885, called by Bridgwoods 'Porcelain Opaque' to compete with French china in North America. It is decorated with a blue-grey Argyle pattern transfer print, underglaze, on a very sharply moulded trellis border with reserves. This moulding matches that of the bone china tea service illustrated in Plate 5. The Dukes of Argyll (*sic*) were chiefs of the Campbell clan and members of the Scottish aristocracy, like the Sutherlands and Rosslyns (see Plate 5). Diameter 10 in., mark Argyle / Porcelain Opaque / Trade (Shield) Mark / Bridgwood & Son. See pages 65 and 77. *Private Collection* A (different) Argyll pattern is still made by Churchill Hotelware at the Bridgwood factory

Colour Plate 7
An 1887 colour advertisement by Bridgwoods, showing six different teacup shapes. The numbering is not clear, as 2722 occurs twice, for different shapes with different patterns. 2700, top row centre and 2722, bottom row right appear to be purely transfer printed, whilst all the others have background prints and enamel colour. In the middle row, 2722 and 2719 are the same shape and pattern, with different colour combinations. The advertisement appeared in the *Pottery Gazette and Glass Trade Review* 1 January 1887, supplement, 2. See page 76

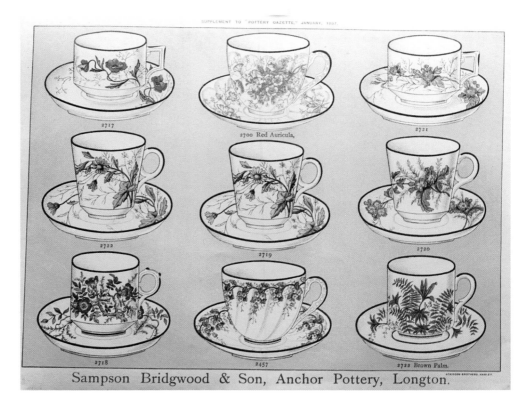

Colour Plate 8
Another 1887 colour advertisement by Bridgwoods, showing a new 'Alpha' tureen shape in P. G. (Parisian Granite) ware, with four different patterns and gilding. Like 'Porcelain Opaque' in Plate 6, 'Parisian Granite' was so-named to compete in North America with imported French china. These two expensive advertisements show how Bridgwoods promoted their new designs to wholesalers and retailers at a critical time for them. *Pottery Gazette and Glass Trade Review* 1 January 1887, supplement, 1. See page 76

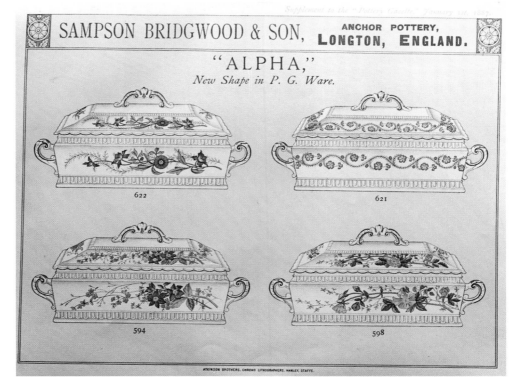

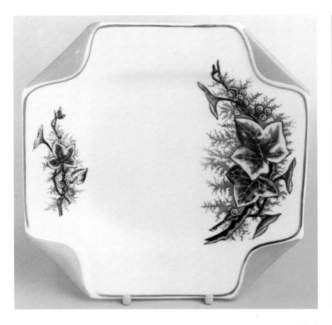

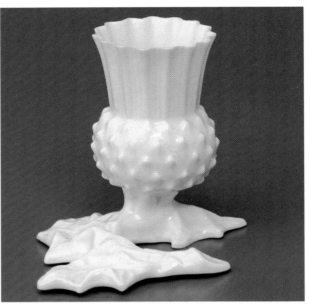

Colour Plate 9 An octagonal dessert plate in bone china, moulded with 'folded' corners which are coloured with pale blue slip. The pattern is transfer printed in brown, filled with turquoise, brown and cream enamel, and finished with a gold line. Bridgwoods advertised this unusual design in 1883, and also offered it as a china dinner service. Diagonal 7 in., stamped mark S B & Son over an anchor in an oval, impressed diamond registration mark for design no. 399135, 9 June 1883, pattern no. 1248. See page 75. *Churchill China Collection*

Colour Plate 10 A 'Thistle' vase in bone china, a design registered by Brigwoods in 1900, a difficult shape to make. Height 4 in., stamped mark Rd. 357636 / S Bridgwood & Son. Bridgwoods resumed making bone china in 1897. Although the American tariff acts had required imports to be marked with the country of origin since the 1890s, this piece is not marked 'England', so presumably was not for export. See page 98. *Churchill China Collection*

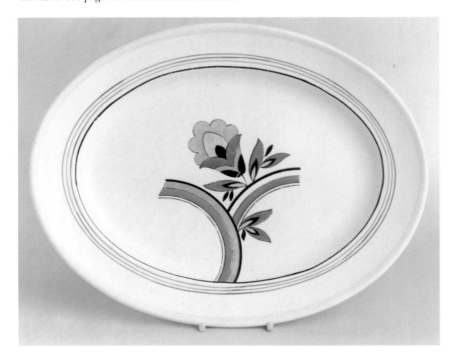

Colour Plate 11 Oval serving dish, ivory earthenware, made by Bridgwoods in a conventional shape in 1935, and enamelled in a style to suit contemporary taste. Length 12½ in., impressed Ivory Bridgwood 3-35, stamped mark Bridgwood / (Anchor) / England, painted pattern no. a/3791. '3-35' is the month and year of production, March 1935. See page 101. *Churchill China Collection*

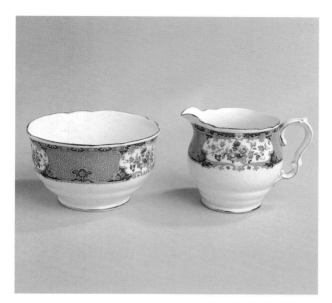

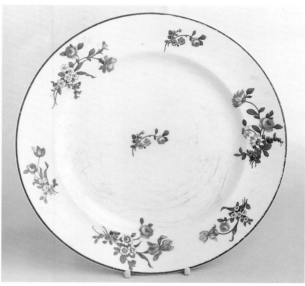

Colour Plate 12 A bone china cream jug and sugar bowl of the 1930s, in a traditional shape. Bridgwoods continued to sell in a good-class market, but by this time used lithograph and gold line decoration, rather than expensive enamelling. Jug height 3½ in., stamped mark Anchor China / Bridgwood / England. See page 101. *Churchill China Collection*

Colour Plate 13 White earthenware dinner plate, decorated with lithographed sprays of roses and a green edge line. The marks show that it was made in August 1927 by Bridgwoods for Harrods Ltd., London, an important customer whom Churchill are again supplying in 1994. Diameter 9½ in., impressed mark Bridgwood & Son / 8-27, stamped Bridgwood / (Anchor) / England, and in a oval laurel wreath Harrods Ltd. / London. See pages 101 and 131. *Churchill China Collection*

Colour Plate 14 Part of a large combined tea and dinner service, made by Bridgwoods in 1936 for another important customer, Waring & Gillow, Oxford Street, London. The cups and saucers are bone china, whilst everything else is Bridgwoods' Ivory earthenware, all decorated with lithographs and gold lining. Apart from their stores, firms such as Harrods and Waring & Gillow included high-class tableware in catalogues for provincial and overseas customers. Length of largest oval dish is 18 in. Most of the earthenware pieces are impressed Ivory Bridgwood / 3-36, and stamped Bridgwood / (Anchor) / England. The largest oval dish is also stamped Waring & Gillow / Oxford Street / London in an oval wreath. The china cups are 2½ in. high, and the cups and saucers are stamped Anchor China / (Anchor) / England. See page 101. *Churchill China Collection*. The pattern has much in common with Churchill Hotelware's 1990s Brantwood Green

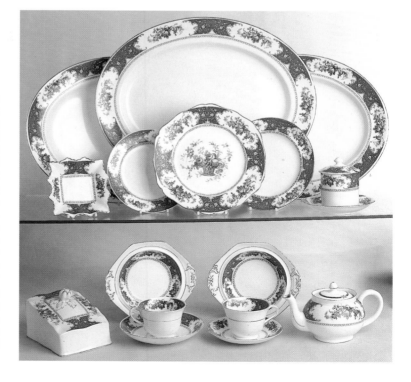

Colour Plate 15 A Bridgwood teapot in white earthenware, supplied through Harrods to the Connaught Hotel about 1930, an example of Bridgwoods' move into hotelware in the 1920s. The pattern is Indian Tree, which continues to be made in the same factory, sixty years later. This example has a brown printed outline, filled with red, yellow, green, and light and dark blue enamel, and is gilded. Length overall 7¾ in., stamped marks Bridgwood / (Anchor) / England / Indian Tree / Connaught Hotel, and Harrods Ltd. / London in an oval wreath. See pages 101,102 and 131. *Churchill China Collection*

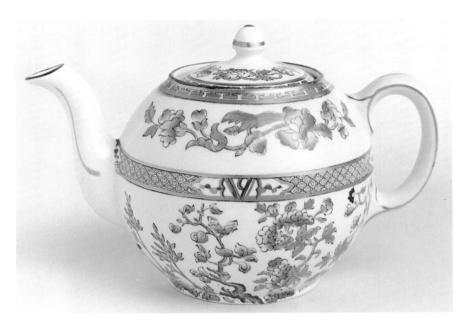

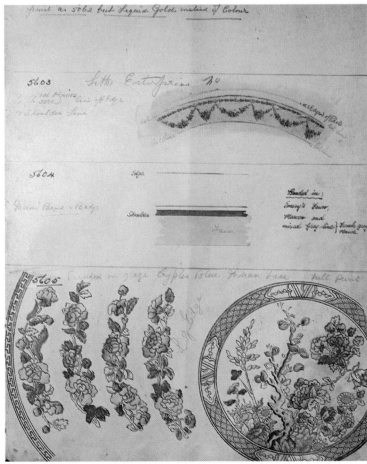

Colour Plate 16 A page from Bridgwoods' 1930s pattern book, showing another version of 'Indian Tree', this one to be printed in 'Cyples Blue'. See page 102. *Churchill China Collection*

Colour Plate 17 Part of a 1927 Bridgwood white earthenware Malayda Lily dinner service, printed underglaze in blue and filled with underglaze red, green, blue and orange. This type of decoration is very durable, being protected by the coating of glaze (glass). The oval dish is 14 in. long. The marks include impressed Bridgwood / 7–27 (July 1927); stamped Malayda Lily / Bridgwood / (Anchor) / England; and painted pattern no. 2135. See page 101. *Churchill China Collection*

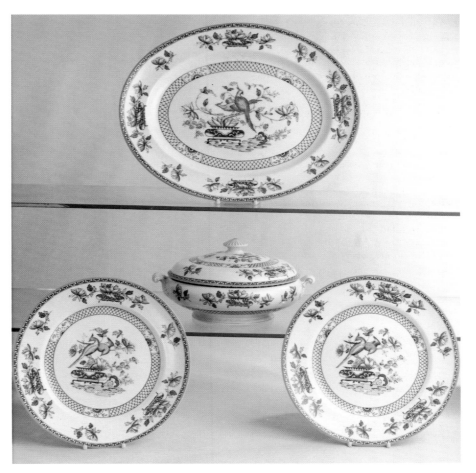

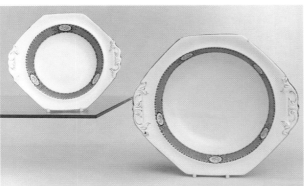

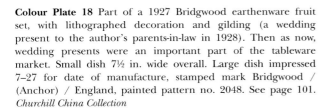

Colour Plate 18 Part of a 1927 Bridgwood earthenware fruit set, with lithographed decoration and gilding (a wedding present to the author's parents-in-law in 1928). Then as now, wedding presents were an important part of the tableware market. Small dish 7½ in. wide overall. Large dish impressed 7–27 for date of manufacture, stamped mark Bridgwood / (Anchor) / England, painted pattern no. 2048. See page 101. *Churchill China Collection*

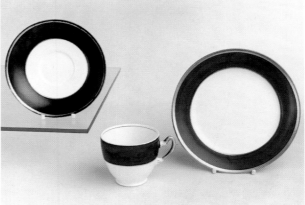

Colour Plate 19 Teacup, saucer and dessert plate from a Bridgwood bone china service of the 1930s. With its underglaze solid blue wide border and gold band, it is an example of elegant simplicity. Cup height 2¼ in., stamped Anchor China / (Anchor in an oval) / Bridgwood / England, painted pattern no. 716. See page 101. *Churchill China Collection*

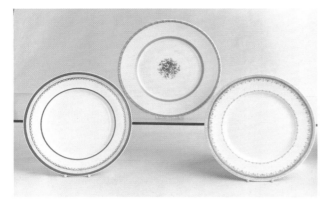

Colour Plate 20 Three Myott 10 in. diameter cream earthenware plates, 1930s-50s, showing a variety of restrained decorative treatments. *Left*, a dinner plate, with underglaze green band and line, on-glaze lithographed yellow and black border, stamped mark (Crown) / Myott Son & Co. / Made in England, and a lithographed mark (Crown) / Royal / Myotts / Crown / Staffs England. *Centre*, a dessert plate with a moulded rim, decorated with an underglaze deep cream wash and underglaze bands and an on-glaze lithographed floral spray. Stamped mark (Crown) / Myott, Son & Co. Ltd. / Made in England, lithographed mark Myott / (Shield) / Staffordshire England. *Right*, a dinner plate with on-glaze lithographed border, yellow, green and brown. Mark as centre plate, together with 'Hostess', the name of the pattern. See page 128. *Churchill China Collection*

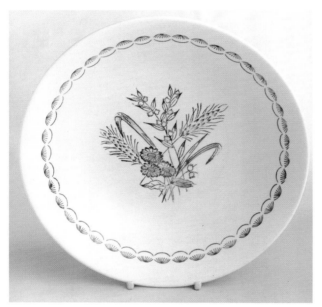

Colour Plate 21 Cream earthenware Harvest pattern fruit bowl made by Broadhursts in the 1950s, an example of their successful 'stamp and fill' decorating technique. The black outlines were applied to the unglazed body with simple rubber stamps, and then 'filled' with hand-painted colours as appropriate. The subsequent coating of glaze ensured that the 'colour is detergent and dishwasher proof' as claimed on the backstamp. Diameter 9 in., stamped mark Broadhurst / Staffordshire / England / Harvest. See page 42. *Churchill China Collection*

Colour Plate 22 Gravy boat and 8¾ in. diameter lobed plate in cream earthenware, with the same decorating technique as in Plate 21. This is 'Revel' pattern, an all-over design which was extremely successful from 1958. Stamped mark Broadhurst / England / Hand painted / Fast Colour / Revel. See page 46. *Churchill China Collection*

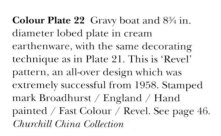

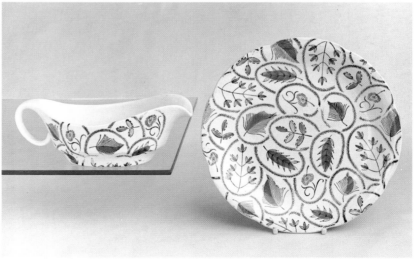

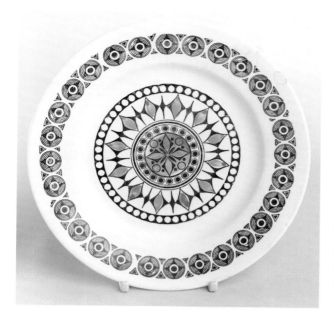

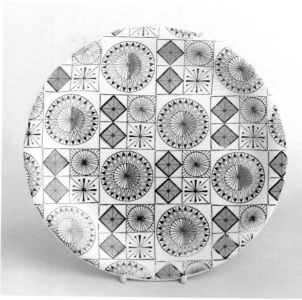

Colour Plate 23 This plate shows the noticeably whiter Ironstone body of the 1960s, still with 'stamped and filled' decoration. The mark credits the Roulette design to Broadhursts' successful designer, Kathie Winkle. Diameter 6½ in., stamped mark Ironstone / Broadhurst / Staffordshire / England / A / Kathie Winkle / Design / Roulette. See page 110. *Churchill China Collection*

Colour Plate 24 Another 1960s plate, with Compass, an all-over stamped and filled pattern designed by Kathie Winkle, on the Ironstone body. The coupe shape reflects the trend to more casual dining habits. Diameter 9½ in., stamped mark Ironstone / Broadhurst / Staffordshire / England / A / Kathie Winkle / Design / Compass. See page 110. *Churchill China Collection*

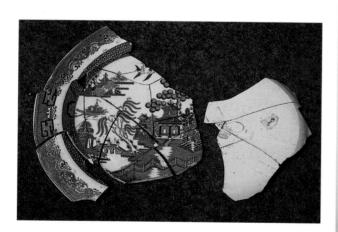

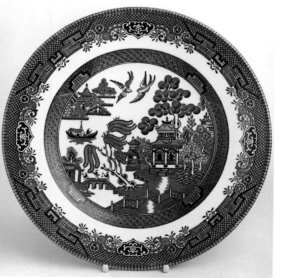

Colour Plate 25 These fragments of c.1820 Bridgwood earthenware Willow Pattern plates were excavated at the Gladstone Pottery Museum site in Longton in the 1970s. The same pattern, first designed by Thomas Minton, and perennially popular, is still made by Churchill, both at Marlborough Works and at the Bridgwood factory in Longton, 175 years later, see Plate 26. Diameter 10 in., transfer printed under glaze, impressed mark Bridgwood. See pages 53 and 133. *Gladstone Pottery Museum*

Colour Plate 26 Current Churchill Tableware dinner plate, decorated under-glaze with almost the same Blue Willow Pattern as was used by Bridgwoods in 1820, see Plate 25. Diameter 9½ in., stamped mark (Lion) / Churchill / England / Willow / Dishwasher / & microwave / Safe. See pages 53 and 133

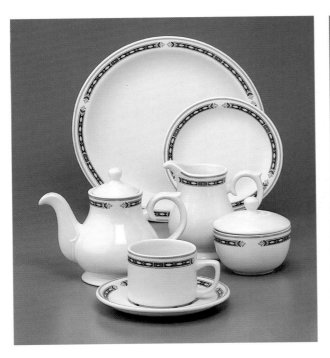

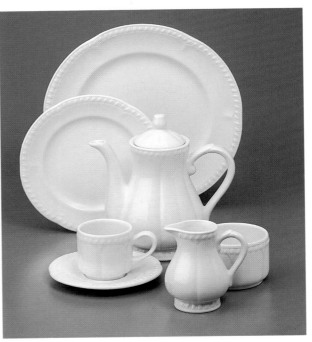

Colour Plate 27 Examples of 1990s Churchill Westminster pattern Hotelware, on a super-vitrified body. See page 135

Colour Plate 28 Churchill Hotelware's current Buckingham shape, an elegant lobed shape with a rope embossed edge. Made in Churchill's super-vitrified body, its graceful shape belies its strength. See page 136

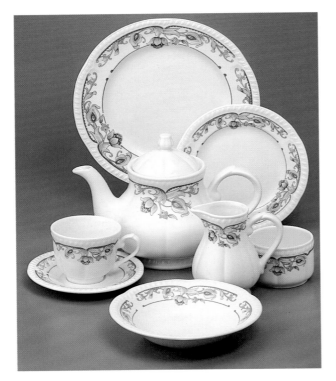

Colour Plate 29 Sumatra pattern on Churchill Hotelware's 1990s Buckingham shape. Hand application of the decoration is seen in Plate 36. See page 136

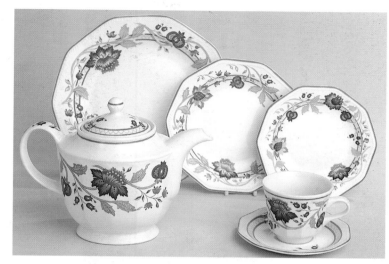

Colour Plate 30 One of Churchill Tableware's 1990s Chartwell Collection, Tamarind, a Jacobean-inspired pattern on facetted Meridian shape, made in English earthenware. Largest plate 10½ in. diameter. See page 132

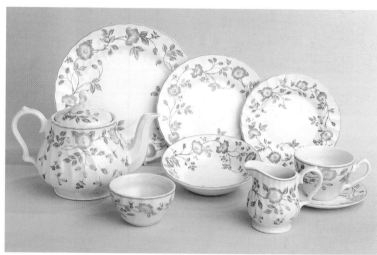

Colour Plate 31 Briar Rose, a delicate floral pattern on Churchill Tableware's current spiral-fluted Chelsea shape, giving the elegance of bone china in earthenware. Teapot 9 in. in length. See page 132

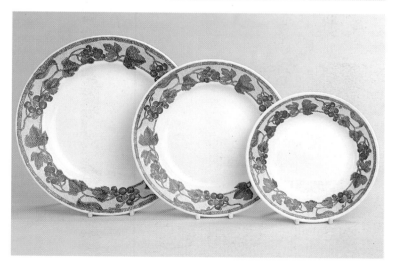

Colour Plate 32 Churchill Tableware's Tuscany, a classical pattern, based on traditional mosaic decoration, on Minton shape. Largest plate 26 cm. diameter. See page 132

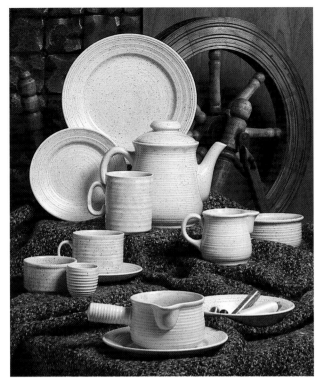

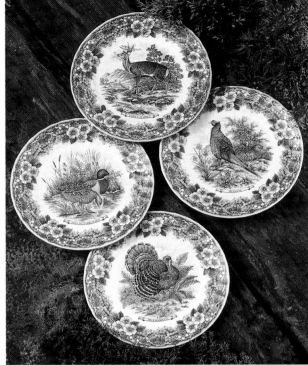

Colour Plate 33 1980s Homespun Stoneware, begun as Broadhurst Homespun earthenware in 1979 and developed into Homespun Stoneware, with an oatmeal glaze on Sampsonite vitrified body. A mug of this design is on display in the Victoria & Albert Museum's 20th century Gallery, as an example of successful industrial production of a 'hand-made' style. Height of mug 3¾ in., moulded mark Churchill / Homespun Stoneware / England. See pages 119 and 131

Colour Plate 34 Churchill Tableware's 1990s Wild Life plaques, in a series which also includes six 'Herring's Hunt' English fox-hunting scenes and four 'Currier & Ives' famous American sailing-ships. The subjects shown are a stag deer *Cervus Elaphus*, a pair of wild duck *Anas Platyrhynchos*, a pair of pheasants *Phasiana*, and a turkey *Meleagridiana*. The series is decorated with Churchill's advanced four-colour underglaze printing process. Diameter of plaque 10 in. See page 132

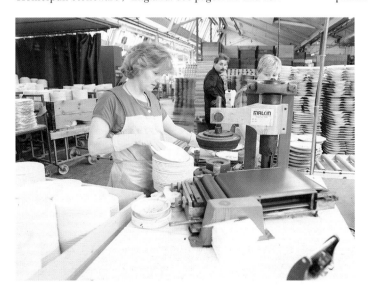

Colour Plate 35 Decorating Broadhurst ware with a Malkin rubber stamping machine. This method was the backbone of Broadhursts' decorated output in the 1950s and 1960s. The stamping technique, although fast (even by today's standards), had a restricted colour palette and poor definition, and was phased out in the early 1980s. See page 110

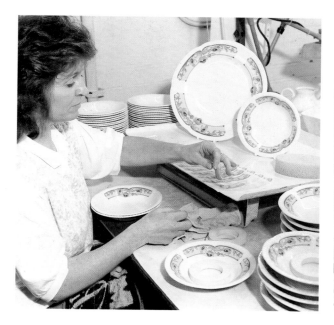

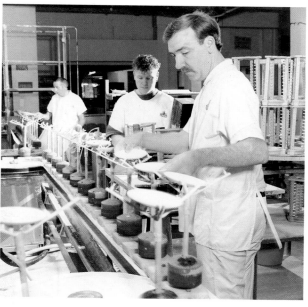

Colour Plate 36 Skilful hand application of Sumatra decoration to Buckingham shape hotelware, in the 1990s. The yellow background burns away in the subsequent firing. Churchill Hotelware, Anchor Works, Longton. See page 136

Colour Plate 37 Unloading saucers from a glaze spraying machine and placing onto glost kiln cranks, seen on the right, ready for glost firing. Churchill Hotelware, Anchor Works, Longton, 1990s. See page 136

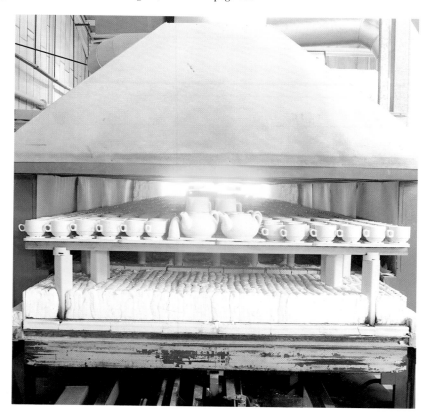

Colour Plate 38 Fast firing vitrified ware in Churchill Hotelware's Anchor kiln, Longton, 1990s. See pages 119 and 136

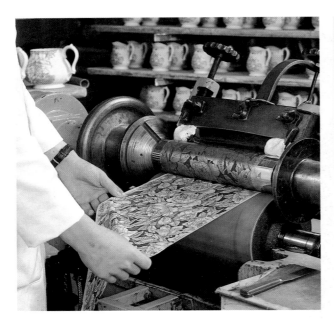

Colour Plate 39 Printing Bermuda pattern tissue with an engraved roller, in the traditional way, at Churchill Tableware's Alexander Works, Cobridge, 1990s. See page 132

Colour Plate 40 Applying printed Bermuda tissue by hand to a Windsor shape teapot, Alexander Works, 1990s. See page 132

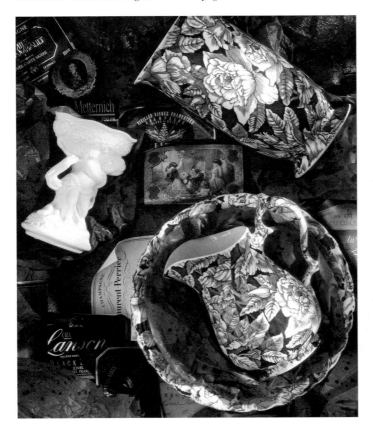

Colour Plate 41 A traditional earthenware ewer and basin, tissue printed with Churchill's Bermuda pattern in cobalt blue, 1990s. See pages 131 and 132

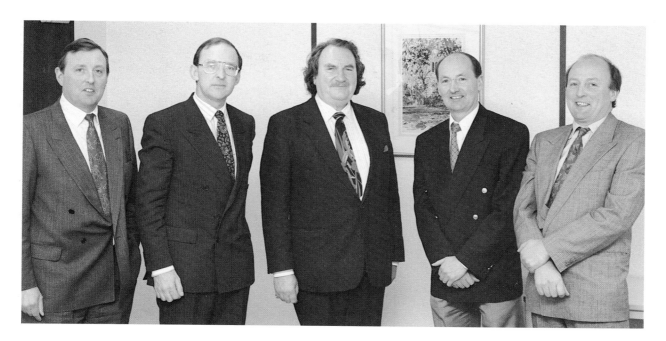

Colour Plate 42 Sir John Harvey Jones, 'Trouble-shooter', seen with Churchill top management on his return visit in 1991. Left to right: Stephen Roper, Churchill Group Chief Executive; Peter Siddall, Non-Executive Chairman; Sir John Harvey Jones; Michael Roper, Group Production Director and Andrew Roper, Managing Director, Tableware. See page 121

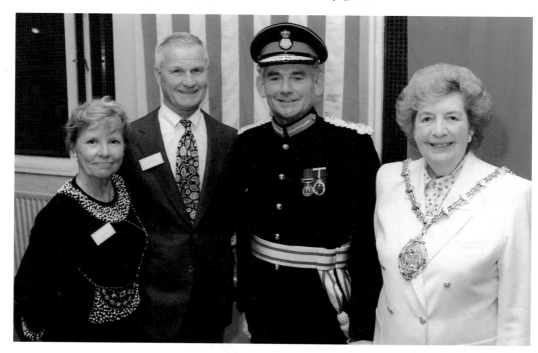

Colour Plate 43 Seen at the presentation to Churchill Tableware of the Queen's Award for Export Achievement in 1993: Joyce and Dale Wright of Heritage Mint of USA, Churchill's principal American customers; the Lord Leiutenant of Staffordshire, Mr. James Hawley and the Lord Mayor of Stoke-on-Trent, Mrs. Marian Beckett. See page 133

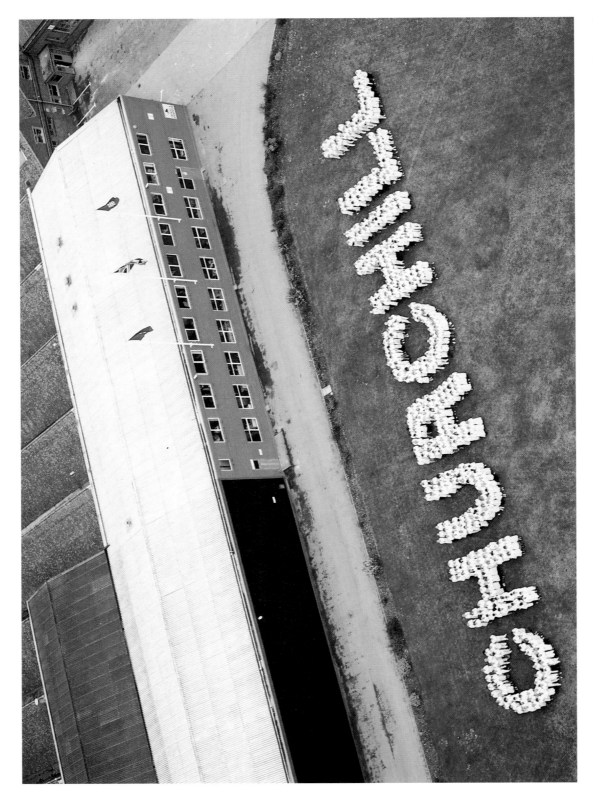

Colour Plate 44 Churchill Tableware staff on the lawn at Marlborough Works, celebrating the Queen's Award for Export Achievement, won by the firm for the second time in 1993. See page 133

John Aynsley was then aged 68, at the peak of his activities as a capitalist and public man of affairs: magistrate, four times Mayor of Longton, and instigator of Longton Park and Cottage Hospital, with interests in coal, brick-making and other industries besides pottery manufacture.[7] In 1903, on his eightieth birthday, John Aynsley demonstrated his personal skill by throwing a number of china loving-cups at Bridgwoods 'for the home trade' i.e., as souvenirs for his family. One of them still exists, beautifully enamelled and gilded, with roses and a view of the Aynsley Memorial Fountain in Longton Park, and with a suitable inscription on the base (Figure 32).[8] When John Aynsley died 7 February 1907, aged 83, Bridgwoods was not named as being owned by him, suggesting that he had already passed the firm on to one of his sons, John Gerrard Aynsley.[9]

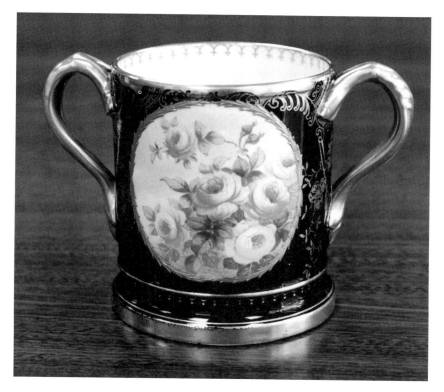

Figure 32 China loving cup, thrown at Bridgwoods' Anchor Pottery on 11 December 1903 by John Aynsley, to mark his eightieth birthday. *Private Collection*

James Aynsley, another son, was reported as 'leaving for New York during the month' (January 1892).[10] Bridgwood's London pattern best quality semi-porcelain tableware was featured in the 1895 catalogue of the American mail order company, Montgomery Ward (Figure 33), handsomely moulded, decorated with pink and canary roses, with bright gold handles, an early connection with the mail order trade.[11] An 1896 advertisement in England shows typical late-Victorian ornate

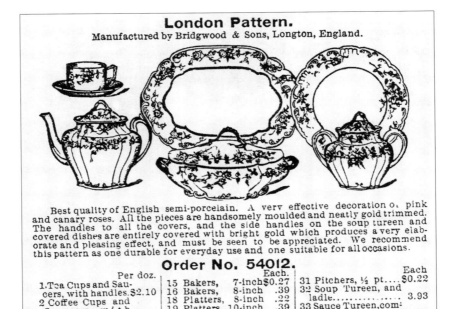

Figure 33 Sampson Bridgwood and Son's London pattern earthenware dinner service featured in an 1895 American mail order catalogue. *Montgomery Ward & Co. Catalogue and Buyer's Guide No. 57, Spring and Summer 1895* (reprinted by Dover Publications, New York, no date) 528

shapes of vases, urns, toilet and table ware, lavishly decorated. A trade 'write-up' of 1897 speaks of imposing shapes, richly enamelled. 'Victoria' shape and 'Florence' pattern are mentioned,[12] and later in the same year 'Gadroon' shape, 'Duke' pattern and a new printed colour 'Congo blue'. Their London agent then was Arthur J. Powell (a surname that recurs in the firm's history), based at 9 Charterhouse Street, E.C.[13]

By 1897 china was again named as a product,[14] confirmed by a china 'thistle' vase to a design registered in 1900 (Colour Plate 10).[15] A 1903 advertisement (Figure 34), offering china and earthenware, stated that Bridgwoods were contractors to leading steamship companies, 'Badges of all kinds a speciality'.[16] Although many potteries offered badged ware at this time, it was a hint of the later specialisation in hotel ware. A most elegant 'Royal' ewer and basin in sweeping *Art Nouveau* shape and decoration was illustrated, confirming that Bridgwoods lived up to their claim to provide the 'latest styles'. Mr. Stockton was their London representative at 9 Bartlett Buildings.

John Aynsley died in 1907, aged 83, but Bridgwoods had probably been supervised if not owned by his son John Gerrard

Aynsley for many years. John Gerrard Aynsley was born in 1855 and married a Miss Walker of Longton, but no connection with the 'Bridgwood' Walker family has been traced. Unlike his flamboyant father, John Gerrard Aynsley was a quiet and unassuming man who held no public office except that of magistrate, but was respected in the trade as 'one of our ablest practical potters and a most level headed man, whom you would always go to for advice on pottery and other matters'. He was also head of the family firm of china manufacturers, John Aynsley and Sons.[17]

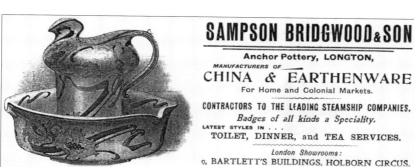

Figure 34 Sampson Bridgwood and Son's 1903 advertisement, illustrating a ewer and basin in contemporary *Art Nouveau* shape. *Pottery Gazette*, 1 July 1903, 637

A William Bailey was a partner in Bridgwoods from 1891 to 1911. Born c.1857, he was a self-made man who was first an oven-man at Broadhursts at Fenton and then a fireman at John Aynsley & Sons' Portland Works, Longton. It seems likely that Aynsleys had found him extremely capable, and promoted him to manage Bridgwoods' Anchor Works when they took it over in 1891. His son, Ernest Bailey, also worked at Bridgwoods, but left in 1909 to start his own business at Park Hall Works. William Bailey also left Bridgwoods, in 1911, and joined his two sons in William Bailey & Sons. He died in 1913 aged 57; Baileys had failed by 1915.[18]

Another member of Bridgwoods' staff was more successful. Mr. F. J. Ray started at Bridgwoods aged 14 and rose to be head warehouseman there, before going to Collingwoods about 1900 and eventually becoming sole proprietor of Jackson and Gosling.[19] Production of both earthenware and china continued, and 1909 and 1910 'write-ups' name Oxford, Cambridge, Trent and Eton shapes, and a Chinese pattern. Mr. A. J. Powell was again appointed London representative.[20]

About 1916, Bridgwoods attempted a technical improvement by installing a Dressler gas-fired tunnel oven for firing glost flat and hollow-ware, one of several installations in the Potteries at that time. Besides the savings in fuel and saggar costs, it was found that placing could be done by young girls, and that the bottom cavities of the kiln trucks could be used for hardening-on and enamel firing whilst glost firing took place above.[21] Like Mr. Hirji at Broadhursts some forty years later, Mr. C. P. Shah from Bombay spent time at Sampson Bridgwoods in 1916 as part of his training at the Clay and Pottery Laboratory at Stoke. He presented a paper to the Ceramic Society on 'The Effect of Magnesian Glazes on Underglaze Colours' and referred to practical working conditions, aerographing, and use of the Dressler kiln.[22]

Bridgwoods did not usually exhibit at fairs, but did so at the British Industries Fair in 1919, showing domestic earthenware in services and fancies, as well as badged ware suitable for hotels and restaurants, and a line of fancies and novelties specially roughened for the use of electroplate mounters.[23] A 1923 advertisement listed their agents in South America, Canada (W. Smith, also agent for Broadhursts), South Africa, Australia and New Zealand, with A. J. Powell at 68–9 Shoe Lane, their London agent; and stressed that Hotel, Ship and Restaurant ware was a speciality.[24]

John Gerrard Aynsley died 30 October 1924 aged 69. He had lived at Blurton House, and was buried at St. Bartholomew's Church, Blurton. Mourners from the Anchor Works included Mr. George Reynolds, general manager of the Anchor works, A. Swift, J. Winkle, H. P. Powell and A. J. Powell. Wreaths were sent by the office staff, by the employees in the china clay department, the glost ovens and biscuit warehouses, the earthenware clay department and the glost warehouses, and by the printers and transferrers, tributes which reflect JGA's 'ready sympathies and generous spirit'. He owned Bridgwoods, and two of his sons, Gerrard and Wilfred, were at the Anchor Works. Another son, Kenneth, was his partner at the Portland Works.[25] John Gerrard Aynsley left £103,871.[26]

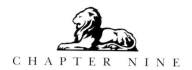

BRIDGWOODS UNDER GERRARD AYNSLEY
1924–1964

Following the death of John Gerrard Aynsley in 1924, owner-ship of the Anchor Works and business passed to his son, Gerrard. Born c.1880, Gerrard Aynsley was apprenticed in the family business of John Aynsley & Sons. He served in the Boer War and in the Great War, and farmed in Australia.[1] Horse riding was his passion: he was a keen member of the North Staffordshire Hunt, and rode each day the six miles to the Anchor Works from his home at The Spot, Hilderstone.[2] The packing place where his horse was stabled is still called 'the barn'.[3]

A private limited company was formed 11 November 1932: Sampson Bridgwood and Son Ltd., registered number 270,153, with capital of £15,000 in £1 shares. The object was to acquire the business of the china and earthenware manufactory carried on by Gerrard Aynsley at Anchor Pottery, Wharf Street, Longton, as 'Sampson Bridgwood and Son'. Gerrard Aynsley, aged about 52, was director for life, and the other directors were Arthur Robert Swift, then about 39, of 40 Princes Road, Hartshill; George William Sterndale Sherratt of Sandhurst, Star & Garter Road, Longton; and Eric George Hendry Powell of Draycott, Beddington, Surrey, a pottery agent. No other directorships were held.[4] The property, including a steam engine, boilerhouses, grinding and crushing places and a smithy, was leased from Gerrard Aynsley from 1932 until 1944.[5]

Both china and earthenware production continued in the inter-war period: ranging from the refined dignity of blue and gold china and pretty lithographed designs and gilding on both china and earthenware, to the brash boldness of contemporary Art Deco design (Colour Plates 11, 12, 17, 18 and 19). As was done a century earlier to the former Rockingham artists, whiteware was supplied to A. E. Gray & Co. Ltd., Hanley, for them to decorate.[6] A patent teapot spout was registered in 1928.[7] Both Harrods and Waring & Gillow were important London customers, and hotelware was an established part of Bridgwoods' range of products (Colour Plates 13, 14 and 15).

At the start of the 1939–45 war, Bridgwoods were members of the Earthenware Manufacturers Association which warned customers that orders would be sent at prices ruling at date of despatch, allowing cancellation if there was an increase of over 15%.[8] Much more stringent measures followed: in 1941, a 'Concentration Scheme' was instituted by the government, and many pottery firms were closed down.[9] Bridgwoods was selected as a 'nucleus' firm to remain in production, and took on the business of another Longton maker, Mayer and Sherratt, a 'concentrated' (closed down) firm. Bridgwoods proposed to:

> concentrate on the manufacture of earthenware to the partial exclusion of china, which will only be supplied by them in connection with their stock china patterns, and that as far as the quota will allow they will endeavour to give satisfaction to their general trade customers in earthenware dinner sets in addition to their stock china patterns.
>
> Regarding hotelware, of which Sampson Bridgwood are one of the leading suppliers, owing to the present heavy demand for this class of ware, this side of their business is receiving particular attention. Like other manufacturers, however, they are finding an acute shortage of workpeople, which makes it impossible to give deliveries as in the past, in consequence of which they find themselves unable to open any new accounts. They would like to assure their old friends, however, that they are doing their utmost to meet their particular demands.

Exceptionally, Bridgwoods advertised in 1942: high-class hotelware, china and earthenware, and their enamelled Indian Tree Design 'known throughout the world' (Colour Plates 15 and 16).[10] A canteen and an air raid shelter were built; and part of the works was used by the Ministry of Supply for storing boxes.[11] Mr. Powell, then living at Porthcawl in South Wales and presumably retired, resigned his directorship in 1944.[12]

As the end of the war approached, the Anchor Works was essentially a typical large potbank, only a little changed since its building ninety years earlier. A plan drawn up by the firm's architects, Wood, Goldstraw and Yorath of Tunstall, shows eight of the 1860s nine bottle ovens and the tall sliphouse chimney still in place, the courtyards still open and the old colliery tramway running across the front of the works. At that time there were three steam engines on the site. The capital of the firm was increased from £15,000 to £25,000 by creating a further 10,000 ordinary £1 shares, and on 8 August 1944, Sampson Bridgwood & Son Ltd., tenants until then, bought the buildings of the Anchor Pottery from Gerrard Aynsley.[13]

At the end of the war, the government set up working parties for various industries, to report on schemes for improvement; and that for the pottery industry included Mr. Yorath.[14] When the report was published 24 May 1946, it commented that the industry's own reconstruction plans were generally well conceived, and included plans for a pottery factory 'as existing' and 'as suggested' (Figures 35 and 36). The works was not named but was in fact Bridgwoods' Anchor Works. The second plan showed a comprehensive scheme of modernisation, adapting the existing buildings for 'flow-line' production and providing a tunnel biscuit kiln on the east of the works and a tunnel glost kiln on the south (railway) side. Only one (china) bottle oven was to be retained. An exercise on tax allowances used Bridgwoods as an example, suggesting that five biscuit bottle ovens rebuilt for £5,000 in 1938 would cost £10,000 to replace in 1948, whereas one continuous biscuit kiln would cost £20,000. A very serious consideration for such an investment is that a tunnel kiln must be used to full capacity for maximum economy, implying constant production and constant sales volume. In fact, most of the five bottle ovens were still standing in 1961.[15] As is so often the case, neither the entire 'Yorath' master plan nor several of the subsequent planned improvements were carried out.

Plans for a Gibbons Dressler glost earthenware kiln and a three-storey decorating shop with a Gibbons gas-fired decorating kiln were drawn up in 1945;[16] and 69 square yards of land was bought from the railway company.[17] The share capital was doubled to £50,000 by the issue of 25,000 £1 5% preference shares. Mr. Neville Nathan Peck of 58 Thistley Hough, Stoke, a chartered accountant, was appointed as director and secretary 11 April 1946;[18] and a mortgage of £20,000 was raised from the officially sponsored Industrial and Commercial Finance Corporation (ICFC) on 24 May.[19]

Bridgwoods' 1946 scheme for enlargement and reconstruction, approved by the Board of Trade and the Factory Inspectorate, included the following items which had already been done out of revenue:

paving the works, conversion of old making shops into a large shop for cup-making with an output of 4,000 dozens per week;

conversion of an old warehouse into a canteen;

a conveyor from the biscuit ovens to the biscuit warehouse;

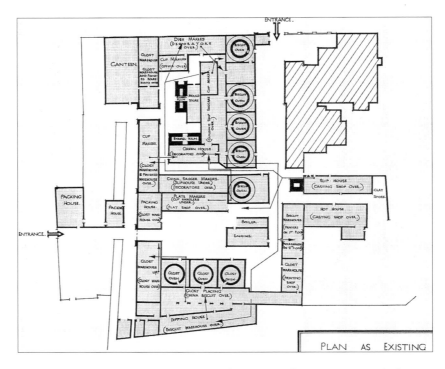

Figure 35 'Plan as Existing' of un-named pottery factory, 1945, included in Board of Trade *Working Party Reports Pottery* (London, 1946); identified as Sampson Bridgwood and Son's Anchor Works. See Figures 24, 25 and 36

new floors in the sorting warehouse and some potters' shops;

new office furniture.

Work then in hand was the rebuilding of a three-storey building with new floors and windows, and strengthening of the fabric; and the rebuilding of some potters' shops. The further proposals included:

a tunnel glost kiln estimated at £7,125;

demolition of existing three glost (bottle) ovens and building a two-storey house for kiln, £7,000;

new sliphouse with new machinery, £5,000;

new dipping house, £3,000;

tunnel enamel kiln, £3,750 (to be built at first floor level, involving strengthening of existing building for £2,125).

With the contemporary difficulties in obtaining labour and materials, and the need to maintain production meanwhile, the work was expected to take two years, for completion by the end of 1947 at a total cost of £28,000.[20] Bridgwoods borrowed

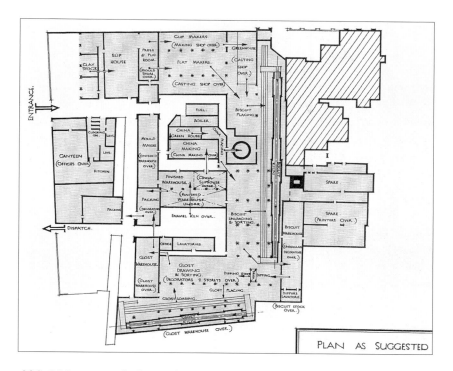

Figure 36 'Plan as Suggested' of un-named pottery factory, 1945, included in Board of Trade *Working Party Reports Pottery* (London, 1946); identified as Sampson Bridgwood and Son's Anchor Works. See Figures 24, 25 and 35

£22,000 toward financing the operation and an additional £13,000 for working capital from the ICFC on 17 September 1946.[21] A plan was made for a Gibbons Dressler open-flame biscuit kiln;[22] and 720 square yards of land at the corner of Goddard Street and Wharf Street (now Bridgewood [*sic*] Street) was bought from the Mossfield Colliery Company.[23]

Further capital was raised in 1947: the share capital was increased to £65,000 by creating 15,000 £1 5% preference shares on 29 October; and £15,000 was borrowed as a second mortgage from ICFC at the end of the year.[24] Mr. A. R. Swift became managing director, and his nephew, Charles Vaughan Prince, was appointed an additional director at the beginning of 1948.[25] A Gibbons Dressler gas-fired kiln, 96 feet long, for decorating earthenware, was installed and in operation by October 1948 (Figure 37).[26] From the 1939–45 war onward, production of china seems to have ceased, although the 'Yorath' plan had provided for retention of one china biscuit oven.[27] In the 1950s, Bridgwoods concentrated on hotel-ware: the 'badged ware' sideline of the 1900s, important because customers returned for replacement, had developed into the main product.[28]

On 22 November 1949, share capital was increased again, to £80,000, by the issue of a further 15,000 £1 5% redeemable preference shares.[29] Existing mortgages to ICFC totalling £35,000 were satisfied by a new mortgage of up to £44,000,

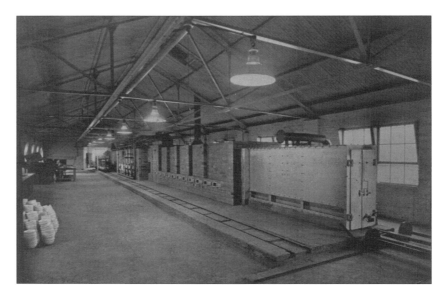

Figure 37 Gibbons Dressler Decorator Kiln, 96′ 0″ long, installed at Sampson Bridgwood and Son's Anchor Works, October 1948. *Pottery Gazette and Glass Trade Review* February 1949, 181

itself finally cleared on the 9 June 1964.[30] New offices, a canteen, a packing house, rebuilding of the upper storey of the casting shop and an electricity sub-station were all planned in 1949.[31] All these post-war changes were paralleled in the industry generally: Staffordshire Potteries, Meakins and Swinnertons built new works; Minton and Maddock made major reconstructions; and less dramatic improvements, like those of Bridgwoods, went on in many of the two hundred or so domestic ware factories.[32]

A new sliphouse was planned in 1950, to be built over the old tramway tunnel; with the machinery designed by Service Engineers on the weight/volume principle. When installed it was considered the most uptodate in the Potteries, shades of the 'best slip kiln in the Potteries', bought by Mrs. Kitty Bridgwood in 1814![33]

Through the 1950s, there were no more plans for improvement or alterations in capital; although the Anchor Mill, sold off in 1890, was re-acquired in 1953.[34] The end of the decade was marked by the loss of the two senior directors: both Mr. Arthur Robert Swift and Mr. Gerrard Aynsley died suddenly in 1959.[35] Aged 79, Mr. Aynsley had probably taken little active part in management in recent years. He was said to be always more interested in rural pursuits, and Mr. Swift had been the active managing director from about 1948. In some ways, the situation resembled that of 1876, when the titular head of the old family firm, Sampson Bridgwood, and his son, Samuel, died within five months of each other. This time, the deaths were even closer together: Mr. Swift died 21 September 1959, and Mr. Aynsley died five weeks later, on 29 October. Dramatically, as in 1876, the business was deprived of its experienced leadership.

Mr. Swift, born at Hartshill about 1893, had worked for George Jones & Sons Ltd. at Stoke, before coming to Bridgwoods in 1919 in charge of the office. His wife had died in 1954 and he later moved to The Leasows, Hilderstone, where he could follow his hobby of keeping dairy cattle. His only daughter, Miss J. E. (Betty) Swift, was a personnel manager for Shell Petroleum Ltd. in South America. Mr. Swift's funeral at Hilderstone Church was attended by many of the works staff.[36]

Gerrard Aynsley, then living at New Trees, Windmill Hill, Meir Heath, died 29 October. His funeral at Carmountside Crematorium was also well attended. Works mourners named included Mr. N. N. Peck, the new managing director, and his fellow director, Mr. Prince; Mr. F. Massey, the works manager and his assistant Mr. G. W. Ellis; Mrs. Bernice Harrison, company secretary; Mrs. M. Talbot, cashier; and over eighty works staff. Mr. Aynsley left a widow, Mrs. Irene Aynsley. They had no children.[37]

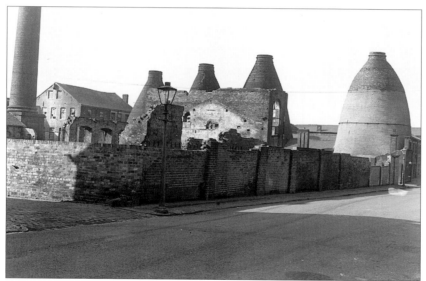

Figure 38 View of Sampson Bridgwood and Son's Anchor Works from Goddard Street in 1961, showing partial demolition of the mill building. *University of Keele, Warrillow Collection of Photographs*: 1383

In 1961, the mill chimney and several of the old bottle ovens were still standing,[38] and several parts of the works presented a derelict appearance (Figure 38).[39] Bridgwoods planned and installed a group of four intermittent electric 'top hat' kilns with their eight bases and 6-ton crane, about 1962. Roller making machinery had been installed before 1965.[40] Capital was reorganised in 1962: the £50,000 of preference shares, all held by ICFC, were redeemed by a mortgage of the same amount to ICFC.[41] In 1965, Sampson Bridgwood and Son Ltd. was sold to James Broadhurst and Sons Ltd. of Portland Pottery, Fenton, but continued to trade under the old name until 1984. Thus was completed a remarkable sequence:

Bridgwoods helped to set up Aynsley at Sutherland Road in 1861
Aynsley helped to set up Broadhursts at Fenton in 1870
Aynsley took over Bridgwoods in 1890
Broadhursts took over Bridgwoods in 1965.

The adjoining Anchor Mill, part of Sampson Bridgwood's 1860 'complete manufactory', had been sold off in 1890, and by 1896 it was occupied by W. Lockett & Co. In the twentieth century it was operated by Potters Mills Ltd. to 1907; then by Stephen Mear until 1916.[42] It was bought back from China and Earthenware Millers Ltd. 3 July 1953.[43]

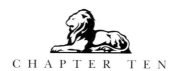

THE GROUP AT FENTON AND LONGTON

—————— 1965–1978 ——————

The acquisition of Bridgwoods was announced in the *Pottery Gazette* of April 1965:[1]

> James Broadhurst and Sons Ltd. have acquired the whole of the ordinary shares in the old established firm of Sampson Bridgwood and Son Ltd. The new directors are Mr. E. P. Roper, Mr. M. J. Roper and Mr. E. S. Roper. It is the intention of the directors to continue to expand the hotelware side of the Sampson Bridgwood business along with the introduction of table lines in general earthenware.

Bridgwoods brought with it a site over three times the size of the Portland Pottery and an old factory with some post-war modernisation, the extra capacity which Broadhursts so badly needed.[2] All the bottle ovens had been cleared; a glost tunnel kiln and four 'top-hat' kilns had been installed; and roller making machinery, new to Broadhursts, was in use. The factory was making mostly hotelware and a little earthenware.[3] Some of Bridgwoods' management stayed on a little while (Mr. Dawson, the works manager and Jack Askey) but Broadhursts' staff quickly took charge.

Michael Roper, director and technical manager, made a six-months sales trip to Canada in 1964, visiting Vancouver, Montreal and Toronto with Mr. Willis of Staffs Sales Ltd., Toronto.[4] Following his visit to Australia in 1964, Stephen Roper took over Broadhursts' sales representation for the Midlands, Northern England, Scotland and Northern Ireland in June of the same year.[5] In 1965, the company's turnover was £300,000, a figure which was to rise five-fold to £1.5 million by 1973.[6] By 1969 sales arrangements of the two firms were combined: British Pottery Ltd. continuing as agents for London and the south of England, whilst Mr. S. C. C. Bond covered the rest of the United Kingdom. Abroad, agents were shared except in New Zealand and South Africa: Australia (Peter Marich), Canada (E. I. Willis), Denmark (Trent Glass), Finland (Armus Kuula), New Zealand (Andrew Hawley for Broadhursts and

Hart for Bridgwoods), Norway (Bjarne Vike), South Africa (Hamlin for Broadhursts and Van Flyment for Bridgwoods) and Sweden (Bo Brandt). At the Portland Pottery, Mr. Morgan continued as decorating manager, Mr. Ray Colclough was works engineer and Mr. R. Evans was secretary.[7]

When Stephen Roper went to Australia in early 1964, he took with him 'four new geometrical patterns'[8] very much in the style of the time, and very much the type of decoration at which Broadhursts could excel. Hand stamping and colouring had long been a speciality, and Broadhursts were well placed to meet the demand for popular earthenware in bright colours on simple shapes. Hand stamping was supplemented by Malkin's stamping machine, developed by Broadhursts and Biltons (Colour Plate 35).[9] Broadhursts found their own in-house designer in Kathie Winkle, who had been a paintress at Portland Pottery since 1950. Her bold, simple designs were popular, and the 'A Kathie Winkle Design' backstamp was as well-known in America as at home (Colour Plates 23 and 24).[10] Besides stamped designs, lithographed patterns from Mattheys, Cappers and Baileys were used.[11]

Advertised designs for the 1965 trade fair were Mikado in a gift box, Rosetta in a carry-home pack, Pomella shown as a two-tier cake stand and Orchard.[12] Other patterns of the period included Geneva, Ascot, Regency, Michelle, Concord and the very successful Rushstone.[13] A 1968 export price list named many more patterns: Corinth, Mandalay, Seattle, Barbados, Corfu, San Tropez, South Seas, Teneriffe, Monte Carlo, Fiji and Lyndhurst. 66-piece Connoisseur 'Rushstone' Sets included matching cutlery and table-linen; 88-piece 'Homemaker' sets included glassware in addition. 'Kofti' pots, for serving both tea and coffee, were offered, and there were 23-piece 'Kofti' sets for South Africa.

The 'Pronto' set, a 12 piece pack of blue or brown Concord pattern, was advertised in 1969 (the pattern bought in from Bennetts).[14] The advertisement clearly spelled out the specialities of the two firms: low-priced tea and dinner earthenware in contemporary patterns from Broadhursts; hotel ware in lithographed and banded designs from Bridgwoods, with a new lower priced range.

The Anchor Works received attention, at last acquiring its tunnel biscuit kiln. A Drayton kiln was planned in detail in 1968 and installed on the east side of the works, where the Gibbons Dressler kiln had been proposed in 1946.[15] The mill site was sold to Stoke-on-Trent City Council for housing; whilst the former Mossfield Colliery coal wharf in Bridgwood Street was bought in 1971 for car parking.[16] In 1973 a 20 cwt. goods and passenger lift was planned, the actual lift being purchased from British Home Stores, Hanley, and brought to Longton by Mr. Colclough on a fork lift truck. In 1974, the boilerhouse was demolished and the factory building extended.[17]

An information sheet of 1973 showed how busy the two factories were: together, the annual turnover was almost £1.5 million. Six hundred and thirty employees produced almost 50,000 dozen pieces a week of white 'Ironstone' earthenware, fired biscuit at 1200°C and glost at 1060°C. Ware was still mostly decorated under-glaze, an advantage for detergent and dishwasher wear resistance. Strong transit cartons, gift packs and polystyrene fittings had replaced the casks, crates, wood-wool and straw of yester-year, and the firm was proud of its reputation for fast and reliable delivery worldwide. Kathie Winkle produced the complete range of designs, frequently changed to keep up-to-date, but three of the most popular patterns (Rushstone, Renaissance and traditional Indian Tree) were 'open stock' and guaranteed to be available for five years.

Broadhursts made a speciality of 'Premium Incentive Offers' and 'Dealer Loader Schemes'; and a mail order catalogue for 1974 shows their share of that important market. Indian Tree, Viscount, a 24-piece Calypso service retailing at £4.75 and a 100-piece Olympus table set for £15.99, including cutlery were all on offer.[18]

Mr. Morgan's notebooks provide details of production at the Portland Pottery through the 1970s.[19] Annual production was:

Year	Dozens	Year	Dozens
1970	818,000	1976	972,000
1971	860,000	1977	894,000
1972	891,000	1978	996,000
1973	938,000	1979	873,000
1974	1,025,000	1980	874,000
1975	880,000	1981	758,000 (46 wks.)

Between 1973 and 1981, the highest weekly production was 75,178 dozens in June 1979. Mr. Morgan recorded wages: a labourer's effective hourly rate, 49 pence an hour in February 1973, increased by 83% to 90 pence an hour in November 1975, and by another 15½% to 104 pence in March 1977, altogether 112% in four years. Incidental information from Mr. Morgan's notebooks is that production of larger dinner plates, 10¼″ diameter, started in 1977.

Wage increases were not the only sign of the times. One side of a broadsheet issued in 1975 reminded customers of the problems shared by all pottery firms in 1974: restricted oil supplies and coal miners on strike, resulted in a one-third reduction in electricity supply. There was also a shortage of timber for packaging, and shortage of shipping space and containers for the export of ware. Despite all these problems, Broadhursts proclaimed with pride that 'we still delivered the goods' and in fact Broadhursts achieved their highest output for the decade, with over 1 million dozen pieces in that year. The other side of the leaflet (Figure 39) told how Broadhursts had installed their own electricity generator in anticipation of the power crisis; and how foresight and persistence had coped with packaging and shipping shortages. On the positive side, Broadhursts had installed three automatic ginnetting (glost-ware cleaning) machines, two new automatic plate-making machines and four new Dekram printing machines. A new 25,000 square feet building for automatic making, a biscuit kiln and under-glaze decorating, had been erected.

The Dekram machines were used for printing Constable designs, reproductions of the famous artist's work, issued to coincide with the 200th anniversary of his birth in 1776.[20] Seven of his best known paintings were reproduced in single-colour engravings, first in blue then in brown, pink or green, so successfully that Broadhursts guaranteed replacements up to seven years. 'Castles' prints, designed by Roy Durber, were also issued, using the Dekram machines, with series to suit individual countries, Danish Castles and Austrian Schlosses amongst them.[21]

Because of Broadhursts' stated aim of keeping up-to-date, there is an amazing range of different patterns in this period, all by Kathie Winkle, including: Calypso, Carousel, Mexico (for the 1970 Olympic Games held there) Michelle (originally for Canada), Olympus, Roulette, Seychelles, Silver Dawn, Vanity Fair, Viscount and Zodiac; with Ashington, Country Lane, Fortuna, Hillside, Moorland, Muscouri and Snowdon in the Sandstone range of matt glaze designs; and Cordoba, Kimberley and October in Ironstone. These were all in bold colours on a black outline, on the standard shapes shown in the 1973 leaflet. Marrakesh, from the Harmony range of Sampson Bridgwood, was also on the same shapes, co-ordinated with enamelled pans, roasting pan and casserole. A printed pattern, 'English Scene', and other designs were sold in 'Copperfield' packs, gleaming copper finish display cartons.[22]

Bridgwoods' range in 1975 was hotel, catering and hospital ware, decorated, banded and white, in addition to domestic ware. Carton packing of hotelware was commenced in 1976.[23] Silver Jubilee mugs were made in 1977, screen-printed on clay.[24]

Mr. Morgan's notebooks show Broadhursts' customers' names and patterns ordered. In six months, between November 1975 and May 1976, he recorded:

Ahlstrom [Sweden]	– Clare, English Scene
A/S Andersen [Sweden]	– English Scene
A/S Oceka	– October
A/S Difa [Denmark]	– Clare
Blundells [U.K.]	– Clare
BMOC [U.K., mail order]	– Tashkent
British Pottery Ltd.	– Viscount
Dansk Supermarket [Denmark]	– Tudor Village
Dargue Hardware	– Clare
David Jones [Australia]	– Clare
Eatons [Canada, mail order]	– Fleur, Tashkent
Elof Hansson [Sweden]	– English Scene, Clare
Frank	– English Scene
Gift Shop	– Rushstone
Goldberg [U.K.]	– Sombrero
Great Universal Stores [U.K., mail order]	– October
Hayward & Warwick [Canada]	– October
Kalle Antilla [Finland]	– Calypso
Kesko [Finland]	– Clare, Indian Tree, Calypso, Tudor Village
Kingsley & Forrester [U.K.]	– Verdi Green
La Loza	– English Scene
Leisure Arts [U.K.]	– Constable, pink
Littlewoods [U.K. mail order]	– Agincourt, Clare, Fleur, Tashkent
McEwan [Australia]	– Constable, pink, Clare
McLaughtons	– Rushstone
Mortier	– English Scene
Nock & Kirby [Australia]	– Lemon Grove, Tashkent
Parkstone Pottery	– Clare
Penney [U.S.A.]	– Clare
RMOC	– Fleur
Roma Pottery	– Verdi Brown
School Meals	– green band and line
SENW Lieshout	– English Scene, Lemon Grove, October
Simpsons Sears [Canada, mail order]	– Agincourt, Lemon Grove, Rushstone, October
SOK [Finland]	– Agincourt
Taska	– Viscount
Tupperware	– English Scene
Zironi [Italy]	– English Scene

The orders which he dealt with at Portland Pottery show the patterns actually in demand then, from the traditional 'band-and-line' for the school meals service to the newly introduced Constable, first mentioned 17 March 1976 for McEwan. The spread of customers' countries show the world-wide range of sales: Sweden, Denmark, Finland and Italy in Europe; further was needed. For Portland Pottery, the old Montrose Works in Fenton was used in the 1970s to pack ware,[25] and for the first time, a works van was employed. A similar arrangement was

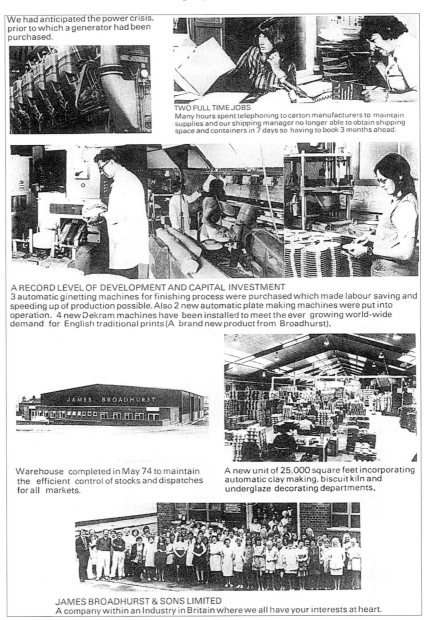

We had anticipated the power crisis, prior to which a generator had been purchased.

TWO FULL TIME JOBS
Many hours spent telephoning to carton manufacturers to maintain supplies and our shipping manager no longer able to obtain shipping space and containers in 7 days so having to book 3 months ahead.

A RECORD LEVEL OF DEVELOPMENT AND CAPITAL INVESTMENT
3 automatic ginetting machines for finishing process were purchased which made labour saving and speeding up of production possible. Also 2 new automatic plate making machines were put into operation. 4 new Dekram machines have been installed to meet the ever growing world-wide demand for English traditional prints (A brand new product from Broadhurst).

Warehouse completed in May 74 to maintain the efficient control of stocks and dispatches for all markets.

A new unit of 25,000 square feet incorporating automatic clay making, biscuit kiln and underglaze decorating departments.

JAMES BROADHURST & SONS LIMITED
A company within an Industry in Britain where we all have your interests at heart.

Figure 39 Publicity Broadsheet issued by James Broadhurst and Sons Ltd. in 1975. *Collection of Mrs. K. Barker*

afield, U.S.A., Canada and Australia are mentioned, besides domestic British customers.

With the continuing expansion of production, more space made for Bridgwoods in May 1974, using a modern building in Sutherland Road, Longton for warehousing, later to become an independent pottery, Crown Trent. Both buildings ceased to be used when new facilities at Sandyford became available about 1980.

A more permanent acquisition was the Crown Clarence Works in King Street, Longton, in 1974 (Figure 40). The Duke of Sutherland had leased the 4,086 square yards site to Thomas

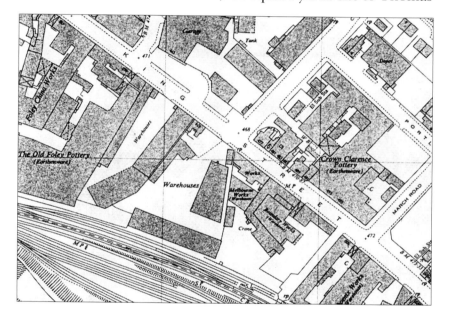

Figure 40
Reproduced from Ordnance Survey 1/2500 Plan SJ 9043, showing Crown Clarence Pottery in 1969

Parker Ratcliffe, Alfred Bailey Jones and John Siddall of Gold Street, Longton, earthenware manufacturers, for 300 years from 25 March 1895, and they built the Clarence Works.[26]

Ratcliffe and Co. had made earthenware there until Charles William Bradley, a Longton outfitter, bought the works in 1921, for ceramic production. Bradleys (Longton) Ltd. was formed in 1922.[27] Mrs. Whitehouse, who worked at Broadhursts between 1931 and 1936, started at Bradleys straight from school, first doing gold stamping and then biscuit banding and lining.[28] A Dressler tunnel kiln was installed about 1936, for both biscuit and glost earthenware.[29] Bradleys went into receivership in 1939[30] and the Cooperative Wholesale Society took over the lease on 16 May 1940, purchasing the site from the Duke of Sutherland on 12 November 1962. C.W.S. Ltd. produced its 'Crown Clarence' earthenware there until 1970.[31] Jon Anton Ltd. ran the works until 22 March 1974 when it was sold to

Toonmain Ltd., a company owned by the Roper brothers, and finally to Churchill China Ltd., a subsidiary of Broadhursts, on 19 January 1976.[32]

Expansion required more managerial staff. Mr. Peter Roper's third son, Andrew David Roper, a chartered accountant, joined the family firm in 1973, and was appointed to the Board on 1 February 1977 as commercial director.[33] Mr. M. S. Robins was sales manager in 1975,[34] and there was a thorough re-organisation of sales in 1976, when the long-standing arrangement with British Pottery Ltd. for the Midlands and Southern England sales ended.[35] Christopher Poole took charge of London and south-east England sales; and Winston Hulme, who had formerly represented Broadhursts in Northern England, took Lancashire, the Midlands and southern and western England. Bob Armstrong's territory was Derbyshire, Notts. and Lincolnshire, north-east England and Scotland, whilst John Seabridge covered the rest of England and hotel sales in Scotland and northern England. Luis da Silva became Export Sales Executive, for North America, Australia, Africa and Europe.[36]

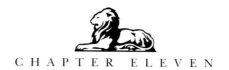

THE GROUP AT LONGTON AND SANDYFORD

—— 1979–1991 ——

In 1979, a new office block and showroom was built at the Anchor Works, Longton, and the Group's commercial operations were centralised there. Mr. Peter Roper was chairman of the Group; Michael Roper was managing director with responsibility for production and technical planning; Stephen Roper was in charge of sales; and Andrew Roper was commercial director supervising Group finance and assisting with sales.[1] Christopher Poole was sales manager, with Mrs. Doreen Amison at Anchor Works and Mrs. T. Brookfield at Portland Pottery in charge of sales administration.[2] The Group had three main firms: Broadhursts, making tableware at Portland Pottery; Bridgwoods producing hotelware at the Anchor Works; and Churchill China, making mugs, figurines and recently horticultural ceramics at the Crown Clarence Works. Wessex Ceramics was formed in 1979, a company importing planters, glassware and cutlery for volume and specialised outlets under the brand name 'Royal Wessex'. The Group was also associated with Stratford Fine Bone China, makers of bone china florals and other giftware, formed in 1978 by John Hinks.[3]

At a time of deep depression, Broadhursts boldly acquired new premises in 1979. Sandyford Works, High Street, Tunstall was bought from Myott-Meakin Ltd., a large modern production unit of 120,000 square feet, standing in 11 acres of ground, some thirteen times the 4,161 square yards of the original Portland Pottery from which the Group had grown.[4] The objectives of this purchase were to develop a self-contained efficient production centre and provide a site for a new 20,000 square feet building to centralise warehousing, packaging and dispatch for Broadhursts, Bridgwoods, Churchill China, Wessex Ceramics and Stratford Bone China. The earlier history of the Sandyford site is to be found in Chapter 12. At the time of purchase, the Sandyford Works was a fully equipped but unstaffed factory. It was initially used for packaging and despatch, and then gradually glazing and decoration of brought-in biscuit ware was commenced, followed by clay manufacture. The sliphouse and kilns were retained, but all other equipment was disposed of. Most of the making machines were brought from the Portland Pottery, but new dryers were installed in the 'clay end'.[5]

As production facilities were developed at Sandyford, the old Portland Pottery was closed down. The company's registered office had already been transferred to Anchor Works in 1978.[6] Mr. Morgan's notes end on 22 November 1981, and that probably signified the end of production at Fenton. The buildings were sold and the old factory demolished, to be replaced by Victoria Court, sheltered accommodation for the elderly, built by The Beth Johnson Housing Association. The post-war Victoria Road building is now a retail supermarket, Kwik Save Discount Store. As a symbol of continuity, the factory chimney foundation stone has been preserved at the Sandyford site. The 'Portland Vase', which had graced the pediment over the entrance, was also preserved at the home of Mr. Peter Roper.[7]

In 1979, the sales force was divided into four territories for home domestic ware sales, with separate representation for hotelware. Abroad, Friedrich Graf Schaffgotsch was the Group's full-time representative for West Germany, Austria and Switzerland, at Parkalle 1, 2 Hamburg 13;[8] and there were local agents in Australia, Belgium, Canada, Denmark, Finland, Greece, the Middle East, New Zealand, South Africa, Spain and Sweden.

Mr. E. Orme, Mr. N. Adlington and Mr. T. Boulton were appointed directors of Churchill China in 1984, continuing to produce mugs and figurines as well as horticultural wares (flower arranging pieces and planters) at the Crown Clarence Works, with Mr. R. Parrish administering sales.[9]

Pattern leaflets and other sales literature, preserved by Mrs. Brookfield at Sandyford, list the innumerable named shapes and patterns of tableware produced by the Group in the 1970s and 1980s, a diversity contributed to by the 'in-house' design department created in 1982 and led by Mr. M. Rogers.[10] Examples almost at random include 'Kaffee' and 'Kombi' (combination tea and dinner) sets for the German market; the seven Constable scenes; Group wares featured in a French mail-order catalogue; Prince Charles' Wedding souvenirs; Edwardian lady and gentleman figurines; as well as the Royal Wessex imported bone china, glassware and cutlery. Bridgwoods' vitrified 'Sampsonite' hotelware body was used for domestic 'Homespun Stoneware', with Briar, Trellis, Romance

Brown and Pink patterns (Colour Plate 33). In 1981 650 staff converted 20 thousand tons of clay into 35 million pieces of ware.[11]

Warehousing developed to keep pace with production. The original 20,000 square feet, built at Sandyford in 1981, had been doubled and then trebled by 1988 to 60,000 feet, capable of loading the largest vehicles inside.[12] Investment was made in improved kilns. In 1984, the Group was the first in Britain to install a Drayton 'once-fired' 'fast-fire' kiln for earthenware mugs and cups, at the Marlborough Works, under the government's Energy Conservation Demonstration Project scheme, reducing firing time from 17 to 4½ hours.[13] In 1987 two more fast-fire kilns were commissioned. A fast-fire kiln was installed at Bridgwoods in 1983 (Colour Plate 38),[14] and a Secomak fast-fire kiln booster was added to an existing DIS electric enamel kiln at the Anchor Works in 1988, increasing firings by four per week, reducing electricity costs by 12% per firing and increasing production capacity by 36%.[15] In 1985, a Drayton fully computerised automatic kiln was installed at the same works for once-fired and biscuit ware.[16] 'Once-fired' ware has become an important part of the industry's ability to produce quality decorated ware for a mass market. Other improvements in equipment included a semi-automatic holloware casting plant installed in 1987, increasing casting capacity by 40%;[17] and a five-colour mug decorating machine which was commissioned in 1990.

A major change to the Group's public image took place in 1984 when the name of Churchill was officially adopted for the whole Group. The name had already been in use within the Group for Churchill China since 1975 and for general publicity.[18] James Broadhurst and Sons Ltd. became Churchill Tableware Ltd., the holding company,[19] and Sampson Bridgwood and Son Ltd. was renamed Churchill Hotelware Ltd.[20] A couchant lion, after the style of the Landseer lions added to the Nelson monument c.1868, was adopted as the Group's logo.[21] The Sandyford Works had already been renamed Marlborough, the family name of Sir Winston Churchill.

Subsidiary companies then were Churchill China, Stratford Bone China, W. Moorcroft, Wessex Ceramics and Staffordshire Crystal. Staffordshire Crystal was started in 1983 by Mr. M. Cartwright, formerly of Webb Corbett, Tutbury, cutting and sandblasting glass to individual orders in premises at the Gladstone Pottery Museum, Longton. Statistics published in November 1984[22] include:

Group turnover £ 13 million, including:
   Staffordshire Crystal turnover £150,000
   Stratford Bone China turnover £700,000
   Wessex Ceramics turnover £1 million
Production of 1 million pieces per week, including:
   Marlborough Works 600,000 pieces per week
780 staff employed by the Group
Over 50% of production exported
Export markets included Germany, USA, Canada, Australia, South Africa and Scandinavia.

The 70% interest in W. Moorcroft of Cobridge was sold in 1986 to a London solicitor, Hugh Edwards, and a London antiques dealer and publisher, Richard Dennis.[23]

Space was again in demand, and by 1985 the Group had bought the old British Anchor Pottery works, opposite the Anchor Works.[24] (A hundred years earlier, Bridgwoods had entertained ambitions to build a works on the eastern half of this site.) British Anchor Pottery Ltd. was formed in 1884[25] to take over the business of J. T. Hudden, in liquidation,[26] who had built the original works by 1875.[27] In the twentieth century the company was owned by Hoods, Birmingham pottery wholesalers,[28] who sold the works to the Alfred Clough Group in the 1970s. The works was closed and sold in 1982 to D. L. Construction, developers,[29] who refurbished the interior for industrial units,[30] leasing space to the Group. Wessex Ceramics, Stratford Bone China[31] and Churchill Housewares, dealing with co-ordinated glassware, cutlery and linen,[32] were all accommodated there.

On the hotelware side, the brand name 'John Maddock Hotelware' was bought from Royal Stafford China, Burslem in 1985;[33] and both high-alumina Sampsonite and Maddock vitrified hotelware were marketed.[34] A new, lighter and thinner Churchill Classic hotelware in more elegant shapes,[35] was recognized by the granting of the Catering Equipment Distributors Association 'best light equipment' award to Churchill's Classic Nocturne pattern, designed in-house and used by Newcastle-upon-Tyne City Council.[36] Large-scale Tableware business continued with the leading mail order companies (Littlewoods, Great Universal Stores and Kays, Marshall Ward, Empire Stores and Texplant (Freeman's)),[37] together with the newer catalogue stores such as Argos.[38] In West Germany, Churchill was the largest selling brand in hypermarkets and mail order catalogues,[39] recognised as early as 1984 by the leading German mail order house's award of the Certificate Otto Versand for excellent cooperation, high quality, punctual delivery and good working relations.[40]

Success in Germany was matched by improved exports in other areas, export values almost doubling from £4.6 million between 1984 and 1986, leading to the coveted Queen's Award for Export Achievement in 1988, with the Group accounting for 8.6% of UK exports in tableware. The patterns at the time were Willow, Trees, Shades, and various traditional landscapes.[41] At the end of the decade, 71% of the Group's production was being exported.[42]

The 1980s saw personnel changes: Miss Olivia Green took over from Mr. Richard Harding as company secretary at Broadhursts 6 March 1981 and from Mr. R. Boulton at Bridgwoods 1 September 1984.[43] Mr. Peter Roper's daughter, Mrs. Diana Swift, ceased to be a director of the Group in 1985[44] and his grandson, another Peter, joined the firm in 1986.[45] Mr. David Fisher was appointed to the board in 1988, taking over as company secretary in 1989.[46] Mr. Dennis Heywood, hotelware chief executive, became a director in July 1989.[47] In that year Mr. Peter Roper senior completed sixty years with the company, and was appointed its first president. Mr. Peter Siddall, a management consultant who had already advised the Group for a number of years, became chairman in his stead,[48] Mr. Stephen Roper was managing director, Mr. Michael Roper production director and Mr. Andrew Roper commercial director. Michael Roper was president of the British Ceramic Manufacturers Federation in 1990.

The Group was divided into three divisions: hotelware, tableware and mugs.[49] Each division operated independently with the three Roper brothers and David Fisher, Group Financial Director, on all three divisional boards. New directors were appointed to the individual boards. For Churchill Tableware at Sandyford, Bernard Burns came from Dorma Ltd. in January 1988 to be sales and marketing director; Edward Orme, production control manager, on the staff for fifteen years, was made manufacturing director; and Melvyn Robins was promoted to be special accounts director.[50] Dennis Heywood, the chief executive, was joined on the Hotelware Board by Thomas Boulton, ten years in hotelware sales, as export sales director. Neil Adlington was confirmed as Chief Executive of Churchill China Mug Division. Both Mr. Orme and Mr. Adlington have been presidents of the British Pottery Managers Association.

In 1989 the Group courageously allowed itself to be publicly scrutinised by Sir John Harvey Jones, former head of ICI, before BBC television cameras, to make one of six 'Troubleshooter' programmes (Colour Plate 42).[51] Sir John's mission was to examine the Group and recommend ways of increasing the return on capital employed. He found possibilities of further automation, a lack of design investment and under-use of senior management (the new directors). Sir John concentrated on tableware production and sales, and his principal recommendation was to 'Make the Dogs Bark' (the title given to the subsequent BBC2 1 May 1990 television programme): allow the new managers enough space to show their capabilities, whilst top management stood back and dealt with long-term development and strategy, setting objectives and insisting on achievement.[52]

Exposure to the candid eyes of Sir John and the television cameras stimulated Churchill: less than a year after their visit, tableware production was profitably up from 85% to full capacity, and the new up-market Mille Fleurs design had been successfully launched. Investment in design had markedly increased[53] and Edward Orme's proposals for cost-saving further automation were being implemented.[54] The Group's first consumer advertising campaign was launched in the autumn of 1990.[55] Over the decade from 1981, production had increased by almost fifty per-cent, from 35 to 51 million pieces of ware a year.[56]

By the end of 1991 Group turnover was £30m. Total exports were 60% of production, with major customers such as Heritage Mint Limited in the USA, and Ikea worldwide. Other important export markets included Germany, France, Spain, Sweden and Australia, where Churchill had long-standing agents such as Friedrich Schaffgotsch, Roger Scherpereel, Russell Willmoth, Elof Hansson and Peter Williams.

Small but consistent sales were still being made to Greece and Israel, where Demetriades and Ravitz have handled Churchill products for many years. The Hotelware Division in particular flourished on its policy of offering a range of patterns and ex-stock service considered to be second to none in the industry, supported throughout the UK by an army of distributors both small and large.[57]

Peter Roper senior, who had joined his father in the company in 1928, resurrected it after the 1939–45 war and overseen its development to a Group employing over a thousand people, died aged 79 on 25 January 1991.[58]

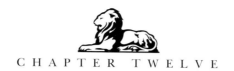

CHAPTER TWELVE

THE ACQUISITION OF
MYOTT MEAKIN IN 1991

The Churchill Group acquired the former Myott Meakin factory, the Alexander Works, Cobridge, in June 1991, for £1.5 million.[1] Besides the additional factory space, making equipment, patterns and customers, the Group also acquired a site with a pottery history reaching back almost two hundred years. The business was bought from the administrators of the failed Myott Meakin concern, a firm whose predecessors had been on the site for some ninety years.

The absence of title deeds makes the early history of the site less than certain, but the site was owned in the late eighteenth century by the Bucknall family.[2] They had been potters and carriers in Cobridge since about 1710,[3] making first 'mottled ware', later white salt-glazed stoneware, and then cream-coloured ware;[4] and also carrying with horse-drawn waggons between Manchester, North Staffordshire, Birmingham and Coventry.[5] Thomas Sherwin was their tenant on the 'Alexander' site in 1783 and William Mayer from 1787 to 1792.[6] There is no evidence that either was a potter at those dates, so they may have been farmers renting the land, or occupants of houses on the site. Ralph Bucknall had the site in 1794 and 1795,[7] and he was a potter at that time.[8] The tenants from about 1800 were also potters: John Blackwell who died 27 August 1804[9] and Andrew Blackwell who had died by 1808.[10]

Robert Bucknall, the owner in 1808, took a Mr. James Stevenson as a partner to run the works,[11] and it is said that the 'Cobridge Works' (fore-runner of the Alexander Works) were erected then, at a time when there was a temporary lull in the Napoleonic Wars.[12] They were certainly built by 30 December 1811, when Waterloo Road and Hope Street, Hanley, were planned.[13]

Charles Stevenson and Sons had been potters in Burslem as early as 1784,[14] and Ralph, James and Andrew Stevenson (presumably the 'sons') were pottery merchants in Glasgow in 1799.[15] James Stevenson, Bucknall's first partner,[16] died in 1813 aged thirty-eight.[17] By 1811 Andrew Stevenson was in the partnership: a letter of that year from him, in the Wedgwood archive[18] inquiring about 'boiled plaster', is signed on his behalf by 'J. Clews'. Ralph and James Clews were to be tenants of the same works from 1828 to 1834.

The partnership between Andrew Stevenson and Robert Bucknall ended 25 August 1816,[19] and Andrew Stevenson continued the business alone until 1827. Like many of his fellow potters, he made blue-printed earthenware ('English Views' and 'American Views' patterns are known)[20] using the mark of 'Stevenson' over a three-masted ship,[21] suggestive of his large export trade. Other designs used include the 'Medallion Portraits' showing Jefferson, Lafayette, Washington and Clinton, above a sheep shearing scene, an obvious American export engraving.[22] Andrew Stevenson went out of business about 1827,[23] and died in Westchester, New York on 28 February 1855.[24]

By 1828, Andrew Stevenson had become the owner of the Cobridge Works, and his tenants were Ralph and James Clews,[25] James being his former clerk of 1811. They were sons of John Clews of Newcastle, who was first a hatter[26] and then also a maltster.[27] Ralph was baptised 12 March 1788 and James 2 September 1790.[28] John Clews was mayor of Newcastle in 1809,[29] and died 31 October 1819,[30] in the year when his son Ralph was also mayor.[31]

James Clews obviously gained pottery experience as Andrew Stevenson's clerk in 1811; by 1813 he and his brother Ralph are said to have started in business for themselves at Bleak Hill Works, Cobridge, owned by Warburtons.[32] They made cream-colour and other wares, and also possibly china.[33] In 1817 the two brothers rented a second works, the twentieth-century 'Globe' works, also at Cobridge.[34] Their father's will in 1819 revealed that they owed him £938, evidence that he had helped to finance their ventures.[35] Like Andrew Stevenson, they traded with the United States,[36] and like him, produced a Lafayette pattern in 1825.[37]

The Clews brothers were bankrupt for £13,419 in 1827,[38] and gave up their Bleak Hill Works.[39] Remarkably, they then leased the larger Cobridge (Alexander) Works, and continued their large American trade. Printed patterns such as 'Tuscan Rose', 'Genovese', 'Domestic Scenes', the 'Dr. Syntax' series, 'Indian Sport' and 'Millenium' were turned out in enormous quantities, in blue and other colours.[40] In 1830, the Clews brothers were alleged to be 'truck-masters', paying their workers in goods, not money. Besides being potters, they also owned the American and Washington Hotel in Waterloo Road, and operated the Jackfield Colliery at Burslem, a brewery at Shelton and a flint mill at Tunstall. Ralph Clews lived at Marsh Street, Newcastle, with a maltster's business, whilst James Clews farmed at Hilderstone and Draycott. All of these properties were up for sale when the Clews brothers were again bankrupt in 1834.[41]

James Clews went to the United States, and took thirty-six potters with him to found the Indiana Pottery Company at Louisville, Kentucky.[42] He was there until 1842, then moved to New York, but was back at Hilderstone by 1849. He died 7 July 1861 aged seventy. Both Clews' flint mill and their colliery at Jackfield seem to have been bought by their brother-in-law, John Bennett of Dimsdale. Ralph Clews continued to manage them until the late 1850s,[43] and was also in business as a maltster in Newcastle until 1863.[44]

From the 1790s, the master potters on the Cobridge works site had been inter-connected: Bucknalls, Blackwells, Stevensons and Clews; but there was a clean break in control from 1834 to 1837 when the works stood empty, a time of strife in the pottery industry, culminating in a two-months-long lock-out at the end of 1836. Despite the gap and troubles, it seems likely that many of the Clews employees would gladly resume work at the same benches with the new masters.

The Cobridge Works were re-opened in 1837 by Noah Robinson and John Wood, moving from a works at Howard Place, Shelton. They took their traveller, William Brownfield, into partnership, the start of a business that was to last for over sixty years.[45] Robinson died in the same year, and his widow withdrew in 1841, leaving Wood and Brownfield as owners.[46] They made earthenware and ironstone tableware.[47] In 1846 they took over the New Hall Mill, now within the Century Oils complex, to grind their own materials.[48] Wood retired in 1850, leaving William Brownfield as the sole owner.[49]

Brownfield was an energetic and ambitious businessman, chief bailiff of Hanley in 1844[50] and mayor in 1858,[51] a friend of John Ridgway, and a director of the North Staffordshire Railway Company.[52] It was he who gave the fountain in Fountain Square, Hanley.[53]

William Brownfield added stoneware and parian to his production,[54] and showed at exhibitions in 1862, 1867 and 1871.[55] In that year, he decided to make bone china, and built a new china works on the south of Crane Street.[56] Also in 1871, Brownfield took his eldest son William into partnership[57] and hired Louis Jahn from Minton to be his art director.[58] William Brownfield died in 1873, aged only 61, leaving a widow and three young sons to continue the business.[59] By then he was a magistrate and Deputy Lieutenant for the county, living at Barlaston Hall.[60]

Louis Jahn proposed that the firm should make the biggest china vase ever, to put Brownfields on the map as china makers.[61] The vase was modelled by a French sculptor, Albert Carrier Belleuse, to be eleven feet high when fired, made of white and celadon green bone china.[62] An oven was reconstructed to provide an even heat, and slip was piped into the oven to cast the vase.[63] During firing it was supported with brickwork. After great difficulties, it was finally produced in 1884, and put on show, first at the works and then at the Crystal Palace. The great vase was damaged whilst being shipped to the Paris exhibition in 1889,[64] and destroyed in a fire at the works in 1894.[65]

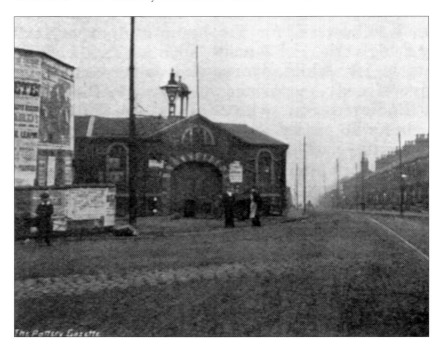

Figure 41 The main entrance to the Cobridge Works, at the junction of Blackwell's Row (now Douglas Street) and Waterloo Road, before demolition in 1900. *Pottery Gazette*, 2 May 1927, 829

During the 1880s two of the brothers left the business, William to go to Australia[66] and Douglas to run the New Hall Mill,[67] leaving Arthur Brownfield in sole control. He invented a sparkling aventurine glaze,[68] and had eight ovens adapted to Minton's Patent, with lower and upper chambers.[69] By 1891 Arthur Brownfield employed six hundred staff with a turnover of £30,000 a year.[70] In 1892 he converted the business into a workers' co-operative,[71] but it failed by 1897.[72] A limited company, Brownfield Pottery Ltd., ran the firm until 1900, when it was wound up.[73] That ended sixty-three years of Brownfield involvement in the works. Again, as in 1834, there was a clean break in management, but no doubt many of the workers resumed employment with the two new firms who took over the works.

The works had originally extended to Waterloo Road (Figure 41), but most or all of the 1808 buildings were demolished in 1901, and three rows of houses, on Waterloo Road, Douglas Street and Arthur Street (now Crane Street) were built.[74] The two streets were named after the Brownfield brothers. The rest of the works was offered for auction in two lots.[75]

The china works, Lot 2, were re-opened in April 1902 as the Upper Hanley Pottery Co. Ltd.'s Brownfield Works.[76] The owner was Mr. J. Hollinshead, who appears to have been previously in a works in Town Road, Hanley, as Stonier and Hollinshead,[77] and had formerly dealt solely with America.[78] The firm continued in name until at least 1912,[79] but from 1906 it was part of the Grimwade syndicate, which also manufactured at the Stoke, Winton and Elgin Potteries.[80]

In 1920, Mr. J. Hollinshead was a director of Grimwades, in charge of the Upper Hanley Pottery's Brownfield Works.[81] By 1922, the factory had been extended east to the railway cutting and west to the back of the houses on Waterloo Road (demolished in the 1980s).[82] Grimwades still owned it in May, 1925, when they were prosecuted for smoke nuisance there,[83] but by December 1927 they no longer claimed ownership in their advertisements.[84]

At some time after 1926, the Brownfield works was absorbed by Myott, Son and Co., who had taken Lot 1, the earthenware works, in June 1902.[85] Ashley Myott, son of a Newcastle draper,[86] was apprenticed to George Thomas Mountford at the Alexander Works, Wolfe Street, Stoke in 1895.[87] Mr. Mountford died in 1897 and Ashley Myott, aged nineteen, took over the works, so successfully that he was able to move to Brownfield's Cobridge Works in 1902. The young Ashley Myott had started a business in 1897 that was to endure, under his own control, for over sixty years.

Publicity spelt out that increasing trade had compelled the erection of an entirely new five-oven works at Cobridge, launched in August 1902 as 'the new Premier Factory of the Potteries'.[88] Its new name was the Alexander Works, a title taken from Myotts' former works in Stoke-upon-Trent. By 1922, the works had been extended eastward over the railway tunnel.[89]

Ashley Myott was Vice-Chairman of the British Pottery Manufacturers Federation in 1930, and took an active part in the Wedgwood Bi-Centenary Celebrations.[90] A keen supporter of Stoke City Football Club, he presided over the successful 'Stanley Matthews must not go' public meeting at Stoke Town Hall, in 1938.[91]

In 1937, the firm made ironstone, white granite, and semi-porcelain tableware, decorated with lithographs and hand-painting, for both home and foreign markets (Colour Plate 20).[92] At the British Industries Fair that year they showed a special light-weight teaset with a turned foot, and a dual purpose vegetable dish, the cover decorated inside and out so that it could be used as a fruit bowl.[93]

Myotts continued business as a nucleus firm during the 1939–45 war, with Adderleys of Daisy Bank, Longton, concentrated upon them, although no Adderley wares were made.[94] Still involved in public affairs, Ashley Myott was a member of the Pottery Working Party set up to advise on reconstruction of the industry in 1946.[95] For his work as chairman of various wages and conciliation committees in the pottery industry, he was awarded the C.B.E. in 1953.[96] At that period, his firm, a limited company since 1949,[97] exported two-thirds of its production. After the war, Myotts made art wares for themselves and also for Marcel Goldscheider, an Austrian refugee figure modeller, but this ceased in 1950 in view of reconstruction of the works.[98]

At the end of 1960, the board of directors of Myott, Son and Co. Ltd. was reconstituted. Sydney Myott, brother of Ashley Myott; Geoffrey Myott, son of Ashley; and C. W. Noake resigned; John Sadler and E. J. Sadler, both of Sadlers, Burslem, became Chairman and Vice-Chairman respectively; and Mr. S. Brooke and Mr. R. C. Hodgkinson became joint managing directors. Ashley Myott, then aged eighty-one, continued as a consultant director. The two firms had for many years shared North American sales agents.[99] Mr. B. J. Vickers became chief engineer in 1965 and Mr. J. G. Glover joined in 1967 as works manager; both became directors in 1969.[100]

In October 1969 an offer by the Interpace Corporation of Parsippany, New Jersey, U.S.A., of £400,000 for the Myott business was accepted by Edward J. Sadler, chairman, and Fred Brookes, managing director. At that date, Myotts employed over five hundred staff, two-thirds of output was still going for export, and major extensions to the works had been made. Interpace was the largest tableware manufacturer in U.S.A., employing over six thousand staff.[101] Ashley Myott died three months later, on 5 January 1970, aged ninety-one.[102] That ended the twentieth century interest of a Newcastle business family in the Cobridge site, similar to that of the Clews family in the previous century.

Seven years later, in 1976, Myott, Son and Co. Ltd. was merged with Alfred Meakin (Tunstall) Ltd., also owned by Interpace, to become Myott-Meakin Ltd.[103] A 1976 announcement of a £1.5 million export order to New Orleans included confirmation that the firm still exported much of its production – 60% to U.S.A. alone, besides Canada and Germany.[104]

Myott-Meakin was in financial difficulties in January 1980. It was proposed to make seven hundred of the nine hundred staff redundant, and the Tunstall factories were probably closed at that time. In 1982, a new management, including an accountant, Neil Gough, and Stanley Jackson, sales director since 1978, took over the Alexander Works and some two hundred workers.[105] Four shapes were to be made: Chelsea, Regent, Cambridge and Perfection, 90% of production being exported. In the mid-eighties, bone china made in Pakistan with the Myott-Meakin back-stamp,[106] and matching table accessories (glass, cutlery, linen) were marketed.[107]

The firm was confident enough in 1988 to install expensive Dorst dust-pressing equipment for flat-making,[108] but a year later it was only saved from closure by a takeover by Melton Modes of Nottingham,[109] becoming Myott Meakin Staffordshire Ltd. In early 1991 the management bought out Melton Modes, but in March the firm was put into receivership and offered for sale in April.[110] At that time the firm had a 4.5 acre leasehold site, 230 employees and an annual turnover of £6.5 million.[111]

The Churchill Group bought Myott Meakin from the receivers in June 1991.[112] In doing so, the Group bought the descendant of the firm from which it had bought its modern Marlborough Works at Sandyford in 1979. The Sandyford site had been bought and the original modern factory built by Alfred Meakin (Tunstall) Ltd., the firm linked with Myotts in 1976.

The Alfred Meakin concern had a history going back to Longton in 1845, when James Meakin, of farming stock, took on the new Newtown Works in Uttoxeter Road, Longton for five years[113] before moving to Hanley. Two sons, James and George Meakin, built up a huge business in Hanley, whilst another son, Alfred, opened the Victoria and Albert Works in Tunstall in 1874. Alfred Meakin died in 1904,[114] and was succeeded by his son, Alfred John, who died only four years later, aged thirty-three.[115] Alfred John Meakin's uncle, Robert Johnson, bought the business for £100,000 in 1908 for his son, Stuart Johnson.[116] He ran the firm until at least 1969,[117] jointly with his son Reginald S. Johnson from about 1952.[118]

By 1949 they had proposed building a new works opposite their Newfield Pottery.[119] They had bought the 46 acre Holly Wall Farm, once part of the Keele Estate, and another farm from the Williamson estate by 1950, a house and land at Broadfield in 1956, and possibly the old Boston Pottery site, making some one hundred and fifty acres in all.[120] Part of their new works on this site was opened in 1957,[121] for underglaze decorating and glazing, with a huge glost kiln. In 1966 a new sliphouse was built, and making and biscuit firing was in operation, using Service cup-making machines and an open hearth Gibbons gas-fired kiln.[122] This was the genesis of the Churchill Group's Marlborough Works.

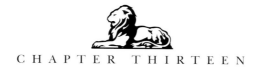

CHAPTER THIRTEEN

CHURCHILL TODAY

In October 1992, the Group was registered as a public limited company, Churchill China PLC, ready for flotation on the Stock Market at an appropriate time.[1] The operating companies were re-formed into two divisions: *Tableware*, operating from Marlborough, Alexander and Crown Clarence Works; and *Hotelware* at the Anchor Pottery.[2] The 1970s Churchill China *Ltd.*, the Group's subsidiary running the Crown Clarence Works, was renamed Crown Clarence Ltd.[3]

Andrew Roper is now Managing Director of Churchill Tableware,[4] leading the move into the 'middle market', which retails dinner sets between £30 and £100, a market principally supplied by Denby, Johnson Brothers, Poole and Portmeirion.[5] Churchill currently ranks fourth amongst British tableware suppliers, after Doulton, Wedgwood and Staffordshire Tableware; the four firms together holding over 50% of sales in the United Kingdom.[6] The 'up-market' strategy will strengthen Churchill's position. Harrods, the prestigious London store (supplied by Bridgwoods in the 1920s, see Chapter 9 and Colour Plates 13 and 15), has become a customer for Tableware's Bermuda (Colour Plate 41), Gingham Patchwork and Tuscany patterns.

Building on Churchill's sound base of reliable products, good packaging and quick, dependable delivery, the move calls for more variety of shapes, more adventurous patterns and more attractive packaging, qualities urged upon the Group by Sir John Harvey Jones in 1989.[7] Good design is not new to Churchill – one of its 1980 'Stonecast' mugs is now on permanent display in the Victoria & Albert Museum's 20th Century Gallery (Colour Plate 33).[8] On a return visit in 1991, Sir John found more automation, more employees and more operating profit. Sales were up 35% on 1989, and operating profit had risen from 2% to 9%, in the midst of the worst trade depression since 1931.[9]

Successful entry to the middle market calls for a change of philosophy, from 'how cheap can you make it?' to 'what do the customers want?'. The answers come from market research, leading to more shapes, more elaborate designs and better packs. In production terms, this means smaller runs and complex stock-holding; assisted by the use of computers and information technology.[10]

The Tableware management team under Andrew Roper includes

Simon Bell, sales and marketing director
Paul Deighton, production director
David Garnett, information technology director
Melvyn Robins, key accounts director
Mary Tavener, financial director

supported by David Taylor, company secretary and Group financial director.[11]

The sales and marketing director, Simon Bell, controls five teams: design, quality (process control and glost selection), sales both UK and worldwide, and a consultant for trade shows and marketing, backed up by good administration.[12] Wendy Morton took sole charge of marketing in 1992, to intensify market research, including trends in household decoration.[13] In March 1993, Candida Kelsall moved from design manager to UK sales executive and public relations manager,[14] and Pam Woodhouse from public relations and marketing to USA sales executive.[15] Karen Tye became design manager in May, and Kate Eardley was appointed a designer.[16] Mrs. Barker (Kathie Winkle), designer from the 1950s to the 1970s, retired in autumn 1992;[17] and Bernard Burns left the group in June 1993.[18]

Designs are now launched for specific markets – examples are Tamarind and Tuscany in bold colours to suit contemporary fashion, and Briar Rose for the bridal market – whilst other designs will be for specific large customers, with guaranteed sales (Colour Plates 30, 31 and 32). Wall plaques reproducing nineteenth century coloured prints have been economically achieved with Churchill's new four-colour printing technique, for Heritage Mint, USA (Colour Plate 34); and traditional tissue printing is used for 'English-style' giftware.[19] A striking 'Stars' range, 'gold' stars on a rich blue background, has been launched for an American buyer, Pier I Imports.[20]

The 1994 range includes the traditional Bermuda design, produced at the Alexander Works, using the old technique of tissue printing (Colour Plates 39, 40 and 41). Bermuda is a faithful reproduction of an archive design.[21] The range has also been segmented into two distinct brand areas: with the Churchill backstamp to attack the middle market, and the Royal Wessex mark for the more competitive mass market.[22]

Almost half the designs in the Tableware catalogue are new, a measure of the pace of design demand. Market demands vary: at home there is a change from formal to casual dining, leading to loose stock and individual items rather than sets, and jumbo cups, pasta bowls and extra large plates.[23] Europe looks for traditional patterns, and Scandinavia, South Africa, Australia and USA respond to multi-colour traditional floral designs.[24] Packaging too, has changed, from corporate identity, emphasising the make, to colour co-ordination to attract the customer.[25] A novel offer is the packaging of tableware in re-usable food containers.[26]

Churchill exhibits at major trade shows: in Britain the NEC in spring,[27] Exclusively Housewares at Olympia in September;[28] abroad, Frankfurt, Paris, and Madrid in Europe; and New York and Chicago in USA.[29] Offices are maintained in Hamburg and Barcelona.

Churchill has maintained a strong presence in the USA over the last ten years through the Wright family, trading as Heritage Mint (Colour Plate 43). Record sales have been achieved, including designs such as Blue Willow (Colour Plates 25 and 26). Country Life and Briar Rose. Churchill's production skills, added to Heritage Mint's design and marketing flare, represent a formidable force.[30]

Despite worldwide competition, Churchill is currently the largest supplier to Ikea, the international store chain. Most of the designs supplied to Ikea are exclusive, and have helped Churchill to counter the extremely low prices offered by Far Eastern producers, who enjoy far lower wage costs.

The same unfair competition has been felt in Europe, causing an estimated loss of up to 1,000 jobs per annum in the European pottery industry.[31] Importers from China into the Common Market are able to evade British, German and Italian quota restrictions by importing through Denmark and Holland, which have no home industry to defend, and set no quotas.

Churchill has responded vigorously. 75% of Churchill Tableware's production was exported in 1993, and that division won the coveted Queen's Award for Export Achievement for a second time (Colour Plates 43 and 44), with exports of over £100 million in the previous five years to fifty countries, USA, Spain, France and Germany being the most significant export markets.[32] Southern Europe, South America and Japan are seen as potential new market areas.[33]

Extensive automation over the past twelve years has provided a sound base for sales expansion. Four-colour printing, introduced for mass market products, has proved as good as lithography, and has enabled new design avenues to be explored, breaking away from traditional border/centre designs.[34] Tableware and Hotelware factories are all progressing towards attaining the quality assurance certificates, British Standard 5750 and ISO (International Standards Organisation) 9000.[35] Currently, a major aim is to improve the flow of work by reducing delays between processes.[36] As a contribution toward staff health, all three factories are now 'No smoking' areas.[37]

The Tableware Division has eight hundred employees,[38] and operates from three factories: Marlborough Works, Tunstall; Alexander Works, Cobridge and Crown Clarence Works, Longton. Marlborough, the largest and most modern plant, has 10,656 square metres of highly mechanized space. It is equipped with handle de-seaming machines, in-line spray glazing machines, four-colour silk screen decorating machines, an automated lithographic transfer application machine and a fast fire tunnel kiln which takes only four hours for 'once-fired' ware. Various automated transfer devices are installed to link the production processes.[39]

The Alexander Works, a recent acquisition of the group, also has in-line spray glazing and four-colour decorating machines, and, most notably, a state-of-the-art Dorst isostatic press, within its 8,003 square metres.[40] This three-head press, with its team of skilled operators, runs continuously. It produces 12,000 dozen pieces of flatware per week, pressing granules prepared by ECC International at Cliff Vale from a special body produced by part-owned Furlong Mills. Plates and dishes are produced, ready for biscuit firing without further drying. As can be appreciated from its chequered history (Chapter 12), the Alexander Works needs, and is receiving, extensive renovation inside and out, to make it fit for modern production methods.[41] A factory shop has been opened at the Alexander Works.

The Crown Clarence Works, with 2,994 square metres of production space, also has appropriate modern equipment: handle de-seaming machines, five colour on-glaze mug decorating machines and automated transfer devices for cup production.[42] It specialises in mug, cup and some biscuit castware production. Tableware production passes through 11,108 square metres of warehouse floor area *en route* to customers world-wide.[43]

Hotelware has also widened its horizons, both in geography and in quality. Agents and distributors cover the entire world, with Europe regarded as part of the home market.[44] Portugese, Spanish, French, Italian and German linguists are employed so that foreign customers are answered in their own language. Lap-top computers linking to a data-base are used by representatives, and a free phone line is provided for Spanish customers.[45]

New markets opened up in 1993 include Germany, Holland, Nigeria, Portugal, USA and Russia.[46]

Under Dennis Heywood, managing director, Alan Miles, sales and marketing director and David Fisher, finance director, an export drive to over forty countries has increased hotelware exports seven-fold since 1989, to 30% of production.[47] They have developed an extremely professional sales team and a global distributor network, offering the same service as in Britain. In January 1993, Christine Harrison, formerly export sales coordinator, was appointed UK sales manager and Jacky Bowen, a fluent French speaker, was appointed export sales manager.[48]

Churchill has the most comprehensive UK distributor network of any British hotelware manufacturer, serviced by a first-rate stock and delivery team. Major UK customers include Autobar of Hemel Hempstead, John Deas in Glasgow, Institutional Supplies at Leeds, Lockhart Catering Equipment at Reading, Ritchie of Stoke, Stephensons of Stockport, V & S Catering Supplies in London, and Walley Tableware in Grays, Essex.[49] In turn, their customers include such well-known names as Forte Hotels, Bass Breweries, P & O and Harry Ramsden. Packing and despatch is from the 4,342 square metres of the former British Anchor Works, adjoining Anchor Pottery, the production unit.[50] In April 1993, a single container with £58,000 of Hotelware was packed and despatched to Spain, the highest value in one package – so far.[51] Churchill Hotelware recently supplied 13,000 pieces of Buckingham pattern for the five P & O passenger ships sailing between Dover and Calais, continuing Bridgwoods' long tradition as 'Contractors to the leading Steamship Companies'.[52]

The 'Churchill Distributor Charter' guarantees UK catering market supply solely through distributors, with ex-stock supply of all items from the top twenty best selling patterns, place-settings from the next twelve, and a maximum four-week delivery of all other items. A five-year life is guaranteed for the top twenty patterns, and five years' notice of discontinuation for any pattern. Distributors are actively involved in canvassing market needs, and supported through staff training and sales publicity.

Several different bodies are produced. Super Vitrified ware, high-fired and made with added alumina for strength, is supplied in some fifty patterns. Many of them are of course traditional catering styles – Greek Key, Indian Tree, Westminster (Colour Plate 27) – but others, such as Chelsea, Kensington and Nocturne, reflect contemporary fashion.[53] Super Vitrified Cookware is supplied in patterns to match other wares, its thermal shock resistant body both freezer-to-oven and freezer-to-microwave proof. (The Churchill 'lion' logo has been discreetly introduced as a practical part of the easy-grip handles.)

As part of Hotelware's move up-market, 'Classic' ware has been introduced, equally strong but thinner and more elegant. The 'Buckingham' shape is currently in production, lobed with rope embossed edge, in both white and in two patterns, Sumatra and the new Sapphire (Colour Plates 28 and 29).[54]

Hotelware production emanates from a single intensively used factory, Anchor Pottery in Longton, with four hundred employees, led by Chris Hammond, production director, turning out some fifteen million pieces a year.[55] Its 7,151 square metres of production area includes handle de-seaming machines, automated backstamping machines, automated transfer devices for cup production and a fast-fire tunnel kiln (Colour Plate 38). A recently installed variable-speed high-output plastic clay extruder is entirely lined in stainless steel to obviate possible contamination of the body.[56]

Alongside extensive automation, traditional skills are maintained: 'jollying' of oval dishes, hand banding, gold lining and lithograph application (Colour Plate 36). The amazing dexterity of hand-dipping continues alongside in-line spray-glazing machines (Colour Plate 37), and at all stages, operatives check the quality of the ware passing through their hands. The vigour with which biscuit plates are tested by banging against the bench before being printed has to be seen (and heard) to be believed!

In 1992, the Group had over 1200 employees, working in eleven acres of floor space, with a wage-bill of £13 million; a turnover of £33 million and a net profit in excess of £2 million.[57] The main board was strengthened in May 1993 by the appointment of Robert Johnson as a non-executive director, bringing with him 34 years experience of the pottery industry, latterly as managing director of Wedgwood's subsidiary, Johnson Brothers.[58] The group board is now:[59]

P. J. Siddall – Chairman	D. P. Heywood – MD Hotelware
E. S. Roper – Chief Executive	M. Swingler – Non-executive
A. D. Roper – MD Tableware	D. J. S. Taylor – Finance
M. J. Roper – Production	R. L. Johnson – Development

Over the next year, Churchill anticipates a major investment in customer service, which will take the form of state-of-the-art computer software systems for production control, inventory, management and despatch. The success of this investment depends on a good management team, and recruitment is currently taking place to strengthen the existing team with experts in operations, systems and financial control.[60] Company policy of recruiting graduate trainees was recently endorsed from the top by group personnel manager Rod Devall's attainment of a Master of Business Administration degree from the Open University.[61]

Customers are rightly demanding faster response times, especially for new designs, requiring product planning to be up-to-date and accurate. Improved response times imply faster turn-around times for decorating equipment in particular. Along with systems investment, massive investment in new equipment and process engineering has been sanctioned.[62]

Churchill is committed to 'quality assurance' through BS 5750 and ISO 9000, so that 'the customers always get a service better than they expected', and above all recognises that its goals cannot be reached without a willing, skilled and motivated workforce.[63] Staff participate in quality 'working parties', and awards are made for workplace improvements and cost-saving ideas. Employees work for charities both individually and in works-sponsored events, and Tableware supports its own successful staff football team.[64]

As befits a long-established company, Churchill can boast numbers of long-serving members of staff. Peter Roper was associated with the firm from leaving school in 1928 to his death in 1991, 63 years, but his achievement was nearly matched by May Flaherty, who worked in the Anchor Works glost warehouse for 59 years, between 1918 and 1977.

Staff who retired in recent years after forty or more years' service include Wilf Morgan (1947–89) and Kath Barker (1950–92) of Tableware, and Ron Boulton (1940–84), May Towey (1946–87), Hilda Stanway (1949–91) and Arthur Stoddard (1949–91) of Hotelware. Other recent retirees with long service include Reg Chilton (1953–86), Francis Bourne (1956–87), Gladys Busby, Bill Busby and Joyce Stoddard, all of Hotelware; and Denis George (1955–88) and Ann Taylor (1966–93) of Tableware.

Thirty-four members of the present staff complete twenty-four or more years service in 1994:

B. M. Allan, Hotelware, 27 years
D. Banks, Tableware, 47 years
M. Birks, Hotelware, 24 years
D. Bold, Hotelware, 24 years
E. Brown, Tableware, 37 years
P. J. Brayford, Tableware, 29 years

M. L. Chappell, Tableware, 27 years
R. Colclough, Hotelware, 43 years
P. M. Condliffe, Tableware, 29 years
D. Cotton, Tableware, 35 years
P. Cotton, Tableware, 26 years
F. Dicken, Tableware, 27 years
I. Dugay, Tableware, 27 years
J. Edwards, Tableware, 24 years
E. Foster, Tableware, 27 years
P. A. Francis, Hotelware, 24 years
D. Frost, Tableware, 24 years
A. Harding, Hotelware, 29 years
B. Kelsall, Tableware, 24 years
G. Mohammed, Hotelware, 28 years
H. Pointon, Hotelware, 26 years
V. Price, Hotelware, 33 years
C. Smith, Tableware, 32 years
D. Stevenson, Tableware, 34 years
D. J. Stevenson, Tableware, 24 years
G. Stevenson, Tableware, 43 years
P. Stokes, Tableware, 24 years
L. Thorpe, Hotelware, 44 years
A. Waterhouse, Hotelware, 24 years
D. Weaver, Tableware, 35 years
E. Weaver, Tableware, 46 years
E. Wilshaw, Hotelware, 29 years
M. Wilshaw, Hotelware, 26 years
P. Wood, Tableware, 25 years

Of the directors, Michael Roper completes 37 years, Stephen Roper completes 34 years and Andrew Roper completes 21 years in 1994.

Looking to the future, Churchill is seeking to widen its customer base into the middle market, by promoting its image as a design-led organisation and exploiting its unique decorative techniques.[65] Flotation on the stock market will provide funds for further expansion, forward to the Group's two hundredth anniversary in 1995 and beyond to the twenty-first century.

CHRONOLOGY

Broadhursts and the Group

1847   James Broadhurst I joined a partnership making earthenware at Green Dock Works, Longton.

1853   James Broadhurst I joined an earthenware partnership at Crown Works, Longton and left the Green Dock business.

1854   James Broadhurst I became sole proprietor of the Crown Works business.

1856   James Broadhurst I took his sons into partnership.

1858   James Broadhurst I died.

1863   James Broadhurst II became sole proprietor.

1870   James Broadhurst II moved his business to a new factory, Portland Pottery, Fenton, making earthenware.

1876   James Broadhurst purchased Portland Pottery from John Aynsley.

1894   James Broadhurst took his sons into partnership.

1897   James Broadhurst II died.

1913   Edward Roper and Llewellyn Meredith started in partnership at Garfield Works, Longton, manufacturing earthenware.

1922   James Broadhurst III formed a limited company, James Broadhurst and Sons Ltd., with himself and Edward Roper as directors. Roper and Meredith's partnership was dissolved.

1928   Edward Roper's son Peter joined the firm.

1929   James Broadhurst III died.

1933   James Broadhurst and Sons Ltd. bought the factory from the Broadhurst family.

1939   The company was re-formed as James Broadhurst and Sons (1939) Ltd.

1941   The factory was closed for the duration of the war. Edward Roper died, and Peter Roper joined the R.A.F.

1945   Peter Roper re-opened the works, and commenced extensive modernisation, resuming making earthenware.

1958   Peter Roper's eldest son, Michael, joined the firm.

1959   The firm reverted to the original name of James Broadhurst and Sons Ltd.

1960   Peter Roper's second son, Stephen, joined the firm.

1965   James Broadhurst bought Sampson Bridgwood and Son Ltd., Anchor Works, Longton, hotelware manufacturers, see below.

1973   Peter Roper's third son, Andrew, joined the firm.

1974   Packing and warehouse space outside the two works was utilised at Montrose Works, Fenton and Sutherland Road, Longton.

1974   The Crown Clarence Works, King Street, Longton, was bought and Churchill China Ltd. (re-named Crown Clarence Ltd. in 1992) was formed to produce mugs.

1979   James Broadhurst and Son Ltd. bought a large modern factory, Sandyford Works, Tunstall to provide warehousing for the group, and later to become a production unit. Wessex Ceramics Ltd. was formed to import china, glass, cutlery &c.

1981   The Portland Pottery, Fenton was closed and production moved to Sandyford.

1984   Broadhursts was re-named Churchill Tableware and Bridgwoods was re-named Churchill Hotelware.

1985   The British Anchor Pottery building at Longton was bought for warehousing and storage.

1989   The group was reorganised into three divisions: tableware, hotelware and mugs. Peter Roper became president and Peter Siddall became chairman.

1991   Peter Roper died, aged 79.

1991   The Group purchased the Alexander Works at Cobridge, see below.

1992   The Group was re-named Churchill China PLC.

1994   The Group bought Crownford China, Longton.

Bridgwoods

1795   Samuel Bridgwood I and Richard Johnson were in partnership as earthenware manufacturers at Wood Street, Longton.

1799   Samuel Bridgwood I was in business alone at Longton, making earthenware.

1805   Samuel Bridgwood I died and his widow Kitty Bridgwood continued his business.

1818   Sampson Bridgwood was his mother's partner as Kitty Bridgwood and Son.

1825   Sampson Bridgwood took over his mother's Wood Street works.

1839   Sampson Bridgwood was first Chief Bailiff of Longton.

1853   Sampson Bridgwood and his son, Samuel Bridgwood II, were in partnership and built the Anchor Works, with a mill.

1860   Anchor Works south extension completed. China and earthenware manufactured.

1866   Samuel Bridgwood II was second Mayor of Longton.

1876   Both Sampson Bridgwood and Samuel Bridgwood died. Two daughters, Mrs. Napier and Mrs. Walker, inherited the works.

1879   Mrs. Walker took over the business completely.

1887   Ceased china production.

1890   Sampson Bridgwood & Son were insolvent. Aynsleys bought the works and business.

1897   Resumed china production.

1924   The owner, John Gerrard Aynsley, died and was succeeded by his son, Gerrard Aynsley.

1932   Sampson Bridgwood and Son Ltd. was formed, with Gerrard Aynsley as life director.

1944   Sampson Bridgwood and Son Ltd. bought the factory from Gerrard Aynsley. The firm came to specialise in hotelware.

1959   Gerrard Aynsley and Mr. Swift, the managing director, both died.

1965   Sampson Bridgwood and Son Ltd. was bought by James Broadhurst and Son Ltd.

Alexander Works (Myott Meakin)

1794   Site owned by Ralph Bucknall, potter.

1808   Cobridge Works built on site, by Bucknall and Stevenson.

1828   Works taken by Ralph and James Clews.

1837   Works taken by Robinson, Wood and Brownfield.

1884   Largest piece of bone china ever made was completed at works.

1902   Works reconstructed and divided into Brownfield Works for Upper Hanley Pottery Co. Ltd. and Alexander Works for Myott, Son and Co.

1927   Works re-united as Myott, Son and Co.'s Alexander Works.

CHRONOLOGY

1969   Myott, Son and Co. Ltd. sold to Interpace Corporation.

1976   Firm became Myott-Meakin Ltd.

1982   Firm went through successive ownerships under 'Myott Meakin' names.

1991   Firm and factory sold to Churchill Group.

SOURCES AND EXPLANATION
OF ABBREVIATIONS

Advertiser: *The Advertiser* (weekly free newspaper, published in Newcastle, Staffs.).

'A History of Co-operation in North Staffordshire' (anonymous typescript in Hanley Reference Library, S 800.334).

Allbut, 1802: Allbut, J. & Son, *The Staffordshire Pottery Directory* (Hanley, 1802).

Allbut, 1822: Allbut, T., *Newcastle and Pottery Directory 1822–23* (Hanley, 1822).

Allbutt, 1800: Allbutt, T., *A View of the Staffordshire Potteries* (Burslem, 1800).

Anderton, P. 'A Trade Union Year: 1864', *Journal of Ceramic History No. 9* (1977).

Andrews, S. *Crested China* (London, 1980).

Argos Distributors Ltd., *Catalogues*.

Art Journal, The.

Bemrose, P. *Nineteenth Century English Pottery and Porcelain* (London, 1952).

Board of Trade *Working Party Reports: Pottery* (London, 1946).

Bridgwood Deeds: Churchill China PLC.

Briggs, J. H. Y. *A History of Longton I: The Birth of a Community* (Keele, 1982).

British Anchor Pottery Deeds: Churchill China PLC.

British Earthenware Manufacturers Association *Home Trade Official Scales 1 January 1923*.

British Parliamentary Papers (year and roman numerals quoted).

British Patent: British Library Science Reference & Information Service, 25 Southampton Buildings, London, WC2A 1AW.

British Telecom Directory Section 226 (and date quoted).

Broadhurst Deeds: The Beth Johnson Housing Association Ltd, title deeds to Victoria Court, Frederick Street, Fenton.

Broadhurst, James & Sons Ltd., publicity leaflets: Churchill China PLC, Marlborough Works, Tunstall.

Brownfield, A. *The Lockout – A Potters Guild* (Hanley, 1892).

Burchill, F. and R. Ross *A History of the Potters' Union* (Hanley, 1977).

Census (and year quoted): National Population Census.

Ceramic Industries Journal (month and year quoted).

Ceramic Society (volume and date quoted): *Transactions of The (British, English, North Staffordshire) Ceramic Society*.

Chaffers, W. *Marks and Monograms on European and Oriental Pottery and Porcelain* (London, 1946).

Chester & Mort, c.1796: Chester & Mort, *The Staffordshire Pottery Directory* (Hanley, no date, but 'publication promised in a few weeks', SA, 26 March 1796).

Church Calendar and General Almanack for the Diocese of Lichfield (and year quoted).

Clarence Works Deeds: Churchill China PLC.

CMAG: City Museum and Art Gallery, Stoke-on-Trent.

Collections for a History of Staffordshire The William Salt Archaeological Society (ed.) (Kendal, year quoted).

Concentration of the Pottery Industry in North Staffordshire (Scott, Greenwood & Co., no date but 1941 from context).

Cox, A. and A. Cox *Rockingham Pottery and Porcelain 1745–1842* (London, 1983).

Cox's Potteries Annual and Glass Trade Year Book A. E. Holdcroft (ed.) (Liverpool, year quoted).

Coysh, A. W. and R. K. Henrywood *The Dictionary of Blue and White Printed Pottery 1780–1880* (Woodbridge, 1982).

Daily Dispatch.

Eatwell, A. *Susie Cooper Productions* (London, 1987).

European Tableware Buyers Guide (and year quoted).

Evening Sentinel, The.

Farmer: *Farmer's New Borough Almanack* (Longton).

Financial Times, The.

Gallimore, P. 'Building Societies and Housing Provision in North Staffordshire' (1850–1880), unpublished M.A. Thesis, University of Keele, 1985.

Gaston, M. F. *Blue Willow An Identification and Value Guide* revised 2nd edition (Paducah, Kentucky, USA, 1990).

Gladstone Pottery Museum, Uttoxeter Road, Longton.

Godden, G. *Encyclopaedia of British Porcelain Manufacturers* (London, 1988).

Godden, G. A. *Jewitt's Ceramic Art of Great Britain 1800–1900* (London, 1982).

Godden, *Marks*: G. A. Godden, *Encyclopedia of British Pottery and Porcelain Marks* (London, 1964).

Gore's Directory of Liverpool 1845.

Green & Stewart: Green, A. T. and G. H. Stewart, *Ceramics a Symposium* (Stoke-on-Trent, 1953).

Grimwades Ltd (Stoke-on-Trent, 1920).

Hampson, Appendix (ref. no.): R. S. Hampson, 'The Development of the Pottery Industry in Longton, 1700–1865 Volume II Appendix', unpublished M.A. Thesis, University of Keele, 1986.

Hampson, R. and E., 'Brownfields, Victorian Potters', *Northern Ceramic Society Journal Vol. 4*, (1980–1981) 177–218.

Hand-painted Gray's Pottery K. Niblett (ed.) (Stoke-on-Trent, 1982).

Harmsworth Encyclopaedia Vol. V, The (London, n.d.).

Harrison's Directory, 1861: *Harrison, Harrod & Co.'s Directory of Staffordshire* (London, 1861).

Harrod, J. G. & Co., *Postal and Commercial Directory for Staffordshire* 2nd Edition (London, 1870).

HBS (and reference quoted): Historic Buildings Survey, records kept in Archaeology Department, City Museum and Art Gallery, Stoke-on-Trent.

Hind, S. R. *Contributions to the Study of Pottery Ovens, Fuels and Firing* (Stoke-on-Trent, 1937).

Holden's Triennial Directory for 1809, 1810, 1811 (London, 1809).

House of Commons *Minutes of Evidence on the Wellington, Drayton and Newcastle Junction Railway Bill from May 8 to 16, 1862*, 342.

HRL (and reference quoted): Hanley Reference Library.

Hulme, G. 'The Wedgwood Bicentenary Proceedings' in *Transactions of the Ceramic Society Vol. XXIX, No. 6* (June, 1930) 481–522.

Huntbach, A. *Hanley Stoke-on-Trent 13th to 20th Century* (Stafford, 1910).

IGI (and county): *International Genealogical Index*.

Ingamells, J. *Historical Records and Directory of Newcastle-under-Lyme* second edition (Newcastle-under-Lyme, 1881).

Instituto Historico e Geografico Brasileiro, Rio de Janeiro, Brazil.

Jewitt, 1878 (volume no.): Jewitt, L., *The Ceramic Art of Great Britain from Pre-Historic Times down to the Present Day* 2 vols. (London, 1878).

John England Spring/Summer 1974 catalogue.

Jones' Directory, 1864: *Jones's Mercantile Directory of the Pottery District of Staffordshire 1864* (London, 1864).

Journal of Ceramic History (no. quoted).

Journal of the Northern Ceramic Society (no. quoted).

Keates's Directory (and year quoted): *Keates's Directory of the Potteries and Newcastle* (titles vary).

Kelly's Directory (and year quoted): *Kelly's Post Office Directory for Staffordshire*.

Larsen, E. B. 'The Truth about Andrew Stevenson' in *English Pottery and Porcelain* P. Atterbury (ed.) (London, 1980) 198–201.

Levitt, S. *Pountneys The Bristol Pottery at Fishponds 1905–1969* (Bristol, 1990).

Lichfield Joint Record Office.

Lidstone, J. T. S. *The Thirteenth Londoniad* (Potteries, 1866).

London Gazette.

Longton New Connexion Methodist Church Register: Hanley Reference Library, Microfilm, Non-Conformist Registers, Reel 2.

Manchester Mercury.

Mankowitz, W. & R. G. Haggar *The Concise Encyclopedia of English Pottery and Porcelain* (London, 1957).

Marryat, J. *A History of Pottery and Porcelain, Mediaeval and Modern* (London, 1868).

Meigh: Meigh, A., *Manufacturers of Pottery in the Staffordshire Potteries 1807–1859 from the Rate Records* (privately, 1940).

Minton MSS: Royal Doulton Tableware Ltd., Stoke-on-Trent.

Montgomery Ward & Co. Catalogue and Buyers' Guide No., 57 Spring and Summer 1895 (reprinted by Dover, n.d.).

Mortimer & Harwood's Directory of Birkenhead 1843.

Newcastle under Lyme Parish Register 1771–1812 (Birmingham, 1981).

Normacott Churchyard: Church of the Holy Evangelists, Belgrave Road, Longton.

Ordnance Survey Maps.

Parsons & Bradshaw's Staffordshire General and Commercial Directory (Manchester, 1818).

People of the Potteries Vol. 1 D. Stuart (ed.) (Keele, 1985).

Pigot, 1841: J. Pigot & Co., *Royal and National Commercial Directory of Staffordshire* (London and Manchester, 1841).

Porter's Directory, 1887: *Postal Directory for The Potteries with Newcastle and District* (Liverpool, 1887).

Pottery and Glass Record.

Pottery Gazette and Glass Trade Review (title varies).

Pottery Gazette Diary.

Pottery Gazette Directory.

Pottery Gazette Reference Book.

Pottery – The Story of Alfred Meakin (Tunstall) Ltd. (Tunstall, 1949).

PRO: Public Record Office, Kew.

Radio Times, The.

Rates 1847: Staffordshire Record Office, D/593/H/14/3/58.

Registrar: Registrar of Companies, Companies House, Crown Way, Cardiff, CF4 3UZ.

Rhead, G. W. and F. A. Rhead *Staffordshire Pots & Potters* (London, 1906).

SA: *Staffordshire Advertiser*.

Scarratt, W., *Old Times in the Potteries* (Stoke-on-Trent, 1906, reprinted Wakefield, 1969).

Sentinel: Staffordshire Weekly Sentinel, Staffordshire Sentinel, Evening Sentinel.

Sentinel Directory (and year quoted): *The Potteries, Newcastle and District Directory* (Hanley, 1907, 1912).

Shaw, History: S. Shaw *History of the Staffordshire Potteries* (Hanley, 1829, reprinted Newton Abbot, 1970).

Shaw, S. *The Chemistry of the several Natural and Artificial Heterogeneous Compounds used in Manufacturing Porcelain, Glass and Pottery* (London, 1837, reprinted London, 1900).

Slater, 1853: *Slater's Classified Directory of the Potteries* (Manchester, 1853).

Somerset House: Principal Registry of the Family Division, Somerset House, Strand, London, WC2R 1LP.

Specimens of Wenger's Collection of Pottery (Stoke-on-Trent, 1914).

SRO: Staffordshire Record Office.

Staffordshire Life.

Staffordshire Porcelain G. Godden (ed.) (London, 1983).

Staffordshire Sentinel.

Staffordshire Weekly Sentinel.

Stefano, F. 'James and Ralph Clews, nineteenth-century potters, Part I: The English experience', in *English Pottery and Porcelain* P. Atterbury (ed.) (London, 1980) 202–06.

Stoke-upon-Trent Parish Register: Staffordshire Record Office, D1188.

Tableware International.

Tableware Reference Book.

Tams Deeds: John Tams Group PLC, Longton, title deeds to Crown Works, Strand, Longton.

Times, The.

Tunnicliff, 1787: W. Tunnicliff *A Topographical Survey of the County of Stafford* (Nantwich, 1787).

UBD: *Universal British Directory* (no date, c.1797).

VCH: *A History of the County of Stafford* J. G. Jenkins (ed.) (London, year of volume).

Venn, J. A., *Alumni Cantabrigiensis Part II, Vol. IV* (Cambridge, 1954).

Ward: J. Ward *The Borough of Stoke-upon-Trent* (London, 1843).

Wedgwood, J. C. *Staffordshire Pottery and its History* (London, n.d., [1912]).

Wedgwood MSS: Keele University Library.

White's Directory, 1834: W. White, *History, Gazetteer and Directory of Staffordshire* (Sheffield, 1834).

White's Directory, 1851: W. White, *History, Gazetteer and Directory of Staffordshire* (Sheffield, 1851).

White, W. *All Around the Wrekin* (London, 1860).

Who's Who 1990 (London, 1990).

Who Was Who 1971–80 (London, 1981).

Williams, B. R. 'The Pottery Industry', in *The Structure of British Industry: A Symposium, Vol. II* D. Burns (ed.) (Cambridge, 1958) 291–330.

Williams's Commercial Directory for Stafford and the Potteries (Manchester, 1846).

Notes

The abbreviations used in these notes are explained in 'Sources and Explanation of Abbreviations'.

Notes for Chapter 1
Pages 1–22

1 Hampson, Appendix, ref. nos. 54, 128, 182.
2 Hampson, Appendix, ref. no. 128; Census, 1841.
3 Longton New Connexion Methodist Church Register, 5 June 1826: William Broadhurst born 5 June 1826, baptised 2 July 1826, 3rd child of Job Broadhurst and Charlotte.
4 *London Gazette*, No. 20935, 12 January 1849.
5 *White's Directory*, 1851; SA, 19 June 1852, p.1, col.6.
6 Census, 1841.
7 IGI, Staffordshire.
8 Longton New Connexion Methodist Church Registers, *passim*; Census, 1841.
9 Hampson, Appendix, ref. no. 128.
10 Godden, *Marks*, plate 5, 307, 317, 319. An earthenware mug with a black print of an early railway train, enamelled over, with the printed mark 'RAILWAY / H & B' (as Godden's Plate 5) was shown on the BBC television programme 'Antiques Road Show' 17 March 1991 (recorded at Gillingham, Kent, November 1990); and attributed to Hampson and Broadhurst.
11 SA, 22 November 1851, p.4, col.6.
12 Census, 1851.
13 *London Gazette*, No. 21526, 24 February 1854.
14 Hampson, Appendix, ref. no. 116; H. Williams, 'The Goodwin Potteries at Longton and Seacombe' *Journal of the Northern Ceramic Society Vol. 7* 1989, 15–26.
15 SA, 13 May 1848, p.5, col.2; 15 November 1851, p.8, col.3.
16 Tams Deeds: 6 May 1851.
17 Hampson, Appendix, ref. no. 53.
18 Tams Deeds, 14 May 1787 – 7 March 1853; Ordnance Survey 1/500 plan OST (20) Longton 1856; Hampson, Appendix, ref. no. 53.
19 *London Gazette*, No. 21526, 24 February 1854.
20 Hampson, Appendix, ref. no. 53; *London Gazette*, No. 21589, 1 September 1854.
21 *Kelly's Directory*, 1856.
22 M. F. Gaston, *Blue Willow An Identification and Value Guide* revised 2nd edition (Paducah, Kentucky, USA, 1990) 19.
23 Somerset House: will of James Broadhurst proved 16 February 1859.
24 *Kelly's Directory*, 1860; *Harrison's Directory*, 1861.
25 SA, 12 October 1861.
26 SA, 6 September 1862, p.8, col.1.
27 SA, 13 December 1862, p.8, col.1.
28 Hampson, Appendix, ref. no. 116.
29 *London Gazette*, No. 22799, 22 December 1863.
30 Jones' Directory, 1864.
31 J. T. S. Lidstone, *The Thirteenth Londoniad* (Potteries, 1866) 31.
32 PRO: BT43/68: 4/197857; 5/243647–8, 5/245605.
33 Letter from the Brazilian Ambassador, n.d. (?4 April 1991), enclosing letter 13 March 1991 and photographs from Instituto Historico e

Geografico Brasileiro, Rio de Janeiro. Letter 25 March 1991 from the Director of the National History Museum, Rio de Janeiro. An oval dish and a cup with Broadhurst's 4 August 1870 design are illustrated in J. Dreyfus *The China used by the Brazilian Aristocracy* (1882) 226, but their present whereabouts are not known.

34 House of Commons, *Minutes of Evidence on the Wellington, Drayton and Newcastle Junction Railway Bill from May 8 to 16, 1862*, 342.

35 *British Parliamentary Papers* 1863, XVIII, 20, 322.

36 *Sentinel*, 28 May 1864.

37 SA, 5 December 1863.

38 SA, 23 December 1865.

39 *Keates's Directory*, 1867.

40 *Keates's Directory*, 1869.

41 Census, 1871.

42 *Pottery Gazette*, August 1897, 1031.

43 SA, 31 July 1869, p.8, col.2.

44 SA, 7 August 1869, p.1, col.3, p.5, col 2.

Notes for Chapter 2

1 HRL: SA-LG-60, Fenton Improvement Commissioners' Minutes, 1865–73, 6 July 1869.

2 SA 7 September 1833, p.3, col.1; 7 November 1840, p.1, col.4.

3 P. Gallimore, 'Building Societies and Housing Provision in North Staffordshire (1850–1880)' unpublished M.A. Thesis, University of Keele, 1985, 210.

4 Broadhurst Deeds: 12 October 1865, 23 June 1866.

5 Broadhurst Deeds: Plan of Land situated at Fenton belonging to the Shareholders of the Fenton Permanent Freehold Land Society 1866; SA 6 June 1866, p.1, col.2; 14 April 1866, p.5, col.1.

6 Broadhurst Deeds: 1 December 1869.

7 Hampson, Appendix, ref. no. 10; HBS: L 206, Aynsley's China factory.

8 Broadhurst Deeds: 21 December 1869.

9 Broadhurst Deeds: 21 December 1869.

10 SA 11 June 1870, p.6, col.6.

11 SA 12 December 1874, p.7, col.7.

12 Information from Mr. R. Colclough.

13 *Sentinel*, 12 November 1870, p.5, col.1.

14 SA, 31 December 1870, p.8, col.4.

15 *Kelly's Directory*, 1872.

16 Tams Deeds: 22 March 1872.

17 *Sentinel*, 4 March 1871, p.1, col.6 to 10 June 1871, p.1, col.7.

18 *Pottery Gazette*, November 1885, 1303; SA 16 November 1872, p.5, col.1.

19 Broadhurst Deeds: 10, 11 April 1876; Mr. J. M. Aynsley: John Aynsley's Securities Deposited book, p.10.

20 Broadhurst Deeds: 1 February 1878.

21 Broadhurst Deeds: 29 May 1883.

22 *Kelly's Directories*: 1872, 1880, 1884, 1892; *Keates's Directories* 1873–4, 1875, 1882, 1889, 1892; *Pottery Gazette Diary*, 1882, 133; 1886, 71; 1890, 58; 1895, 61; 1896, 133; *Porter's Directory*, 1887.

23 G. Bemrose, *Nineteenth Century English Pottery and Porcelain* (London, 1952) 10; and shards found by Mrs. K. Barker.

24 PRO: BT43/73, 5/375054.

25 PRO: BT43/74, 6/395688.

26 Mr. J. M. Aynsley: John Aynsley's Pass Book, 1892–1902.

27 Copy from Mr. J. Smith, Stourbridge, source not recorded.

28   *Pottery Gazette*, November 1885, 1303.

29   *Pottery Gazette*, May 1891, 458.

30   F. Burchill and R. Ross, *A History of the Potters' Union* (Hanley, 1977) 149–50.

31   *Keates's Directory*, 1873–4. The house is now the surgery of Dr. Yates, latterly known as Penton House.

32   Directories, 1876–1896.

33   Census, Blythe Bridge, 1881.

34   Broadhurst Deeds: 10 July 1894.

35   *Kelly's Directory*, 1896.

36   SA 31 July 1897, p.5, col.7; *Pottery Gazette*, August 1897, 1031.

37   Somerset House: Will of James Broadhurst, proved at Lichfield 29 September 1897.

38   Directories, 1897–1921.

39   Broadhurst Deeds: 1 February 1898; *Keates's Directory*, 1892–3.

40   Broadhurst Deeds: 10 February 1903 to 29 January 1918.

41   *Kelly's Directory*, 1900, 1904, 1908.

42   Information from Mr. W. Morgan and Mrs. N. Whitehouse.

43   *Kelly's Directories*:1896, 1900, 1904, 1908, 1912, 1916; *Sentinel Directory*, 1907.

44   *Pottery Gazette*, December 1922, 1819.

45   *Pottery Gazette* 1899 to 1913 *passim*; June 1913, 680; April 1919, 352.

46   *Pottery Gazette*, December 1922, 1819.

47   G. Griffiths, 'Pottery Printing Machines', *Ceramic Society*, Vol. II 1902–3, 49–61.

48   *Pottery Gazette*, December 1922, 1819.

49   *Pottery Gazette*, May 1934, 628.

50   H. W. Edwards and A. Leese, 'The Influence of Grog in Saggar Marls', *Ceramic Society*, Vol. II, 1902–3, 14–30; Vol. III, 1903–4, 26, 29; Vol. IV, 1904–5, 46.

51   A. Leese, 'Unestimated Losses in Pottery Manufacture', *Ceramic Society*, Vol. VXI, 1916–7, 189–94.

52   *Ceramic Society*, Vol. XVII, 1917–8, 115, 134; A. Heath and A. Leese, 'The Effects of Calcination of Flints on Earthenware Bodies', Vol. XX, Part II, 1920–1, 121–6; A. Heath and A. Leese, 'Black and Grey Flints', Vol. XXII, 1922–3, 313; A. Leese, 'Scientific Treatment of Boiler Feed Water, introducing the Colloidial Aspect', Vol. XXV, 1925–6, 205; A. Leese, 'Discolouration of Clays during Firing', Vol. XXVI, 1926–7, 19; Vol. XXVII, 1927–8, 219, 327; *Sentinel*, 15 March 1934, p.3, col.7; 10 April 1934, p.8, col.3; *Pottery Gazette*, May 1934, 628.

53   Information from Mr. Peter Roper.

Notes for Chapter 3

1   *Pottery Gazette*, October 1922, 1543, 1922.

2   Information from Mr. Peter Roper.

3   Census, 1881.

4   Information from Mr. Peter Roper.

5   Godden, *Marks*, 370, 448; *Keates's Directory*, 1875–6.

6   Information from Mr. Peter Roper and Mr. K. Allerton.

7   *Sentinel Directory*, 1912.

8   *Pottery Gazette*, February 1907, 208.

9   *Pottery Gazette*, April 1929, 650.

10   *Kelly's Directory*, 1916; *Cox's Potteries Annual and Year Book, 1924*, 175; *Pottery Gazette*, October 1941, 803.

11   *Pottery Gazette*, November 1922, 1705.

12   Ordnance Survey 1:500 Plan OST (20), 1856.

13   *Pottery Gazette*, June 1919, 545; January to May, September to December 1920; January to August 1921.

14   *Cox's Potteries Annual and Year Book, 1924*, 175.

15   Godden, *Marks*, 548.

16   *Pottery Gazette*, November 1922, 1705.

17   *Pottery and Glass Record*, July 1923, 534.

18   S. Andrews, *Crested China*, (London, 1980) 206.

19   Information from Mr. Peter Roper; *Kelly's Directory*, 1928; *Pottery Gazette*, December 1929, 1964.

20   *Pottery Gazette*, December 1922, 1764, 1819.

21   British Earthenware Manufacturers' Association, *Home Trade Official Scales 1 January 1923; Pottery Gazette*, April 1923, supplement.

22   *Pottery Gazette*, February to August 1923.

23   A. Heath and A. Leese, 'Black and Grey Flints', *Ceramic Society* Vol. XXII, 1922–3, 313.

24   *Ceramic Society* Vol. XXVI, 1926–7, 19.

25   *Pottery Gazette*, May 1934, 628; information from Mr. W. Morgan.

26   Somerset House: Will of Constance Amelia Broadhurst died 24 May 1923.

27   *Sentinel*, 3 November 1924.

28   *Sentinel*, 15 October 1929.

29   Somerset House: Will of James Broadhurst died 13 October 1929, proved 8 February 1930.

30   Broadhurst Deeds: 7 April 1933; *Sentinel*, 20 November 1984, 15.

31   *Kelly's Directories*: 1916, 1921, 1924.

32   Somerset House: Will of Frances Louisa Broadhurst died 3 August 1934.

33   Somerset House: Will of Drusilla Elizabeth Broadhurst died 20 December 1940.

34   Information from Mr. Peter Roper. Although very ill, Mr. Roper was able to give invaluable first-hand information about Broadhursts from the 1920s onward, in reply to written questions in October 1990. Mr. Roper died on 25 January 1991.

35   Information from Mr. Peter Roper.

36   Information from Mrs. K. Barker.

37   Information from Mr. Peter Roper.

38   *Pottery Gazette*, April 1939, 528.

39   Information from Mrs. N. Whitehouse.

40   *Pottery Gazette*, June 1939, 795, 802.

41   Letter 14 June 1939 from Geo. E. Harding, 8 Brook Street, Stoke-upon-Trent to E. R. Roper Esq., and Schedule A enclosed. (Churchill China PLC Records).

42   See S. R. Hind, *Contributions to the Study of Pottery Ovens, Fuels and Firing*, (Stoke-on-Trent, 1937).

43   *Pottery Gazette*, September 1939, 1170.

44   Information from Mr. Peter Roper.

45   *Pottery Gazette*, October 1941, 791; *Concentration of the Pottery Industry in North Staffordshire*, (Pottery Gazette, n.d., 1941 from context).

46   Information from Mr. Peter Roper, Mr. W. Morgan and Mrs. K. Barker.

47   *Sentinel*, 5 September 1941; *Pottery Gazette*, October 1941, 803.

Notes for Chapter 4

1   Information from Mr. W. Morgan.

2   Information from Mr. P. Roper.

3   Information from Mr. W. Morgan.

4   *Pottery Gazette*, November 1945, 4; April 1946, 252.

5   Information from Mr. K. Allerton.

6   Information from Mr. P. Roper.
7   Information from Mr. W. Morgan.
8   A. Eatwell *Susie Cooper Productions* (London, 1987) 101.
9   Information from Mr. W. Morgan and Mrs. K. Barker.
10   Information from Mr. P. Roper and Mr. W. Morgan.
11   Information from Mr. W. Morgan.
12   Information from Mr. W. Morgan.
13   Somerset House: Will of James Broadhurst, 5 Frederick Street, Fenton, died 8 January 1940, administration to James Broadhurst, lorry driver; and information from Mr. W. Morgan.
14   Information from Mr. W. Morgan.
15   *Pottery Gazette Reference Book 1949*, 57; and shards found by Mrs. K. Barker.
16   *Pottery Gazette*, May 1949, 435.
17   Private collection.
18   *Pottery Gazette*, September 1949, 941.
19   *Pottery Gazette*, January 1951, 123; information from Mr. W. Morgan.
20   *Pottery Gazette*, March 1952, 404.
21   Information from Mr. W. Morgan.
22   *Pottery Gazette Reference Book 1952*, 46; information from Mr. W. Morgan.
23   Somerset House: Will of Laura Broadhurst died 16 May 1953; information from Mr. W. Morgan.
24   *Pottery Gazette Reference Book 1954*, 47; information from Mr. W. Morgan.
25   *Pottery Gazette Reference Book 1946*, 73; information from Mr. W. Morgan.
26   *Pottery Gazette Reference Book 1954*, 47; information from Mr. W. Morgan.
27   Information from Mr. W. Morgan.
28   *Sentinel*, 20 March 1990, 20.
29   *Pottery Gazette*, November 1956, 1607–10.
30   *Pottery Gazette*, February 1955, 278.
31   A. T. Green and G. H. Stewart, *Ceramics A Symposium* (Stoke-on-Trent, 1953) 381.
32   Information from Mr. R. Colclough.
33   Information from Mr. W. Morgan.
34   *Pottery Gazette*, November 1956, 1607–10.
35   *Pottery Gazette*, November 1956, 1549.
36   *Pottery Gazette*, May 1957, 593.
37   *Pottery Gazette*, January 1958, 41.
38   Information from Mr. Peter Roper; *Pottery Gazette*, January 1958.
39   *Pottery Gazette*, November 1956, 1607–10; information from Mr. Peter Roper.
40   Information from Mr. Peter Roper.
41   *Pottery Gazette*, November 1956, 1607–10.
42   *Pottery Gazette*, February 1957, 272.
43   Information from Mr. W. Morgan.
44   *Pottery Gazette*, November 1958, 1370; *Sentinel*, 20 March 1990, 24.
45   Registrar, 15 May 1959.
46   *Sentinel*, 20 March 1990, 24.
47   *Pottery Gazette Reference Book 1962*, 39.
48   *Pottery Gazette*, November 1961, 48.
49   *Pottery Gazette*, February 1961, 241.
50   *Pottery Gazette*, November 1956, 1607–10.
51   Information from Mr. W. Morgan.
52   Information from Mrs. Barker.
53   Information from Mr. W. Morgan; *Pottery Gazette*, February 1961, 244.
54   Information from Mr. W. Morgan.
55   *Pottery Gazette*, February 1964, 246.
56   Information from Mr. W. Morgan.
57   *Sentinel*, 11 February 1991, 9.

58   *Pottery Gazette*, February 1961, 244.
59   *Pottery Gazette*, January 1962, 37.
60   *Pottery Gazette*, February 1963, 122.
61   Information from Mr. Peter Roper.
62   F. Burchill and R. Ross, *A History of the Potters' Union* (Hanley, 1977) 228; S. Levitt, *Pountneys The Bristol Pottery at Fishponds 1905–1969* (Bristol, 1990) 10.

Notes for Chapter 5

1   'The Staffordshire Hearth Tax 1666', *Collections for a History of Staffordshire 1921*, 85.
2   Stoke-upon-Trent Parish Register, 9 March 1736/7; Lichfield Joint Record Office: Will of Thomas Barker, 5 May 1737.
3   SRO: D(W) 1742/46, Rate Book, Penkhull ... Longton ... 1740.
4   SRO: D/593/J/22/2, Longton Manor Court Record, 1733.
5   SA, 21 December 1805.
6   Rodney Hampson, Notes of Gravestone Inscriptions, St. John's Church, Longton: Lettice, daughter of Samuel and Kitty Bridgwood died 5 February 1787 aged 2.
7   SRO: Q/RPL Land Tax Returns, microfilm Q/42; UBD.
8   SRO: Q/RPL Land Tax Returns, microfilm Q/42; Hampson, Appendix, ref. no. 96.
9   *Tunnicliff, 1787*, Lane End.
10   *Chester & Mort*; UBD.
11   CMAG: Heathcote Papers (now at SRO).
12   SA, 9 April 1842.
13   *Allbut, 1802*, map reference 131, Johnson & Brough, successors to Johnson & Bridgwood.
14   SA, 11 January 1800; *Pottery Gazette*, February 1885.
15   *Allbut, 1802*, map reference 130, Samuel Bridgwood.
16   SRO: D(W)1742/55, Church Levey Bagnall ... Longton & Lane End Octr. 1802.
17   Shaw, *History*, 171.
18   SA, 21 December 1805.
19   *Sentinel*, 3 June 1876, obituary.
20   HRL: SA/C-C/1.1–13, indentures relating to the Crown and Anchor Hotel, Longton, 1777–1878.
21   SA, 19 June 1813, p.1, col.3.
22   SA, 22 December 1810.
23   SA, 17 September 1814, 2 September 1815.
24   Meigh, 135, 139.
25   Census, 1841, 1851, 1861.
26   IGI, Staffordshire; Census, 1851.
27   *Parsons & Bradshaw's Staffordshire General and Commercial Directory* (Manchester, 1818), Lane End.
28   Gladstone Pottery Museum, Longton: Archaeological excavation, 1976, box 20, layer B146.
29   SA, 23 September 1820.
30   Meigh, 135, 139.
31   *Allbut, 1822*: Bridgwood, Sampson, China Mfr., Market St., Lane End.
32   SA, 6 April 1822.
33   Meigh, 139–175, 1822–1824.
34   SA, 24 April 1824.
35   Meigh, 175.
36   Shaw, *History*, 171.

37   Jewitt, 1878, II, 398.

38   *Allbut, 1822* to *Slater, 1853.*

39   SA, 10 August 1833, p.3, col.1; 26 April 1834, p.3, col.2.

40   Wedgwood MSS, 33/25219–25277.

41   *British Parliamentary Papers 1843 XIII*, Royal Commission on the Employment of Children, Second Report, Trades and Manufactures, Interviews 155, 156.

42   Meigh, 277, 294.

43   Hampson, Appendix ref. no. 108.

44   Shaw, *History*, 75.

45   *Allbut, 1822.*

46   SA, 30 May 1863, letter from William Cyples.

47   Jewitt, 1878, I, 462; A. Cox and A. Cox, *Rockingham Pottery and Porcelain 1745–1842* (London, 1983) 73.

48   W. Chaffers, *Marks & Monograms on European and Oriental Pottery and Porcelain* (London, 1946) 732.

49   W. Scarratt, *Old Times in the Potteries* (Stoke-on-Trent, 1906, reprinted Wakefield, 1969) 166–7.

50   S. Shaw, *The Chemistry of the several Natural and Artificial Heterogeneous Compounds used in Manufacturing Porcelain, Glass and Pottery* (London, 1837, reprinted London, 1900) vii.

51   *White's Directory, 1834; Pigot's Directory, 1841*; Meigh, 283, 285; Census, 1841.

52   SA, 28 December 1833, p.1, col.3.

53   SA, 5 October 1839, p.3, col.2; Ward, 581.

54   SA, 13 May 1843.

55   *Allbutt, 1800, 25.*

56   *Pigot's Directory, 1841, 40.*

57   SA, 30 November 1839, p.2, from *Chambers' Edinburgh Journal* 23 November 1839.

58   SA, 11, 18 May, 22 June, 13, 20 July 1839.

59   SA 26 June 1840, p.3, col.4; Ward, 582–4.

60   SA, 20, 27 August 1843; Ward, 584–9.

61   SA, 16 May 1840.

62   SA, 8 May, 2 October 1841, 4 June 1842.

63   *Pigot's Directory 1841* to *Kelly's Directory 1854.*

64   Rates 1847.

65   Rates 1847.

66   Hampson, Appendix, ref. no. 52.

67   *Mortimer & Harwood's Directory of Birkenhead 1843; Gore's Directory of Liverpool 1845*: 23 Argyle Street, Birkenhead and 4 Hanover Street, Liverpool.

68   Letter from J. W. Michener, 10 September 1990; Hampson, Appendix, ref. no. 115.

69   SA, 22 November 1862, p.7, col.4.

70   Rates 1847; *White's Directory, 1851*, 264.

71   CMAG (Heathcote Papers, now in SRO): Indenture 23 July 1846.

72   *Williams's Commercial Directory for Stafford and the Potteries* (Manchester, 1846).

73   Census, 1851.

74   SA, 20 June, p.1, col.7; 19 September 1857, p.8, col.3; Census, 1861.

Notes for Chapter 6

1   Census, 1851; Slater, 1853.

2   *White's Directory, 1851.*

3   Hampson, Appendix, ref. no. 52.

4   SA, 22 November 1862, p.7, col.4.

5   HRL: SM 18 R.

6   *Slater, 1853*.

7   SA, 1 January 1853, p.4, col.6.

8   VCH, Vol. VIII, 241, note 33.

9   SA, 1 July 1854.

10   Hampson, Appendix, ref. no. 10.

11   Hampson, Appendix, ref. no. 82.

12   Hampson, Appendix, ref. no. 10; HBS: L 206, Aynsleys' China Factory; Mr. J. M. Aynsley: John Aynsley's Securities Deposited book, p.19.

13   SA, 17 November 1860, p.4, col.7; *Sentinel*, 17 November 1860, p.5, col.4.

14   SA, 16 November 1861.

15   *Staffordshire Porcelain* G. Godden (ed.) (London, 1983) 397, plate 560; private collections.

16   Information from The Friends of Blue.

17   J. T. S. Lidstone, *The Thirteenth Londoniad* (Potteries, 1866) 42–3.

18   J. Marryat, *A History of Pottery and Porcelain, Mediaeval and Modern* (London, 1868) 467.

19   *J. G. Harrod & Co's. Postal and Commercial Directory for Staffordshire* 2nd Edition (London, 1870).

20   Jewitt, 1878, II, 406.

21   SA, 26 February 1870, p.4, col.7.

22   Farmer, 1870, 7.

23   *British Parliamentary Papers 1863*, XVIII, 322.

24   *British Parliamentary Papers 1863*, XVIII, 20.

25   P. Anderton, 'A Trade Union Year: 1864', *Journal of Ceramic History No. 9* (1977) 16, 17.

26   SA, 11 January 1868, p.7, col.4; 18 January 1868, p.5, col.1; p.7, col.5.

27   W. White, *All Round the Wrekin* (London, 1860) 372–3.

28   Farmer, 1879, 1887.

29   SA, 22 November 1862, p.7, col.4.

30   Farmer, 1866, 1887; SA, 28 October 1876, p.5, col.7.

31   *Keates's Directory*, 1875–6; *Pottery Gazette* December 1897, 1556.

32   SA, 3 June 1876, p.5, col.7; *Sentinel*, 3 June 1876; gravestone, Normacott Churchyard.

33   SA, 28 October 1876, p.5, col.7; gravestone, Normacott Churchyard.

34   Somerset House: Sampson Bridgwood, will proved 14 December 1876; Samuel Bridgwood, will proved 22 November 1876.

Notes for Chapter 7

1   Somerset House: Sampson Bridgwood, will proved 14 December 1876; Samuel Bridgwood, will proved 22 November 1876; *London Gazette* 10 January 1879, No. 24667.

2   *Church Calendar and General Almanack for the Diocese of Lichfield* 1857, 8; 1858, 5; 1859, 5; 1860, 81; 1862, 82; 1863, 82; 1865, 86.

3   *Pottery Gazette*, July 1890, 632.

4   *London Gazette*, 10 January 1879, No. 24667; *Pottery Gazette*, July 1890, 632–3.

5   *Pottery Gazette*, July 1890, 632–3.

6   IGI, Staffordshire: Stoke-upon-Trent, 22 April 1817.

7   J. A. Venn, *Alumni Cantabrigiensis Part II, Vol. IV* (Cambridge, 1954); *Who Was Who 1971–80; Who's Who 1990; The Times* 2 December 1989, 15f. Mr. H. B. Walker has no family information.

8   SA, 25 August 1883, p.7, col.6; *Pottery Gazette*, September 1883, 862; R. and E. Hampson, 'Brownfields, Victorian Potters', *Northern Ceramic Society Journal Vol. 4* (1980–1981), 182.

9   *Pottery Gazette*, July 1890, 632–3.
10 *Pottery Gazette*, March 1878, 206.
11 Green & Stewart, 365, 367.
12 *Pottery Gazette*, November 1880.
13 Jewitt, 1878, (II), 536; Green & Stewart, 365, 367.
14 *Keates's Directory*, 1879, 13; *Sentinel*, 28 November 1874, p.1, col.6.
15 *Pottery Gazette*, May 1882, July 1890, 633.
16 *Specimens of Wengers' Collection of Pottery ...* (Stoke-on-Trent, 1914) Some Notes on Historical Processes in Pottery, 1873.
17 *Pottery Gazette*, August 1886, 948; September 1886; December 1886, 1416.
18 *Pottery Gazette*, July 1890, 632–3; August 1890, 742.
19 *Pottery Gazette*, November 1880.
20 *Pottery Gazette*, April 1885, 438.
21 British Patent, Provisional Specification 9 November 1885, No. 13,609; Complete Specification 23 July 1886.
22 *Pottery Gazette*, September 1886, 1036, 1073; July 1890, 632.
23 PRO: BT43/72: 3/367549; BT43/73: 3/373541, 7/379767, 5/382407, 5/382408, 2/384160, 2/384161, 3/387958, 3/387959, 3/387960, 2/389894, 1/393107, 3/393418; BT43/74: 3/396056, 2/399135, 2/399136, 5/404329, 5/404330, 4/404571, 4/404745, 3/407624.
24 *Pottery Gazette*, January 1883, 40; April 1883, 344; Jewitt, 1883, 552.
25 Information from Dr. E. E. Collard.
26 *Pottery Gazette* December 1883, 1152–3.
27 *Pottery Gazette*, February 1885, 164.
28 *Pottery Gazette*, March 1886, 431 and January 1887, supplement.
29 Churchill China PLC and private collections.
30 *Pottery Gazette*, November 1882, 1028; February 1887, 177; November 1885, 1303.
31 *Pottery Gazette*, July 1887, supp.2.
32 SA, 19 November 1887, p.8, col.6.
33 *Pottery Gazette*, March 1888, supp.3; June 1888, 545.
34 *Pottery Gazette*, March 1888, 257; April 1888, 353; May 1888, 545.
35 *Pottery Gazette*, February 1889, 120; June 1888, 545; September 1889, 600.
36 *Pottery Gazette*, June 1890, 546.
37 *Pottery Gazette*, June 1890, 554; July 1890, 631–3.
38 *Pottery Gazette*, July 1890, 631–3.
39 *Sentinel*, 9 May 1890.
40 *Sentinel*, 9 May 1890.
41 *Sentinel*, 2 July 1890; *Pottery Gazette* August 1890, 746.

Notes for Chapter 8

1   *Sentinel*, 19 July 1890, p.8.
2   *Pottery Gazette*, August 1890, 742; *Sentinel*, 31 July 1890.
3   VCH, VIII, 241.
4   SA, 15 November 1890, p.8, col.5; *Sentinel*, 21 November 1890, 3.
5   *Pottery Gazette*, October 1890, 931; January 1891, 62; February 1891, 159; April 1891, 343, 447.
6   *Pottery Gazette*, January 1892, 25 and supp.3.
7   J. H. Y. Briggs, *A History of Longton I: The Birth of a Community* (Keele, 1982) 108–9.
8   *Pottery Gazette*, January 1904, 63; Private Collection.
9   *Sentinel*, 7 February 1907.
10 *Pottery Gazette*, January 1892, supp.3.
11 *Montgomery Ward & Co. Catalogue and Buyers' Guide No. 57 Spring and Summer 1895* (reprinted Dover, n.d.) 528.

12 G. A. Godden, *Jewitt's Ceramic Art of Great Britain 1800–1900* (London, 1972) 105.
13 *Pottery Gazette*, July 1897, 890; December 1897, 1546.
14 *Pottery Gazette Diary* 1897, 30, 73.
15 Churchill China PLC Collection.
16 *Pottery Gazette*, July 1903, 637; October 1903, 1006–7.
17 *Sentinel*, 31 October 1924.
18 *Pottery Gazette*, June 1909, 704; June 1913, 668; February 1915, 210.
19 *Pottery Gazette*, December 1922, 1838.
20 *Pottery Gazette*, January 1909, 64–5; March 1910, 287.
21 *Pottery Gazette*, July 1919, 714–6.
22 *Ceramic Society*, Vol. XVI, 1916–17, xiii; C. P. Shah, 'The Effect of Magnesian Glazes on Underglaze Colours', Vol. XVII, 1917–18, 106–110.
23 *Pottery Gazette*, April 1919, 352.
24 *Cox's Potteries Annual & Year Book 1923*, 55.
25 *Sentinel*, 3 November 1924.
26 Somerset House, will of John Gerrard Aynsley died 7 February 1924, proved at Lichfield.

Notes for Chapter 9

1 *Pottery Gazette*, December 1959, 1422; *People of the Potteries Vol. 1* D. Stuart (ed.) (Keele, 1985) 23–4.
2 *Daily Dispatch*, 22 November 1933, 5.
3 Information from Mr. P. O'Reilly.
4 *Pottery Gazette*, December 1932, 1519; Registrar, 11 November 1932.
5 Bridgwood Deeds: Insurance policy 29 September 1932; Debenture 28 November 1932; 8 December 1944.
6 *Hand-painted Gray's Pottery* K. Niblett (ed.) (Stoke-on-Trent, 1982) 57.
7 *Pottery Gazette*, August 1928, 1197, registered no. 292,361.
8 *Pottery Gazette*, October 1939, 1272.
9 *Concentration of the Pottery Industry in North Staffordshire* (Pottery Gazette, n.d. [1941]).
10 *Pottery Gazette Directory* 1942, 36.
11 Bridgwood Deeds, 5 May, 7 July 1943.
12 Registrar: 30 April 1944.
13 Registrar; 25 October 1944; Bridgwood Deeds: 8 August 1944 and letter from Industrial and Commercial Finance Corporation 5 February 1969.
14 Board of Trade *Working Party Reports Pottery* (London, 1946), 48, appendix III, 45, 46.
15 University of Keele, Warrillow Collection: 1383.
16 Wood, Goldstraw & Yorath: Bridgwood plans, 1945.
17 Bridgwood Deeds: 18 October 1945.
18 Registrar: 7 November 1945, 11 April 1946.
19 Registrar: 24 May 1946.
20 Bridgwood Deeds: undated list (1946 from context).
21 Bridgwood Deeds: 14 September 1946; 17 September 1946.
22 Wood, Goldstraw & Yorath: plan 1946.
23 Bridgwood Deeds: 14 September 1946.
24 Registrar: 29 October 1947, 27 January 1948.
25 Registrar: 1 January 1948.
26 *Pottery Gazette*, February 1949, 181.
27 *Pottery Gazette Year Books*, 1946–50.
28 Information from Mr. K. Allerton.
29 Registrar: 22 November 1949.

30   Registrar: 9 June 1964.
31   Wood, Goldstraw & Yorath: plan, 1949.
32   B. R. Williams, 'The Pottery Industry', in *The Structure of British Industry: A Symposium, Vol. II* D. Burns (ed.) (Cambridge 1958) 291–330.
33   Wood, Goldstraw & Yorath: plans: 1950; information from Mr. R. Colclough.
34   Bridgwood Deeds: 3 July 1953.
35   *Pottery Gazette*, November 1959, 1323; December 1959, 1422; *People of the Potteries Vol. 1* D. Stuart (ed.) (Keele, 1985) 23–4.
36   *Sentinel*, 22, 25, 29 September 1959.
37   *Sentinel*, 30 October, 3 November 1959.
38   Information from Mr. D. Morris.
39   Information from Mr. P. O'Reilly.
40   Wood, Goldstraw & Yorath: plans; information from Mr. R. Colclough.
41   Registrar: 23 January 1962.
42   VCH, Vol. VIII, 241.
43   Bridgwood Deeds, 3 July 1953.

Notes for Chapter 10

1   *Pottery Gazette*, April 1965, 468.
2   *Pottery Gazette*, January 1966, 45.
3   Information from Mr. R. Colclough; *Sentinel*, 20 November 1984, 20.
4   *Pottery Gazette*, April 1964, 454; September 1965, 986.
5   *Pottery Gazette*, July 1964, 752.
6   James Broadhurst and Sons Ltd., publicity leaflet 1973.
7   *Pottery Gazette Reference Book 1969*, 53–4.
8   *Pottery Gazette*, February 1964, 246.
9   Information from Mr. W. Morgan.
10   *Pottery Gazette Reference Book 1969*, 140. Kathie Winkle is now Mrs. K. Barker.
11   Information from Mr. W. Morgan.
12   *Pottery Gazette*, December 1964, 1277.
13   Private collection.
14   *Pottery Gazette Reference Book 1969*, 30; information from Mrs. K. Barker.
15   Wood, Goldstraw & Yorath: plans, 1968; information from Mr. R. Colclough.
16   Information from Mr. B. Clarke, Wood, Goldstraw & Yorath; Bridgwood Deeds, 2 October 1971.
17   Wood, Goldstraw & Yorath: plans, 1973, 1974; information from Mr. R. Colclough.
18   *John England Spring/Summer 1974* catalogue, 826–830.
19   Mr. W. Morgan's notebooks, preserved by Mrs. K. Barker.
20   *Tableware International*, June 1976, 17; September 1979, 33–35; information from Mr. W. Morgan.
21   Information from Mr. W. Morgan and Mr. R. Twigg.
22   Leaflets preserved by Mrs. Barker.
23   *Tableware Reference Book 1975*, 3; *Tableware International*, September 1979, 33–35.
24   Information from Mrs. K. Barker.
25   Information from Mr. W. Morgan and Mr. E. E. Orme.
26   Clarence Works Deeds, 1895–1976.
27   *Pottery Gazette,* June 1922, 905.
28   Information from Mrs. N. Whitehouse.
29   *Ceramic Society*, Vol. XXXVI, Part 6, June 1937, vii.
30   *Pottery Gazette*, November 1939, 1376.
31   *Pottery Gazette*, February 1968, 183; *Pottery Gazette Reference Book 1969*, 4.

32 Clarence Works Deeds, 1970, 1974, 1976; information from Mrs. P. Woodhouse.
33 Registrar, 1 February 1977.
34 *Tableware Reference Book 1975*, 4; *Sentinel*, 20 November 1984, 15.
35 *Tableware International*, August 1976, 54.
36 *Tableware International*, May 1976, 43.

Notes for Chapter 11

1 *Tableware International*, September 1979, 33–5.
2 *Tableware Reference Book 1980*, 23.
3 *Tableware International*, September 1979, 34–5; February 1982, 5; *Sentinel*, 20 November 1984, 19.
4 *Tableware International*, September 1979, 33; *Sentinel*, 20 March 1990, 24.
5 Information from Mrs. P. Woodhouse.
6 Registrar, 1978.
7 Information from Mr. R. Colclough, Mr. W. Morgan and Mrs P. Woodhouse.
8 *Tableware Reference Book 1980*, 23; Sales literature preserved by Mrs. T. Brookfield.
9 *Tableware International*, September 1979, 35; *Tableware Reference Book 1979*, 24; *Sentinel*, 20 November 1984, 14.
10 *Sentinel*, 20 November 1984, 17; 20 March 1990, 25.
11 *Tableware International*, February 1982, 5, 8, 9.
12 *Tableware International*, May 1988, 12.
13 *Sentinel*, 20 November 1984, 18; 20 March 1990, 31.
14 *Sentinel*, 20 November 1984, 14.
15 *Ceramic Industries Journal*, October 1988, 23–4.
16 Information from Mr. R. Colclough.
17 *Tableware International*, May 1988, 12; *Sentinel*, 20 March 1990, 27, 31.
18 *Sentinel*, 20 November 1984; *Tableware International*, February 1982, 5–12.
19 Registrar, 17 September 1984.
20 Registrar, 8 February 1985.
21 *European Tableware Buyers Guide 1987*, 17; *Tableware International*, February 1982, 5.
22 *Sentinel*, 20 November 1984.
23 *Sentinel*, 2 October 1986.
24 British Anchor Pottery Deeds: 5 July 1983, 11 September 1985.
25 *Pottery Gazette*, July 1884, 730; August 1884, 1020.
26 *Pottery Gazette*, July 1883, 671; October 1883, 970; February 1884, 190.
27 *Keates's Directory*, 1875.
28 Information from Mr. K. Allerton.
29 British Anchor Pottery Deeds: 22 February 1982.
30 Information from Mr. K. Allerton.
31 Information from Mr. K. Allerton; British Anchor Pottery Deeds: 1 October 1986.
32 *British Telecom Directory Section 226*, June 1987.
33 *Sentinel*, 12 March 1985.
34 G. Godden, *Encyclopaedia of British Porcelain Manufacturers* (London, 1988), 236.
35 *Sentinel*, 20 November 1984, 15; *Tableware International*, May 1988, 12.
36 *Sentinel*, 20 March 1990, 21.
37 Price lists preserved by Mrs. T. Brookfield.
38 Argos Distributors Ltd., Half-annual catalogues.
39 *Staffordshire Life*, December 1989, 41.
40 *Sentinel*, 20 November 1984, 21.
41 *Sentinel*, 20 March 1990, 19, 30; information from Mrs. P. Woodhouse.

42   Information from Mrs. P. Woodhouse.
43   Registrar, 6 March 1981, 1 September 1984.
44   Registrar, 26 July 1984, 3 June 1985.
45   *Sentinel*, 21 March 1990, 29.
46   Registrar, 18 October 1988, 9 June 1989.
47   Registrar, 12 July 1989.
48   Registrar, 22 February 1989; *Staffordshire Life*, December 1989, 41; *Sentinel*, 20 March 1990, 24, 26.
49   *Sentinel*, 20 March 1990, 26.
50   *Sentinel*, 20 March 1990, 46; Registrar, 1 April 1990.
51   *Sentinel*, 20 March 1990, 28.
52   *Tableware International*, August 1990, 48.
53   *Sentinel*, 11 September 1990, 21.
54   *Tableware International*, August 1990, 48.
55   Information from Mrs. P. Woodhouse.
56   *Tableware International*, February 1982, 5, 8, 9; information from Mr. E. E. Orme.
57   Information from Mr. A. D. Roper.
58   *Sentinel*, 26 January 1991, 8; 11 February 1991, 9.

Notes for Chapter 12

1   *Sentinel*, 7 June 1991, 20.
2   SRO: Q/RPL/5/23A-E, Land Tax records for Burslem.
3   J. C. Wedgwood, *Staffordshire Pottery and its History* (London, n.d., [1912]) 52.
4   Shaw, History, 206; Tunnicliff, 1787.
5   *Manchester Mercury*, 22 April, 7 October 1760.
6   SRO: Q/RPL/5/23A-E, Land Tax records for Burslem.
7   SRO: Q/RPL/5/23A-E, Land Tax records for Burslem.
8   UBD, 1797.
9   SRO: Q/RPL/5/23A-E, Land Tax records for Burslem.
10   SRO: Q/RPL/5/23A-E, Land Tax records for Burslem.
11   SRO: 239/M/63, mortgage deed 30 May 1829.
12   Jewitt, 1878, II, 290.
13   HRL: EMT 13/811, Adams papers.
14   W. Mankowitz & R. G. Haggar, *The Concise Encyclopedia of English Pottery and Porcelain* (London, 1957) 269.
15   SA, 20 July 1799.
16   SRO: Q/RPL/5/23A-E, Land Tax records for Burslem.
17   SA, 27 March 1813.
18   Wedgwood MSS 33/25182: quoted by R. Pomfret Esq., lecture to Friends of Blue, 15 October 1989.
19   SA, 7 September 1816.
20   W. Mankowitz & R. G. Haggar, *The Concise Encyclopedia of English Pottery and Porcelain* (London, 1957) 210.
21   A. W. Coysh and R. K. Henrywood, *The Dictionary of Blue and White Printed Pottery 1780–1880* (Woodbridge, 1982) 260, 349, Plate XX.
22   E. B. Larsen, 'The Truth about Andrew Stevenson' in *English Pottery and Porcelain* P. Atterbury (ed.) (London, 1980) 198–201.
23   SRO: Q/RPL/5/23A-E, Land Tax records for Burslem.
24   SA, 24 March 1855.
25   SRO: Q/RPL/5/23A-E, Land Tax records for Burslem.
26   UBD, 1797.
27   *Holden's Triennial Directory for 1809, 1810, 1811* (London, 1809) 368.
28   *Newcastle under Lyme Parish Register 1771–1812* (Birmingham, 1981) 115, 133.

29   J. Ingamells, *Historical Records and Directory of Newcastle-under-Lyme* second edition (Newcastle-under-Lyme, 1881) 80.

30   SA, 6 November 1819.

31   J. Ingamells, *Historical Records and Directory of Newcastle-under-Lyme* second edition (Newcastle-under-Lyme, 1881) 80.

32   Wedgwood MSS33/25182: quoted by R. Pomfret Esq., lecture to Friends of Blue, 15 October 1989.

33   R. Pomfret Esq., lecture to Friends of Blue, 15 October 1989.

34   F. Stefano, 'James and Ralph Clews, nineteenth-century potters, Part I: The English experience' in *English Pottery and Porcelain* P. Atterbury (ed.) (London, 1980) 202–06.

35   F. Stefano, 'James and Ralph Clews, nineteenth-century potters, Part I: The English experience' in *English Pottery and Porcelain* P. Atterbury (ed.) (London, 1980) 202–06.

36   R. Pomfret Esq., lecture to Friends of Blue, 15 October 1989.

37   *The Harmsworth Encyclopaedia Vol. V* (London, n.d.) 3060.

38   F. Stefano, 'James and Ralph Clews, nineteenth-century potters, Part I: The English experience' in *English Pottery and Porcelain* P. Atterbury (ed.) (London, 1980) 203.

39   SA, 19 April 1828.

40   R. Pomfret Esq., lecture to Friends of Blue, 15 October 1989; F. Stefano, 'James and Ralph Clews, nineteenth-century potters, Part I: The English experience' in *English Pottery and Porcelain* P. Atterbury (ed.) (London, 1980) 202–03.

41   SA, 26 April 1834, *passim* to 30 May 1835.

42   F. Stefano, 'James Clews, nineteenth-century potter, Part II: The American experience', in *English Pottery and Porcelain* P. Atterbury (ed.) (London, 1980) 207–09.

43   SA, 19 November 1836, 16 December 1837, 21 March 1857; *Newcastle under Lyme Parish Register 1771–1812* (Birmingham, 1981) 348, 24 August 1812.

44   SA, 16 May 1863.

45   White's Directory, 1834. For a more detailed account of Brownfields at Cobridge, see R. and E. Hampson, 'Brownfields, Victorian Potters' in *Northern Ceramic Society Journal Volume 4* (1981) 177–218.

46   SA, 9 September 1837, 31 July 1841.

47   Pigot, 1841.

48   *Williams's Commercial Directory for Stafford and the Potteries* (Manchester, 1846).

49   SA, 16 November 1850.

50   SA, 16 March 1844.

51   SA, 13 November 1858.

52   SA, 12 July 1862.

53   SA, 23 April 1859.

54   Jewitt, 1878, II, 290–93.

55   SA, 3 May 1862, *The Art Journal New Series Vol. I* 1962, 165, SA, 23 February 1867, *Art Journal Catalogue, 1871*, 187, 301.

56   Jewitt, 1878, II, 292.

57   Jewitt, 1878, II, 290.

58   W. Mankowitz and R. G. Haggar, *The Concise Encyclopedia of English Pottery and Porcelain* (London, 1957) 117–18.

59   *Sentinel*, 14 July 1873.

60   SA, 19 July 1873.

61   *Pottery Gazette*, 1 June 1911, 662.

62   *Sentinel*, 26 April 1884.

63   *Pottery Gazette*, 1 May 1884.

64   SA, 27 April 1889.

65   SA, 10 March 1894.

66 SA, 26 May 1883; Somerset House: Administration, William Etches Brownfield, 20 May 1904.

67 A. Huntbach, *Hanley Stoke-on-Trent 13th to 20th Century* (Stafford, 1910) 37.

68 *Pottery Gazette* 1 December 1881, 1042, 1052; G. W. Rhead and F. A. Rhead, *Staffordshire Pots & Potters* (London, 1906) 308.

69 Minton MSS: 1031 *passim* to 1166.

70 A. Brownfield, *The Lockout – A Potters Guild* (Hanley, 1892).

71 *Pottery Gazette*, 1 October 1892, 916.

72 *Pottery Gazette*, 1 December 1897, 1555.

73 *Pottery Gazette*, 1 October 1900, 1137.

74 'A History of Co-operation in North Staffordshire' (anonymous typescript in Hanley Reference Library, S 800.334).

75 SA, 15 September 1900.

76 *Pottery Gazette*, 1 May 1902, 451; 2 June 1902, 583.

77 Keates's Directory, 1892–93; W. Scarratt, *Old Times in the Potteries*, (Stoke-on-Trent, 1906) 141.

78 *Pottery Gazette*, 2 June 1902, 583.

79 *Kelly's Directory*, 1912.

80 *Pottery Gazette*, 2 April 1906, 589.

81 *Grimwades Ltd.* (1920 booklet in Hanley Reference Library, P738.94246 GRI).

82 Ordnance Survey 1/2500 Plan *Staffordshire XII.9*, revised 1922.

83 *Sentinel*, 1 May 1925.

84 *Pottery Gazette*, 1 December 1927, 1861.

85 *Pottery Gazette*, 1 April 1902, 379.

86 Census, 1881, Newcastle-under-Lyme, District No. 2, Ironmarket.

87 *Pottery Gazette*, March 1961, 400.

88 *Pottery Gazette*, 1 August 1902, 735.

89 Ordnance Survey 1/2500 Plan *Staffordshire XII.9*, revised 1922.

90 G. Hulme, 'The Wedgwood Bicentenary Proceedings' in *Transactions of the Ceramic Society Vol. XXIX, No. 6* (June, 1930) 497.

91 *Sentinel*, 6 January 1970.

92 *Pottery Gazette*, 1 February 1937, 252.

93 *Pottery Gazette*, 1 April 1937, 555.

94 *Concentration of the Pottery Industry in North Staffordshire* (Pottery Gazette, n.d. [1941]).

95 *Sentinel*, 6 January 1970, 16.

96 *Sentinel*, 1 January 1953, 5.

97 *Pottery Gazette Reference Book 1949*, 30.

98 *Pottery Gazette*, September 1950. 1360.

99 *Pottery Gazette*, January 1961, 120.

100 *Pottery Gazette*, June 1969, 521.

101 *Sentinel*, 3 October 1969; *Pottery Gazette*, November 1969, 901.

102 *Sentinel*, 7 January 1970, 3; *Pottery Gazette*, February 1970, 105.

103 *Tableware International*, August 1976, 25.

104 *Tableware International*, July 1976, 18.

105 *Sentinel*, 3 January 1980, 2 June 1982; *Tableware International*, May 1983, 48–49.

106 *Tableware International*, March 1991, 50.

107 *Tableware International*, April 1986, 28.

108 *Sentinel*, 18 March 1988.

109 *Sentinel*, 22 July 1989.

110 *Sentinel*, 18 April 1991.

111 *Sentinel*, 18 April 1991, 37; 7 June 1991, 20.

112 *Sentinel*, 7 June 1991.

113 Jewitt, 1878, II, 395.

114 J. C. Wedgwood, *Staffordshire Pottery and its History* (London, n.d., [1912]) 193.

115 *Pottery Gazette*, 1 July 1908, 819.
116 *Pottery Gazette*, 1 August 1908, 947.
117 *Pottery Gazette Reference Book 1969*, 69.
118 *Pottery Gazette Reference Book 1952*, 77–78.
119 *Pottery – The Story of Alfred Meakin (Tunstall) Ltd.* (Tunstall, 1949).
120 VCH VIII, 89, 92.
121 VCH VIII, 101.
122 *Pottery Gazette*, April 1968, 382–83.

Notes for Chapter 13

1   Letter from Andrew Roper, 1 October 1992; *Evening Sentinel* 5 May 1993, 5.
2   Churchill China PLC, Company Plan.
3   Letter from Andrew Roper, 1 October 1992.
4   *Tableware International* August 1993, 13.
5   *Tableware International* June 1992, 52–53.
6   *Tableware International* June 1993, 4.
7   *Radio Times* 7–13 November 1992, 35–36.
8   *Sentinel* 29 December 1992, 8.
9   *Radio Times* 7–13 November 1992, 35–36.
10 Information from Bernard Burns, May 1993.
11 Information from Wendy Morton, August and October 1993.
12 Churchill China PLC, Tableware Division, Sales & Marketing Structure.
13 *Financial Times* 12 May 1992.
14 *Sentinel* 24 March 1993, 24.
15 *Sentinel* 17 March 1993, 28.
16 *Sentinel* 12 May 1993, 24.
17 *Advertiser* 22 October 1992, 6; *Sentinel* 11 November 1992, 33.
18 *Tableware International* August 1993, 13.
19 Information from Candida Kelsall, May 1993.
20 *Churchill News No. 4* Summer 1993, 4.
21 Information from Edward Orme, September 1993.
22 Information from Wendy Morton, March 1994.
23 *Tableware International* June 1992, insert; June 1993, 15–16.
24 Information from Bernard Burns, May 1993.
25 *Tableware International* June 1992, insert.
26 *Tableware International* September 1993, 14.
27 *Sentinel* 10 March 1992.
28 *Tableware International* June 1992, insert.
29 Information from Simon Bell, May 1993.
30 Information from Wendy Morton, October 1993.
31 *Sentinel* 21 April 1993, 19.
32 *Sentinel* 21 April 1993, 24; 10 November 1993, 26.
33 Information from Andrew Roper, May 1993.
34 Information from Edward Orme, May 1993; *Financial Times* 12 May 1992.
35 *Financial Times* 12 May 1992; *Churchill Tableware 1993* catalogue; information from Alan Miles and Dennis Heywood, May 1993.
36 Information from Edward Orme, May 1993.
37 *Sentinel* 17 March 1993, 25.
38 Information from Wendy Morton, August 1993.
39 Information from Sue Platt, August 1993.
40 Information from Sue Platt, August 1993.
41 Information from Edward Orme, September 1993.
42 Information from Sue Platt, August 1993.
43 Information from Sue Platt, August 1993.

44   Information from Alan Miles and Dennis Heywood, May 1993.
45   Information from Dee Frankish, May 1993.
46   *Churchill News No. 4* Summer 1993, 4.
47   Information from Dee Frankish, May 1993.
48   *Advertiser* 28 January 1993, 16.
49   Information from Dennis Heywood, October 1993.
50   Information from Sue Platt, August 1993.
51   *Churchill News No. 4* Summer 1993, 4.
52   *Sentinel* 2 March 1994, 32; see Chapter 8, Figure 30.
53   *Churchill Hotelware* catalogue, 1993.
54   Information from Alan Miles and Dennis Heywood, May 1993.
55   Information from Wendy Morton, August 1993 and Dennis Heywood, October 1993.
56   Information from Sue Platt, August 1993 and Ray Colclough, October 1993.
57   Information from Wendy Morton, August 1993.
58   *Sentinel* 19 May 1993, 19; Waterford Wedgwood PLC Report and Accounts 1992, 7.
59   Information from Wendy Morton, August 1993.
60   Company statement, August 1993.
61   *Sentinel* 19 May 1993, 22.
62   Company statement, August 1993.
63   Company statement, August 1993.
64   *Churchill News No. 4* Summer 1993.
65   Information from Andrew Roper and Pam Woodhouse, May 1993.

INDEX

Pattern and Shape names are indexed under the heading of *Patterns and Shapes Names*

INDEX

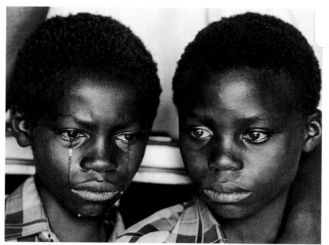

soweto

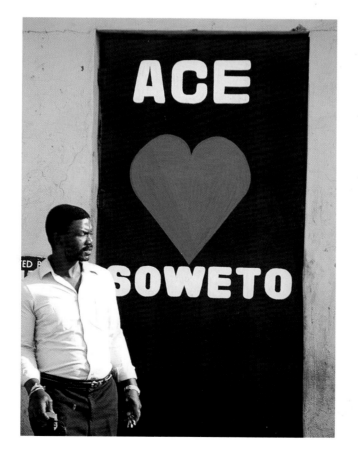

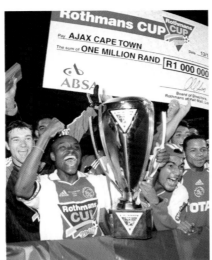
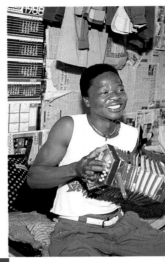
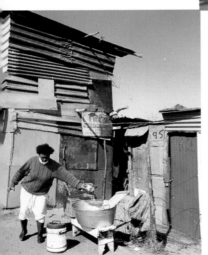
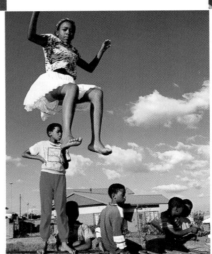
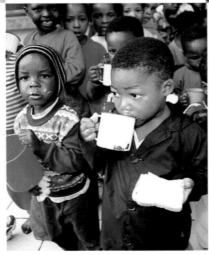
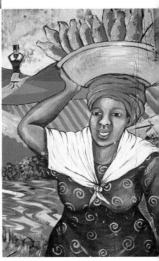

soweto

PETER MAGUBANE

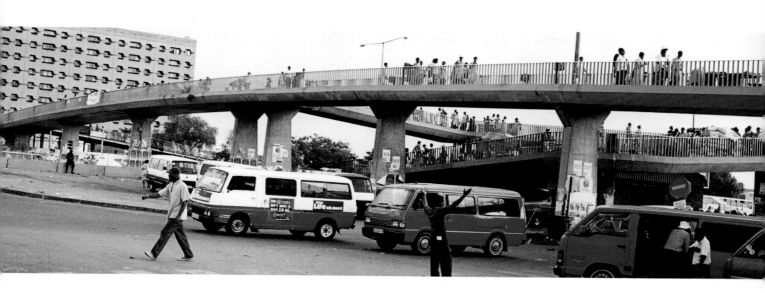

TEXT BY CHARLENE SMITH

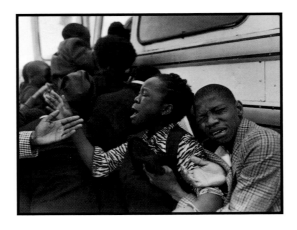

First published in 2001 by Struik Publishers
(a division of New Holland Publishing (South Africa) (Pty) Ltd)
London · Cape Town · Sydney · Auckland

Garfield House
86 Edgware Road
W2 2EA London
United Kingdom

14 Aquatic Drive
Frenchs Forest
NSW 2086
Australia

80 McKenzie Street
Cape Town 8001
South Africa

218 Lake Road
Northcote, Auckland
New Zealand

Website: **www.struik.co.za**

2 4 6 8 10 9 7 5 3 1

Copyright © 2001 in published edition: Struik Publishers (Pty) Ltd
Copyright © 2001 in photographs: Peter Magubane
Copyright © 2001 in text: Charlene Smith
Copyright © 2001 in map on pages 6–7: Struik Publishers

ISBN 1 86872 584 7

Designer: Janice Evans
Managing editor: Lesley Hay-Whitton
Publishing manager: Annlerie van Rooyen
Design assistant: Illana Fridkin
Proofreader: Helen Keevy
Indexer: Sylvia Grobbelaar
Cartographer: John Hall

Reproduction by Hirt & Carter Cape (Pty) Ltd
Printed in Hong Kong by Sing Cheong Printing Company Limited

Front cover: Street child reunited with his mother (*top left*), double-storey shack in Mandelaville Squatter Camp (*top right*), teargas victims, Avalon Cemetery, 1978 unrest (*centre left*), a Soweto woman working in her kitchen (*centre*), singer Mara Louw and her daughter Lerato (*centre right*), child drinking from a communal tap (*bottom*); front flap: Sowetan men in a shebeen; back cover: child labourer with his dog (*top*), a Soweto barber's shop (*centre left*), Soweto women fetching water for the family (*centre right*), mural in Soweto (*bottom*). Page 1: Twelve-year-old twins whose mother burnt to death in a car accident in 1975 (*top*); sign in Soweto (*bottom*); page 2: soccer match at which Ajax Cape Town beat Orlando Pirates 4–1 at the FNB Stadium (*top left*), music is a way of life for Sowetans (*top right*), Mandelaville Squatter Camp (*centre left*), Sowetan children trampolining (*centre right*), school feeding schemes keep children well nourished (*bottom left*), a mural in Soweto depicting a 'mealie lady' (*bottom right*); page 3: the pedestrian bridge and taxi rank at Chris Hani-Baragwanath Hospital. Above: teargas victims at Avalon Cemetery, 1978; opposite page: Peter Magubane in 1955.

Quotations on the cover are from the following sources. Front cover: Louis Rive, *The Significance of Soweto*; back cover: the Freedom Charter (*top*), Nelson Mandela, *Long Walk to Freedom* (*centre right*), Father Trevor Huddleston, *Naught for your Comfort* (*centre left*), Charlene Smith (*bottom*).

This book is dedicated to my dear parents:
my father Isaac, who gave me my very first
camera, a Kodak Brownie, that I used at school,
and my mother Wilhelmina for her strictness.
I also extend my thanks to Cindy Futhane
for her invaluable assistance.

Peter Magubane, 2001

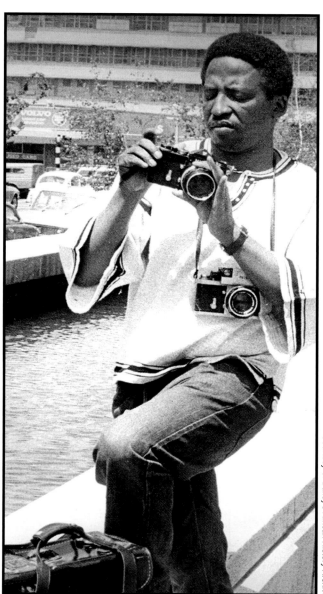

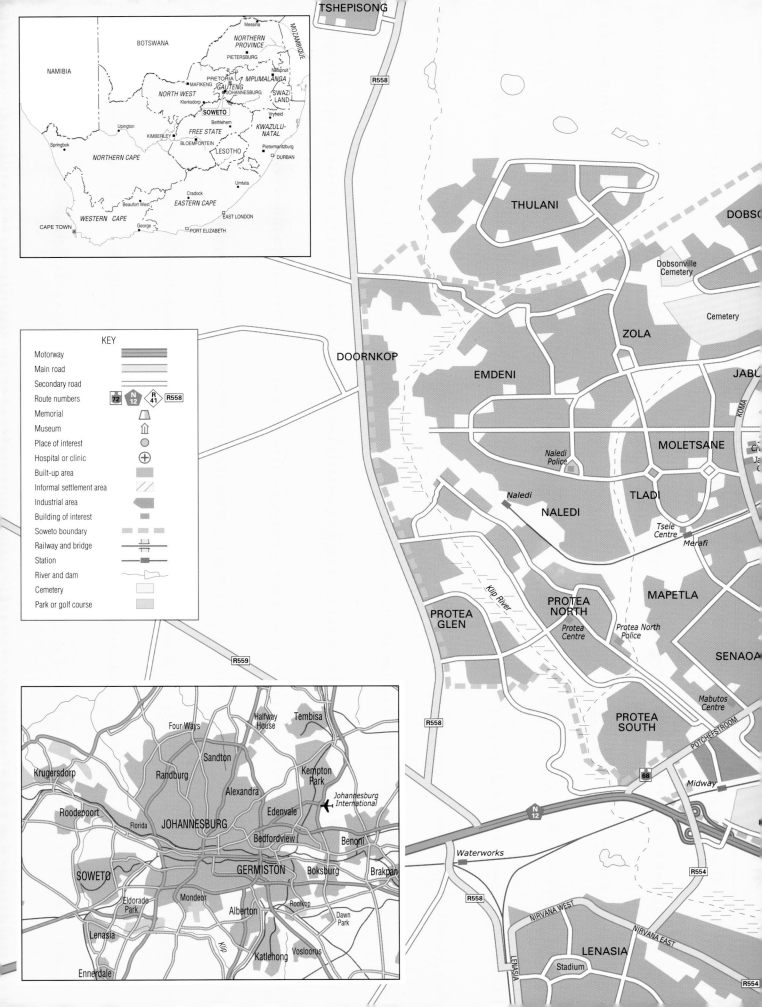

TSHEPISONG

R558

THULANI

DOBSO

Dobsonville
Cemetery

Cemetery

ZOLA

DOORNKOP

EMDENI

JABU

KOMA

MOLETSANE

Naledi
Police

Ci...
Ja...
O...

Naledi

TLADI

NALEDI

Tsele
Centre

Merafi

MAPETLA

PROTEA
GLEN

Klip River

PROTEA
NORTH

Protea
Centre

Protea North
Police

SENAOA

Mabutos
Centre

PROTEA
SOUTH

R558

POTCHEFSTROOM

68

Midway

N
12

Waterworks

R554

R558

NIRVANA WEST

NIRVANA EAST

LENASIA

LENASIA

Stadium

R554

KEY

Motorway	
Main road	
Secondary road	
Route numbers	72 N 12 R 41 R558
Memorial	
Museum	
Place of interest	○
Hospital or clinic	⊕
Built-up area	
Informal settlement area	
Industrial area	
Building of interest	
Soweto boundary	
Railway and bridge	
Station	
River and dam	
Cemetery	
Park or golf course	

R559

Inset map (top left)

BOTSWANA

NAMIBIA

NORTHERN
PROVINCE

Messina

MOZAMBIQUE

PIETERSBURG

PRETORIA MPUMALANGA

Nelspruit

MAFIKENG

GAUTENG
JOHANNESBURG

SWAZI-
LAND

NORTH WEST

Klerksdorp

SOWETO

Vryheid

Upington

FREE STATE

Bethlehem

KWAZULU-
NATAL

Springbok

KIMBERLEY

BLOEMFONTEIN

LESOTHO

Pietermaritzburg

NORTHERN CAPE

DURBAN

Cradock

Umtata

Beaufort West

EASTERN CAPE

WESTERN CAPE

George

EAST LONDON

CAPE TOWN

PORT ELIZABETH

Inset map (bottom left)

Four Ways

Halfway
House

Tembisa

Sandton

Krugersdorp

Randburg

Kempton
Park

Alexandra

Johannesburg
International

Roodepoort

Edenvale

Florida

JOHANNESBURG

Bedfordview

Benoni

SOWETO

GERMISTON

Boksburg

Brakpan

Mondeor

Eldorado
Park

Alberton

Roolkop

Dawn
Park

Lenasia

Klip

Katlehong

Vosloorus

Ennerdale

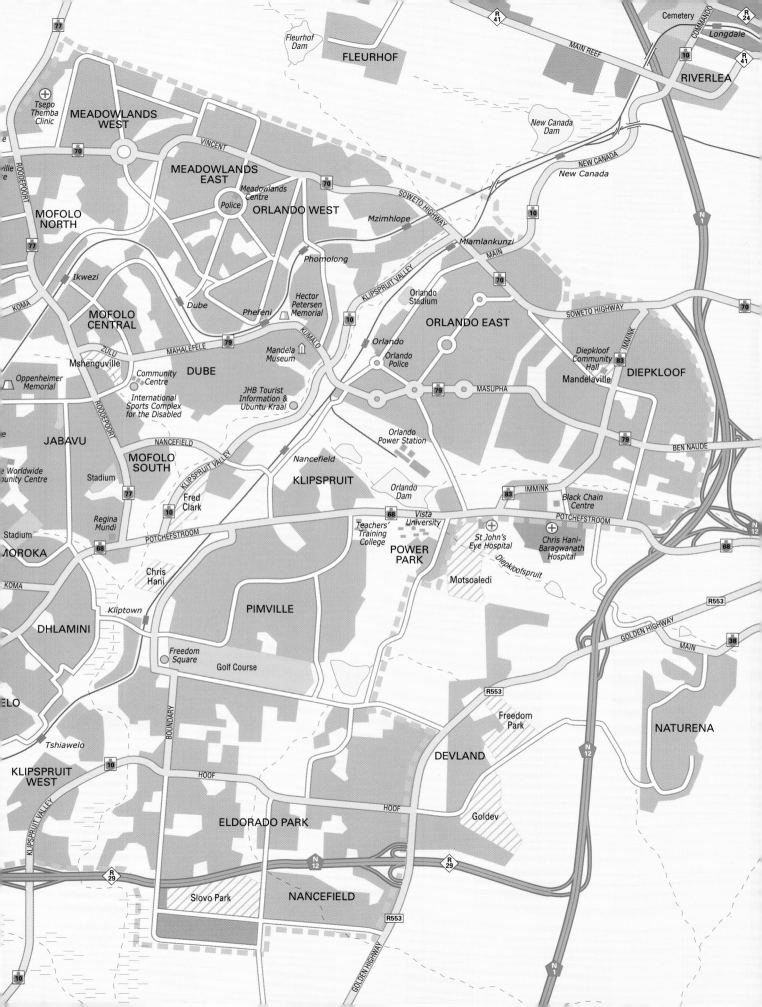

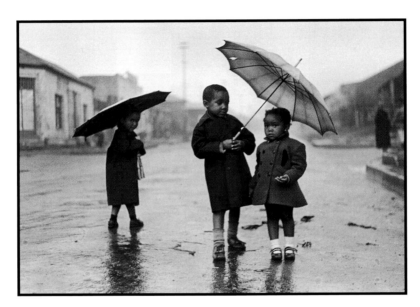

Sophiatown, 1955

And I am certain that ...
all shall be well ...
for the Africa I love,
the Africa of my heart's desire

Father Trevor Huddleston

(*Naught for your Comfort*, 1956)

I shall never forget that winter morning
A rainy November morning
They dismantled our shantytown ...
Morena! I thought I was dreaming
As at the bank of Klip River
Sprawled on the bank; demobbed soldiers
To demob our peaceful camp
In the name of human rights
In the year of allied nations ...
A stinking lavatory hole there,
A heap of rubbish here,
A stray dog there
It's all that is left ...
South, west, we are being driven in circles ...

Modikwe Dikobe

(*Shantytown Removal*, 1948)

SOWETO'S EVOLUTION

Ubucub' obuhle buhamba ngabubili
('Good waxbills go in pairs')

According to this Zulu proverb

two people are always better than one:

they are interdependent, as

Johannesburg and Soweto are.

Less than a century ago, Soweto did not exist. Today's smoky stretch of densely packed people was just another patch of highveld, and few could have predicted the worldwide impact and historical significance that it was to have in the future.

With the discovery of gold in 1886, Johannesburg grew rapidly and haphazardly. It was a wild town of few rules, its economy, ever hungry for cheap labour, dominated by gold, liquor and prostitution. Rural black people flocked to the town, some driven by the introduction of taxes that had to be paid, others drawn by the glinting prospect of wealth. Black men entered short-term contracts on the mines, leaving their families in rural areas while they lived in single-sex barracks on mining property. They also came to supply the other needs of the fledgling town, braving the squalor of the racially mixed slums around the city centre.

In 1904, plague spread among the black residents of Vrededorp, one such suburb hugging the centre of Johannesburg, to the west of its produce market and abattoir. Seeing this as an opportunity to clear out the slums, the Johannesburg Town Council forced the ill to move to a sewage farm more than 10 kilometres to the south-west of Johannesburg. Here they lived in corrugated iron sewage tanks that had been sawn in half (43 years later those people were still living in the tanks). Klipspruit, as this new area was called, was the seed of Soweto, becoming the location of Pimville.

The Land Act was introduced in 1913, dispossessing many black people of their land and increasing the now steady flow of migrants to Johannesburg. By the early 1920s there were more than 20,000 black people living in and around the city, the number doubling before the end of the decade.

Despite their efforts, the town council was unsuccessful in keeping black people from living in the city centre. The council did not possess the finances to set up housing elsewhere for evicted inner-city black people, something that they were obliged by law to do. A change of law and an upswing in the gold price appeared to solve their problem; in 1931, a new area of low-cost housing was created for black people near Johannesburg. Orlando, named after Councillor Edwin Orlando Leake, the first chairman of the Native Affairs Committee, was close to Pimville, the two later forming the heart of Soweto.

Between 1936 and 1946, the black population of Johannesburg increased by more than 100,000, the Second World War having a major impact on urbanisation. Many more people facing poverty and land confiscation moved to the cities with their families. Yet the council built fewer than 4,000 houses for black people during this time, a trend the apartheid government would continue. The rationale was that, if houses were not built for black people, who were not allowed to build in 'white' areas, they would eventually return to rural areas. Orlando rapidly became a sprawl of backyard shanties, as new-comers had no option but to rent space in the yards of those with houses.

In 1944, an Orlando local, James 'Sofasonke' Mpanza gave up petitioning the Johannesburg Town Council for more houses for black people and led a large group of protesters from Orlando to erect shacks on open municipal land in an area that was to become Orlando West. Soon 25,000 shanties had sprung up. Mpanza showed that, if the white authorities refused to listen to black demands, black people would take matters into their own hands.

In the 1940s and 50s, increased pressure by the growing number of squatters on the council forced them to declare new areas for settlement. These included Jabavu and Moroka where people constructed shanties on miniscule plots and lived in highly insanitary conditions. Diepkloof and Meadowlands, with their tiny houses were further additions. Under the Nationalist apartheid government it was ruled that all black residential areas in Johannesburg were to be to the south-west of the city, in the area around Orlando. The racially-mixed suburb of Sophiatown was just one of the casualities in the government's actions to entrench racial segregation and clear out the slums of the city centre; many Sophiatown residents were moved to these two new suburbs.

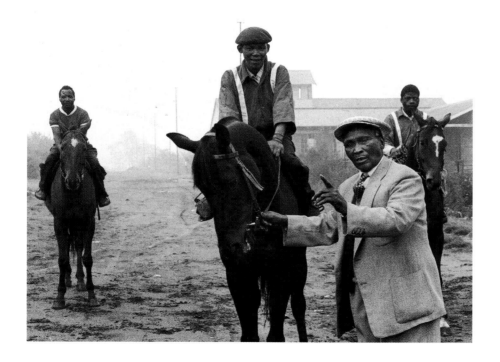

'Sofasonke' Mpanza, one of the great men of Soweto, with some of his race horses. Since black people were not allowed to own race horses, his horses were raced under the names of white people, who acted as fronts.

A young lawyer, Nelson Mandela, considered these matters when, in 1944, he and friends Oliver Tambo, a lawyer, and Walter Sisulu, an estate agent, joined the African National Congress Youth League (ANCYL), led by Anton Lembede. The three lived in Orlando and were acutely aware of the challenges facing inhabitants of the bustling township and surrounding shanty towns. Sisulu sold houses in areas like Dube where freehold title was allowed. (Soon after coming into power in 1948, the Nationalist government removed freehold from black homeowners, and replaced it with 30-year leaseholds.) He was conscious of the housing problems and the barriers to finance for housing that black people experienced. The three discussed these issues, speaking about them on public platforms, and rapidly rising to senior positions in the ANCYL.

In 1955, the Minister of Justice, Hendrik Verwoerd, the architect of apartheid, ordered single-sex hostels to be built in what had officially become known as the South Western Townships. The idea was that men would leave their families in the impoverished rural areas demarcated for black people (only 13% of the country for over 80% of the population), come to the city to work, live in single-sex hostels, and return for vacations and retirement to their rural homes. In 1956 the first men were moved into the hostels: Dube for Zulu-speakers and Nancefield for Sotho-speakers.

Hostel dwellers were discriminated against by township residents, who whispered that they were having sex with young boys. The men in the hostels hated township residents too; they knew they were looked down upon and bitterly resented it. Hostels rapidly became dens of beer drinking and dagga smoking. Their facilities were shocking: they had only cold water; there were no partitions between toilets, and no toilet paper was provided; a single washbasin for clothes, dishes and ablutions was shared by dozens of men; one small coal stove was shared by 20 or more people; and beds were either concrete bunks or rickety steel frames with cheap foam mattresses.

A competition was held in 1959 to find a name for the sprawling community of

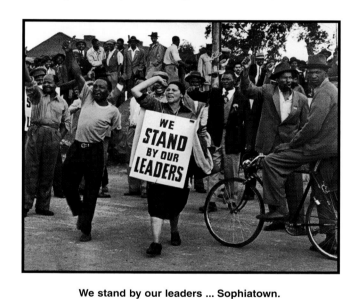

We stand by our leaders ... Sophiatown.

The late 1940s were a heady time in campaigns for black rights. 'We stand by our leaders' was the rallying call for those who supported leaders in the Defiance Campaign led by the African National Congress against unjust laws. Little did these demonstrators in Sophiatown know that in 1948 the Nationalist government would come to power, increasing racial separation and injustice. These people would be forcibly moved from Sophiatown to the burgeoning South Western Townships, later Soweto, and the white rulers would cynically rename the area Triomf (Afrikaans for 'Triumph').

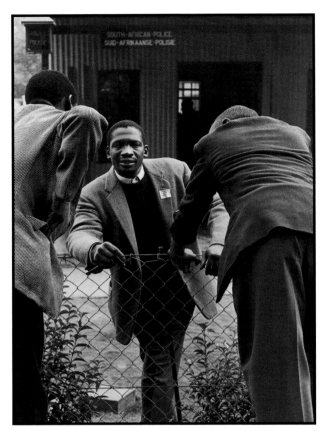

'Africa for Africans' became the rallying cry of the Pan-Africanist Congress under Robert Sobukwe (*centre*). He formed the organisation after breaking away from the African National Congress in the late 1950s in protest at the ANC allowing white membership. On this day, Sobukwe and his followers began burning the 'passes' that controlled their movement, capacity to marry, find work and accommodation, and indeed be a lawful citizen. Sobukwe surrendered himself to the police at the Orlando police station on 21 March 1960, while 100 kilometres away, at Sharpeville, police opened fire on peaceful demonstrators burning their pass books, and killed 69 people. Within a year Sobukwe was jailed in a solitary hut built for him on Robben Island, a bleak windswept prison island in the Atlantic Ocean, just off Cape Town. Sobukwe lived out most of his days in imposed solitary confinement until shortly before his death less than two decades later.

hostels, shacks and tiny houses that sheltered more than half a million people outside Johannesburg, and that the apartheid government saw as its showpiece of slum clearance. Names such as Vergenoeg ('far enough'), Goldella, Dumuzweni ('famous the world round') and Khethollo ('segregation') were submitted. It took four years for the naming committee to settle on Soweto, an abbreviation of South Western Townships.

Willem Carr, the Administrator of Soweto, divided the new city according to ethnicity: Zulu people lived in Zola, for example, and the Baralong and Sotho in Naledi. The closeness of the community was thus shattered and ethnic tensions began emerging.

Finding a place to stay in the designated suburb of the vast township and dealing with the often atrocious living conditions were only a part of the problem faced by black people coming to live and work in Johannesburg. A section 10 stamp in every black person's identity book or pass (known dismissively by African people as a *dompas*, 'stupid pass'), introduced in 1955, determined whom they could marry, where they could live, and whether or not they might work in the so-called 'white urban areas'. Even those people who were qualified by a section 10 stamp to live in urban areas could be endorsed out of the city by another stamp that gave them 72 hours to leave.

By 1959, both the ANC and a break-away wing, the Pan-Africanist Congress, had launched anti-pass campaigns. On 21 March

1960, protesters set fire to their passes outside a police station in a township called Sharpeville, roughly 100 kilometres south of Soweto. Police opened fire, killing 69 people. The demonstrations that followed saw swift and ruthless police action. People were detained, both people and organisations were banned, and there was a massive escalation in the repression of black people.

While political activism appeared to be crushed, interest in the news media flourished, much of it drawing its inspiration from the busy streets of Soweto. Black publications like *Drum*, *Golden City Post* and *Bantu World* had healthy circulations. They encouraged interest in music, with musicians such as Dolly Rathebe and

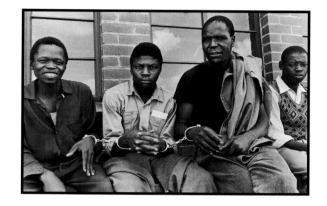

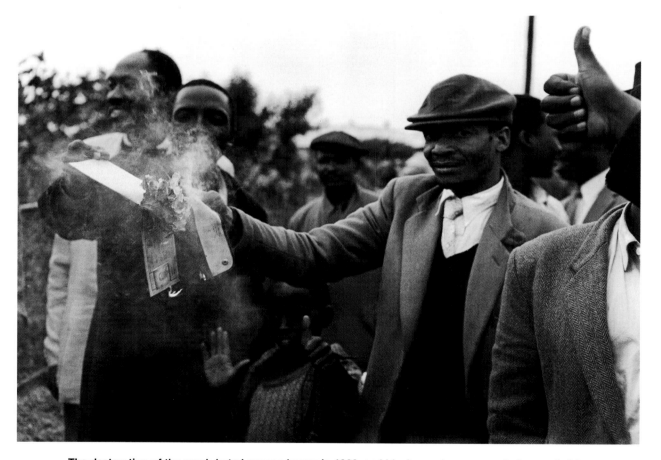

The destruction of the much-hated passes began in 1960, and black people were regularly arrested for 'pass offences' (*top*). A Soweto commuter (*above*) holds his burning pass in his hand while a supporter of his actions gives the ANC thumbs-up salute of the 1950s and early 1960s.

Police dogs growling at crowds became a common scene in the apartheid years. These dogs force back a crowd at Orlando stadium in Soweto in the early 1960s.

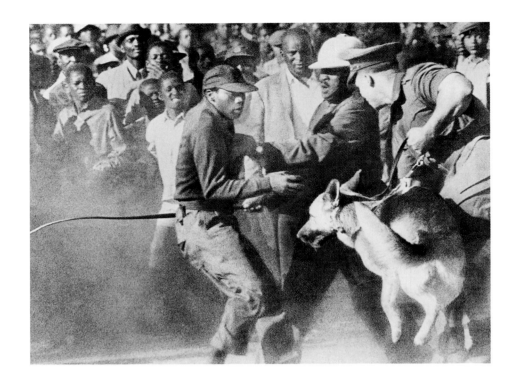

Kippie Moeketsi leading the jazz-influenced scene. There was an intense interest in sports, in particular soccer which drew large devoted followings. Orlando Pirates, Moroka Swallows and the inimitable Kaiser Chiefs are a few of the Soweto-born teams that continue to draw huge crowds.

Soweto's spirit was far from crushed, and oppression always carries with it a necessary ancillary – the spirit of resistance. In July 1969, the match was lit again when the South African Students' Organisation (SASO) was formed at the University of the North. Young people, mostly from Soweto and townships around it, began studying the writings of Frantz Fanon, Kwame Nkrumah and, most of all, Malcolm X. In 1972, SASO fell under the Black People's Convention, which came to embody the Black Consciousness being articulated by a brilliant young medical student, Steven Bantu Biko, who said: 'Black consciousness seeks to instill the idea of self determination, to restore feelings of pride and dignity to blacks after centuries of racist oppression.' Nowhere did the words of this young man have greater resonance than in the streets, shebeens and schools of Soweto.

SOWETO TODAY

When I am old I would like to have a wife and to children
a boy and a girl and a big house and to dogs and freedom.
My friends and I would like to meat together and tok

Moagi (8), Soweto

(*Two Dogs and Freedom*, Ravan Press, 1986)

During the apartheid era, Soweto was dubbed 'the shadow city': a city eclipsing Johannesburg both in size and population, but a place the white rulers tried to pretend was not there – until the Soweto student uprising of 1976 forever ended that. The 1976 uprising against Afrikaans as a medium of instruction (*see* pages 22–35) saw black pupils shot by police after protesting discriminatory and inferior education. It signalled the beginning of the end of apartheid, and put Soweto on the world map.

By 1976 Soweto had a population of some two million people, compared with one million living in Johannesburg.

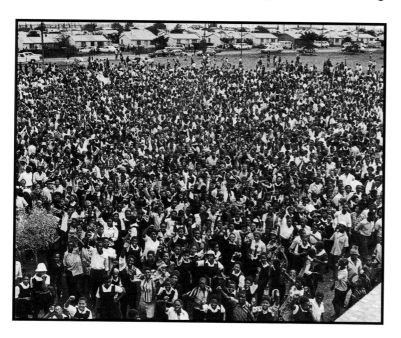

Symbols of the hated white rule of repression in Soweto were all attacked in 1976 by angry students after police opened fire on them. They burned down the beer halls erected to fund the infrastructure of the township and, as young black people perceived it, to enslave their parents with liquor. Schools were burnt down, pass offices razed, even clinics were torched. Students marched on the Soweto administration offices in Jabulani that would soon see 'puppet' black mayors present a façade of black autonomy. Not long after this photograph (*left*) was taken, a heavy police contingent teargassed and scattered the crowd. The entire perimeter of these buildings was then encased in razor wire, high security fencing, watchtowers and, at certain stages over the years, even sandbags to repel the occasional grenade or drive-by AK47 attack by guerrillas.

It had no industrial or commercial infrastructure, only one swimming pool, one park, and many small shops but no shopping centres. It was a place that white people tried to ignore, even though it was crammed with the labour force that kept Johannesburg moving and growing. Soweto was, and still is, a sprawl of small matchbox houses,whose bland exteriors belie the vibrancy of the city.

In winter and summer, it is a red-roofed, red dust sort of place, set among beige highveld grasslands. Occasionally the rains swell the Klipspruit River, but most of the time it meanders lazily through the township, giving the city its lush borders of green. Roadside enterprises offer anything from goats and chickens for slaughter, to wedding cakes and coffins.

Less than 20 years ago Soweto had no pharmacy, no hairstylists, no shopping malls, and a few banks. The burden of women was to trek daily into and out of Johannesburg, braving cramped, often dangerous and unreliable public transport, weighed down by supermarket bags from the city.

Soweto is still a long way from being a shoppers' paradise, but today you can buy live chickens at the roadside or frozen birds from a supermarket refrigerator. Hairstylists range from barbers under trees with a good range of gossip, to chic salons and elegant stylists. Nightlife was formerly restricted to shebeens and one or two clubs. Now residents have a choice of cinemas, restaurants, clubs, taverns and theatres.

The introduction of shopping malls into Soweto in the mid-1990s was not easy. The first major mall at Dobsonville stood for months with huge empty parking lots and unemployed young people shuffling around its corridors. Today the picture has improved. Cinema managers initially complained that township cinemas were being frequented only by young men, and that higher income couples and families were still driving all the way to Johannesburg or Sandton to watch movies, where nightlife was deemed to be more sophisticated than in ghetto malls. There is currently a more settled pattern: rich people still often go into the suburbs of Johannesburg for entertainment, but they also make use of the growing number of facilities available in Soweto.

In the handful of years from the unbanning of black political organisations in 1990 to democratic elections in 1994, restrictions on black movement were lifted and corporations vied with each other to appoint black people to senior management positions. This in turn saw living standards for many black people accelerate rapidly. Higher earning people flocked from Soweto and other townships to the more tranquil suburbs of Johannesburg. But, as one person, noted: 'People are leaving townships and finding life is not better in the suburbs. They find they lose that community spirit and their social life disappears. The middle to upper class will move away and settle in richer suburbs, but, as the townships develop and improve, people will stay in their communities.'

At the time of writing Soweto was ranked seventh among tourist destinations most visited by foreign visitors to South Africa, and is almost unparalleled in terms of the stories it has to tell.

Sydney Phuti, a former executive member of the Soweto Heritage Trust, grew up in Soweto. He was educated at Orlando High, one of the schools that marched on 16 June 1976 against the poor standard of education for black pupils and Afrikaans as a medium of instruction. He was part of the demonstration that saw police open fire, killing a number of school pupils, with Hector Petersen the first child to fall.

Phuti's recollections are those of someone who knows Soweto as home, and not as scenes from video clips. The classroom he was in as a pupil, he recalls, had large holes in some of the walls. Dogs would chase cats through one wall, across the classroom, and out the opposite wall. The tin, ceilingless roof leaked and, when it rained, teachers and pupils alike would sit at their desks under umbrellas. Situations like this were a combination of vandalism and a failure by education authorities in the apartheid era to maintain school premises.

Many schools are now benefiting from aid organisations and wealthy former pupils trying to rehabilitate them. Morris Isaacson, for example, one of the schools involved in the '76 Uprising, now has gleaming computer labs and the Internet to connect it to schools abroad.

But the community still throws up quirks. A black empowerment company, Thebe Investments, that built a new stadium in Soweto in the mid 1990s, was astonished to note, days after laying down the field, that the turf had disappeared. A couple of days later, it all reappeared. A local man, noting the ease with which the lawn was rolled up and unrolled, had borrowed it to cover the dusty earth in the tents at his daughter's wedding. After the nuptials he returned it.

It is estimated that around 1,000 tourists a day visit Soweto, and all of them go to the Mandela Museum. It houses a collection of gifts to Mandela from leaders such as Muammar Qaddafi of Libya, as well as Mandela's prison shoes and his graduation robe. The museum is a stone's throw from the brown and beige mansion Mrs Madikizela-Mandela built before her former husband was released from jail, and in which she still lives. Tourists can often be seen tramping the low ridge of the hill that separates the houses, as they survey both of them.

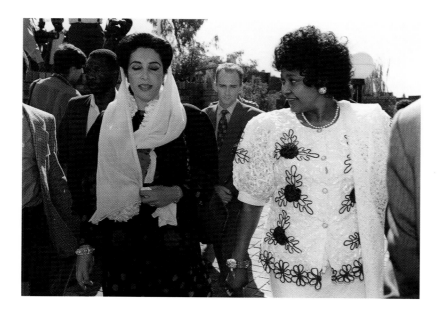

Winnie Madikizela-Mandela in Soweto with Benazir Bhutto, former Prime Minister of Pakistan. Ms Bhutto was the first woman to head the government of an Islamic state.

Tourists who have little interest in the travails of politicians can take a short walk or drive to the nearby Ubuntu Kraal, where they can quaff traditional beer or watch traditional dancing.

Those interested in history may prefer the Hector Petersen Memorial, close to the Mandela homes and to the former house of Desmond Tutu. Like Mandela, Archbishop Tutu is also a Nobel Peace Prize winner, and he lived with his family in Vilakazi Street for many years. The Hector Petersen Memorial, which was dedicated by then US President Bill Clinton on his visit to Soweto in March 1998, will in time be flanked by a museum, a library, art gallery and theatre, as well as a living museum in part of a nearby school.

Not far away is Avalon Cemetery, the final resting place of great South African political figures such as Lilian Ngoyi, Elias Motsoaledi, Helen Joseph, Joe Slovo and Hector Petersen. The Oppenheimer Park in Central West Jabavu, some five kilometres west of the Mandela homes, with its imitation Zimbabwe tower, has the best vantage points across Soweto, and the most comprehensive collection of indigenous plants in the town. These include superb cycads concentrated around the remarkable concrete village built by *sangoma* and African traditional historian Credo Mutwa (*see* pages 120–121). The village is a testimony to African mythology and culture. There are numerous other sites to visit and at each, if you are friendly, Soweto folk will be only too pleased to stop and have a chat.

Most tourists retire to a shebeen for some refreshment and gossip. Shebeens reveal much about the history of Soweto. They were born during the period when the apartheid government denied black people the right to consume liquor unless they could prove they had passed 10 years of schooling. They might then apply for a permit for no more than six bottles of beer and a bottle of spirits a month.

This action in turn saw 'spots' (as early shebeens were known) formed by professional bootleggers. The late Godfrey Moloi, one of Soweto's best known nightclub owners, and a patron of youth football, was one of these bootleggers. Moloi said they would go into the cities and get white hoboes to buy beer or spirits for them. The quantities were small, and the hoboes often tried to drink the goods before handing them over, but it was enough to keep spots going.

Moloi was arrested hundreds of times. During his bootlegging career, a career that continued until liquor restrictions were eased in 1988, he had five cars, nine refrigerators and unknown quantities of alcohol confiscated by police. In 1989, shebeens were licensed and are now run as taverns and nightclubs. Moloi's family and some householders are also turning a profit with guesthouses.

In the decade since black entrepreneurship has been allowed, black owned and controlled companies have proliferated, and they now occupy more than 10% of the Johannesburg Stock Exchange board. Soweto and Johannesburg are located in South Africa's smallest and wealthiest province, Gauteng. The name Gauteng means 'place of gold' in seSotho, one of South Africa's 11 official languages. While Johannesburg is home to some of the world's wealthiest mining houses, its economy has shifted to technology and financial services. Soweto and Johannesburg have arguably the wealthiest, most sophisticated and liberal-thinking population on the continent.

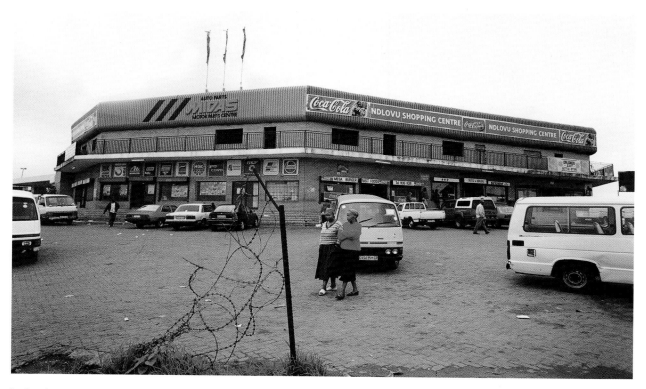

In the decade or more since black people were allowed tenure and free movement, shopping centres have sprung up, urban malls have been created and fast food outlets have flourished in townships. Despite this, Soweto has not met the building and development expectations many property developers and planners anticipated in the early 1990s. Its growth has been modest as many well-to-do residents have relocated to leafier suburbs, and many shoppers still prefer to commute to larger and cheaper malls for their monthly supplies.

Workers still primarily travel from Soweto to Johannesburg to work in one of its two primary business centres. The first is to Sandton, which has the newest financial district in the country, and the most powerful in Africa. The second is the older traditional central business district, a fascinating hub of people drawn from all over Africa, who speak a multitude of languages and dialects. Street traders sell anything from cashew nuts and coconuts, piles of fruit and vegetables on brightly coloured plates, to handbags and shoes – indeed 60% of African visitors to the city say they come to shop.

Motswalle ya amolehileng
('Welcome friend' in seSotho)

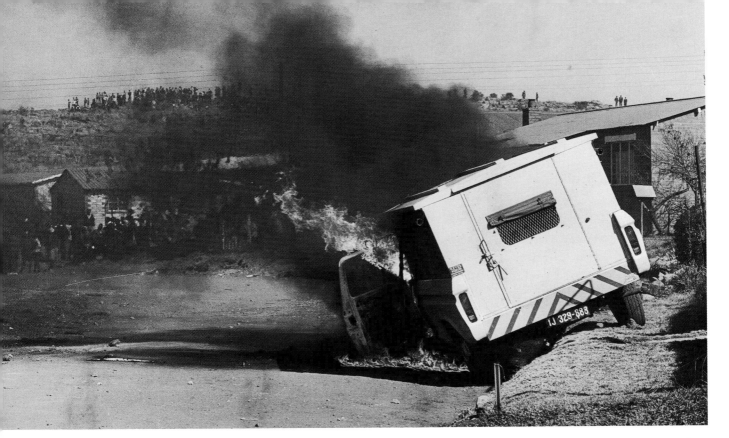

Students from Phefeni (Orlando West) Junior Secondary School were in the fifth week of their boycott against Afrikaans as a medium of tuition on the day Soweto exploded – 16 June 1976. They stood for hours on this ridge (*above*) guarding the bodies of two pupils who had been shot by police (*below*). Other young people torched this police van (*above*) in Vilakazi Street, in response to police opening fire on them. The vehicle burnt out almost exactly halfway between the home of a humble priest, Desmond Tutu, who would later become South Africa's first black Anglican Archbishop, and the home of a jailed lawyer, Nelson Mandela, who would go on to become the country's first democratically elected president. Within a decade Tutu won the Nobel Peace Prize for his efforts to bring an end to conflict and injustice in South Africa; almost a decade later Mandela shared the same award with FW de Klerk for his powerful attempts at reconciliation and at the healing of a brutalised land.

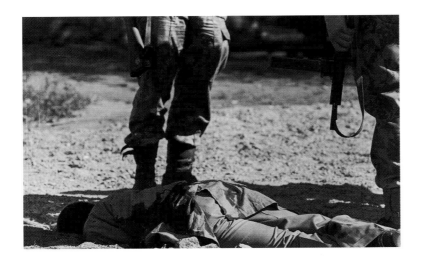

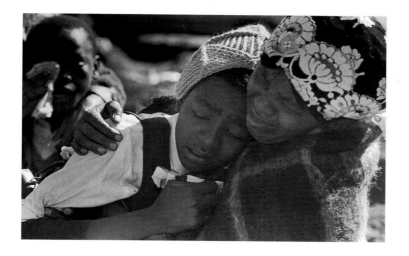

A sister and relatives grieve at the funeral of Hector Petersen, the first child to die in the Soweto uprising of 16 June 1976. His name has become synonymous with the tremendous sacrifices of the 'young lions' – the hundreds of children and young people who laid down their lives in the apartheid struggle.

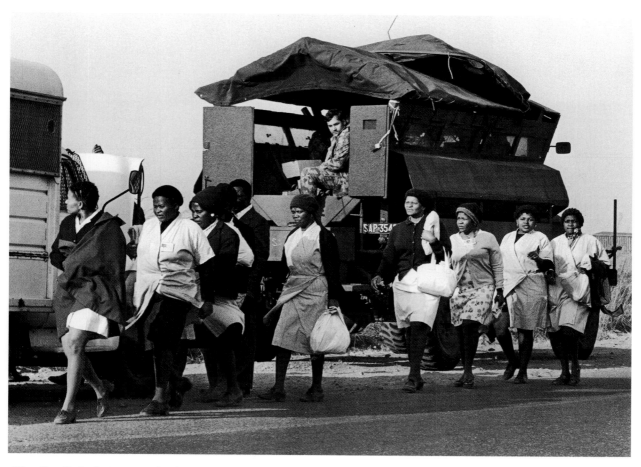

After the first shots were fired early in the morning of 16 June 1976, quelling a student march and provoking unprecedented mayhem in the township, police quickly set up roadblocks at all of Soweto's entry and exit points. White people and journalists were banned from entering the township. Taxis and buses were confined to the perimeters and thousands of people, like these nurses from Baragwanath Hospital, had to walk miles home or to public transport.

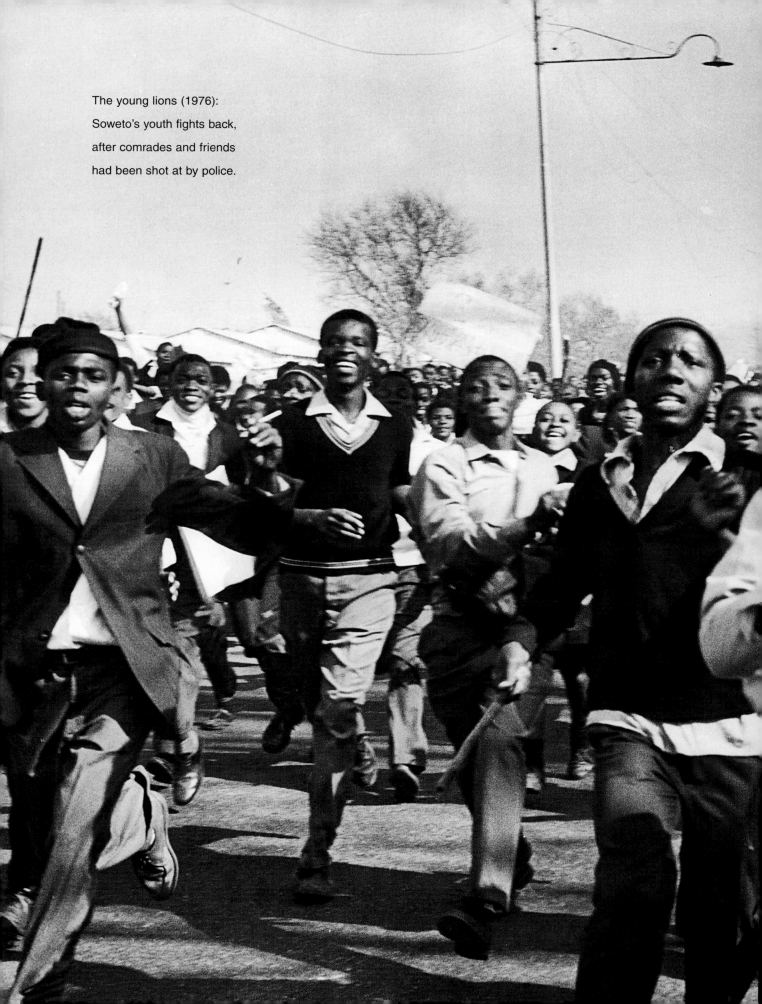

The young lions (1976):
Soweto's youth fights back,
after comrades and friends
had been shot at by police.

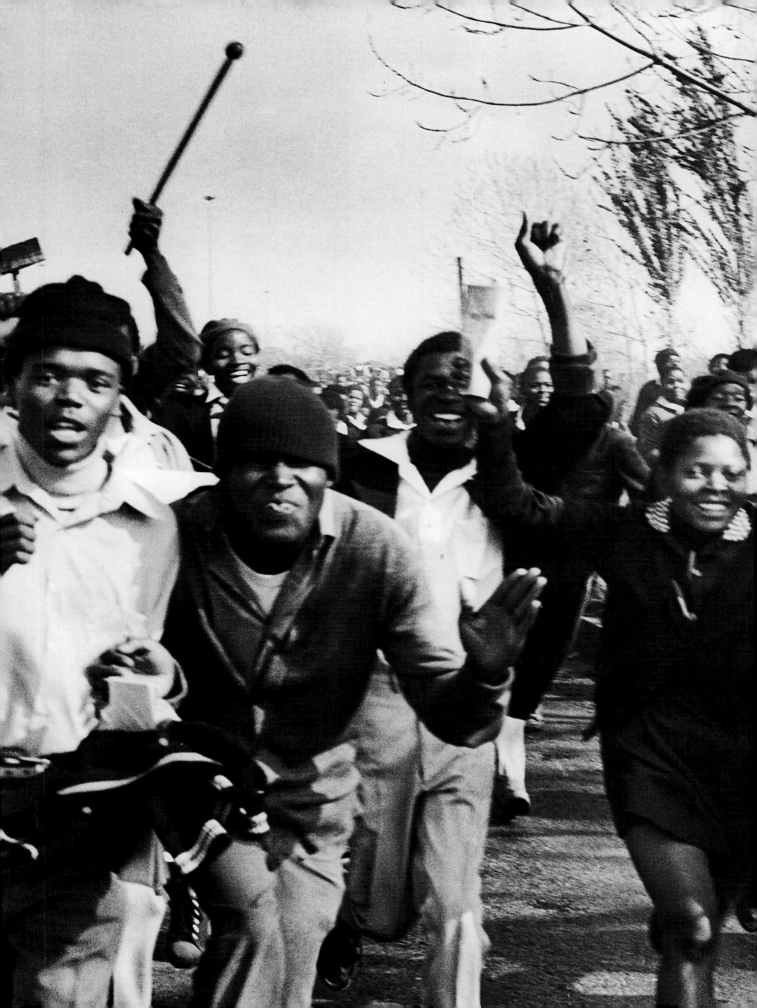

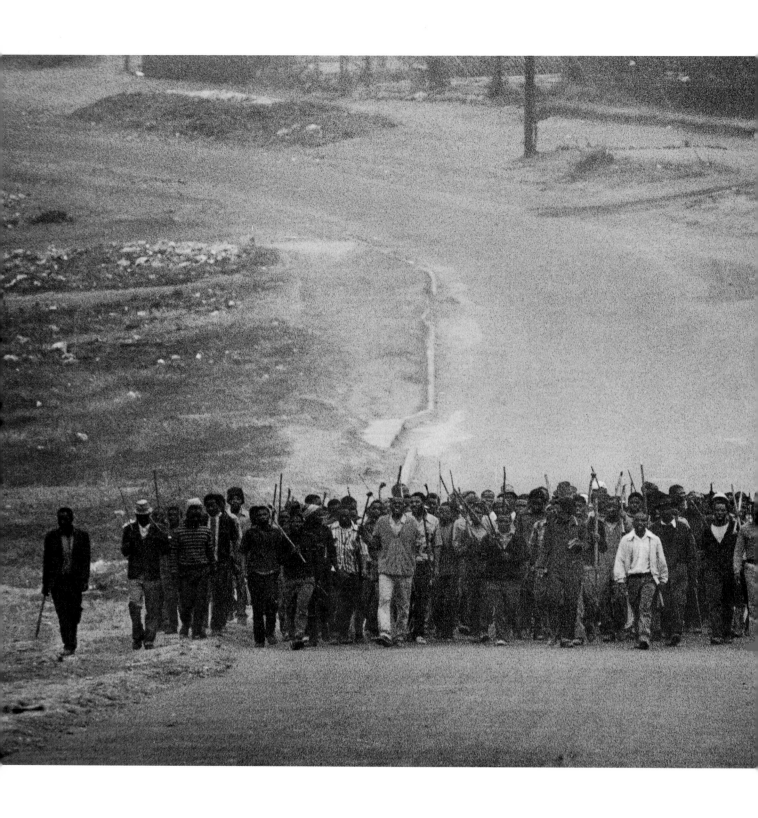

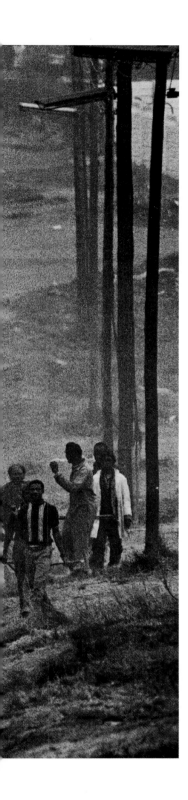

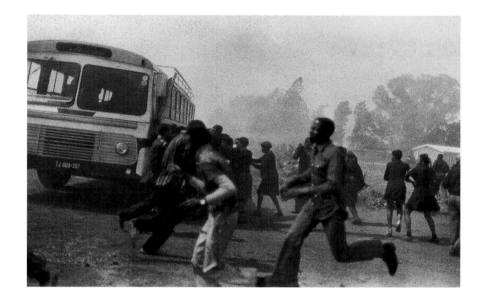

There were few more chilling sounds in the turbulent apartheid days than the chant 'Usuthu, Usuthu', as Zulu hostel dwellers, like these from Mzimhlope hostel (*left*), armed with sticks, knives, pangas and axes, marched in huge phalanxes to attack communities with whom they were at odds.

Another weekend, another funeral, more teargas, more rubber bullets: mourners at Avalon Cemetery flee before clouds of tear-gas smoke (*above*).

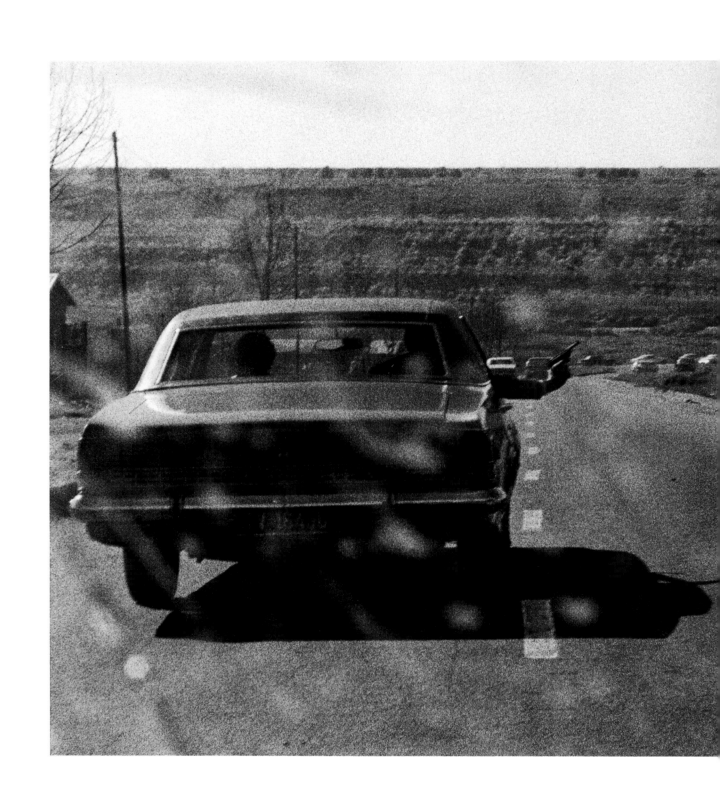

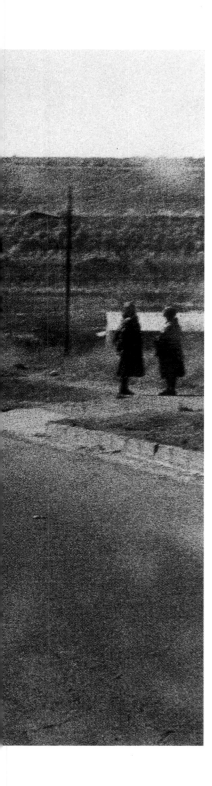

June of 1976 was a month of mayhem in Soweto and townships across
South Africa, as young people began protesting at inferior education
for black children. Police tried to exclude journalists from townships so that
they would not witness scenes like this one (*left*): a police vehicle, a pale
green Chevrolet, cruises along a major Diepkloof thoroughfare with a police
officer taking pot shots at pedestrians.

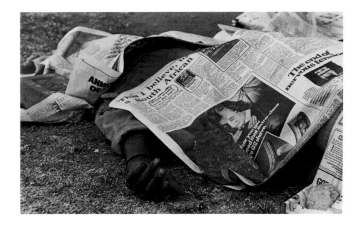

'What would you die for?' a newspaper headline asks as it lies over the body of a young man shot by police officers in Killarney, Soweto, in 1976.

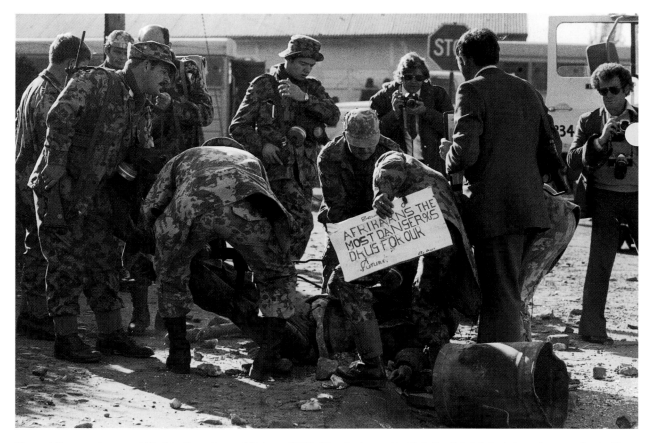

Two white people were killed in Soweto on 16 June 1976. The first was Dr Melville Edelstein (*above*), a medical officer working in the township, who had just received a phone call from someone telling him to leave Soweto. As he prepared to leave, he was attacked in his office and beaten to death. A short distance away, the second man, a West Rand Administration Board official, whose name is lost to history, was forced to stop the truck he was driving. A student later recalled that, as he reached for a firearm, students attacked his vehicle, pulled him out, and beat him with axes and stones, before throwing his lifeless body into a dustbin.

Black Consciousness drew from Malcolm X's dictum, 'Black man, you are on your own', and on the intellectual leadership of a young medical student, Steven Bantu Biko, who led the South African Students' Organisation (SASO). The young people pictured below, on their way to the funeral of a comrade in Soweto, followed Biko's leadership. When giving evidence during the May 1976 trial, during which student leaders of SASO were tried for alleged subversive activities, Biko explained Black Consciousness thus: 'The Black man is first of all oppressed by an external world through insitutionalised machinery, through laws that restrict him from doing certain things, through heavy work conditions, through poor pay, poor education and ... the Black man himself has developed a certain state of alienation. He rejects himself because he attaches the meaning White to all that is good ... this arises out of his development from childhood.' He said schools for white children were better than those for black children: 'Black kids normally have shabby uniforms if any; the White kids always have uniforms ... with sport White kids have uniforms, we have to share uniforms. Their homes are different, the streets are different, the lighting is different, so you tend to begin to feel that there is something incomplete in your humanity, and that completeness goes with whiteness. This is carried through into adulthood ... When you say, "Black is beautiful" you are saying ... "Man, you are okay as you are; begin to look upon yourself as a human being".'

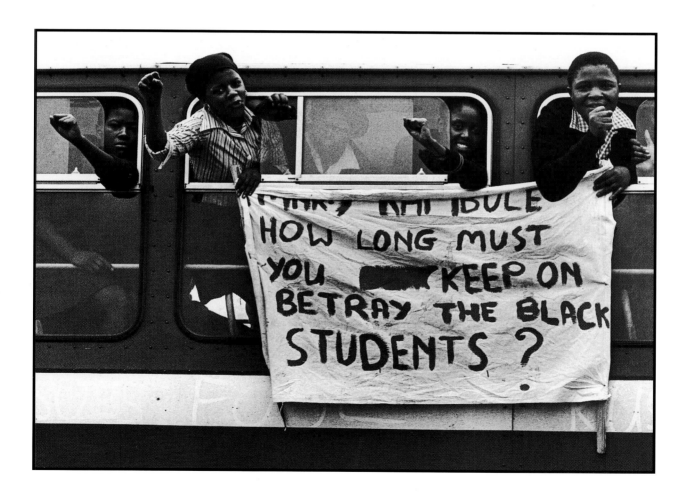

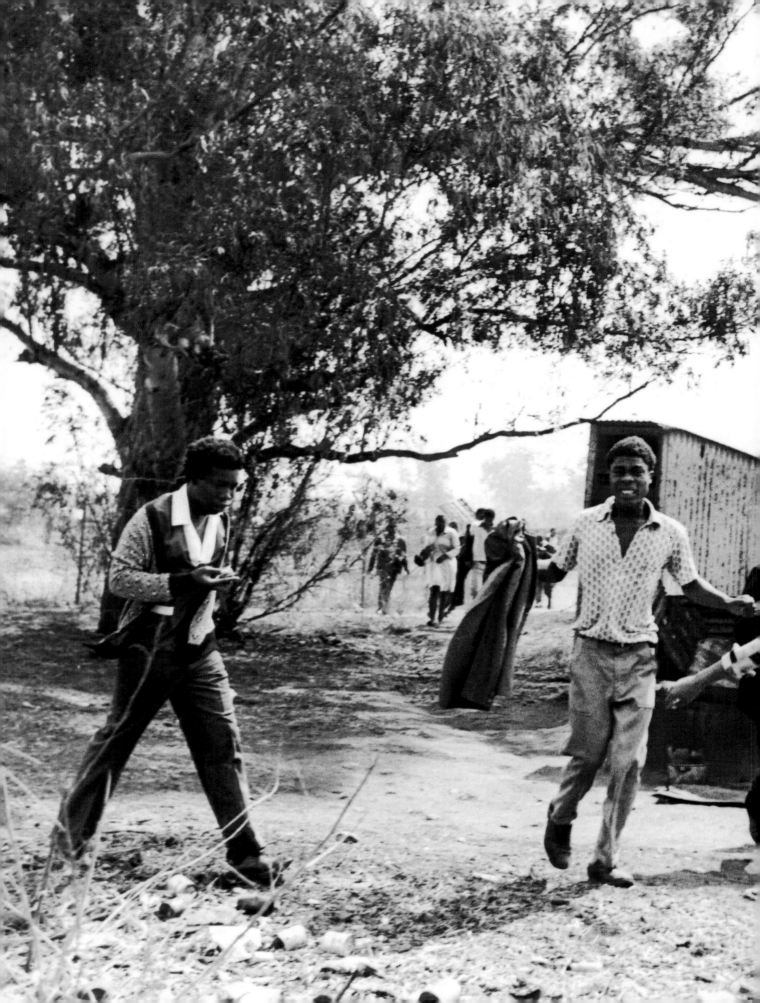

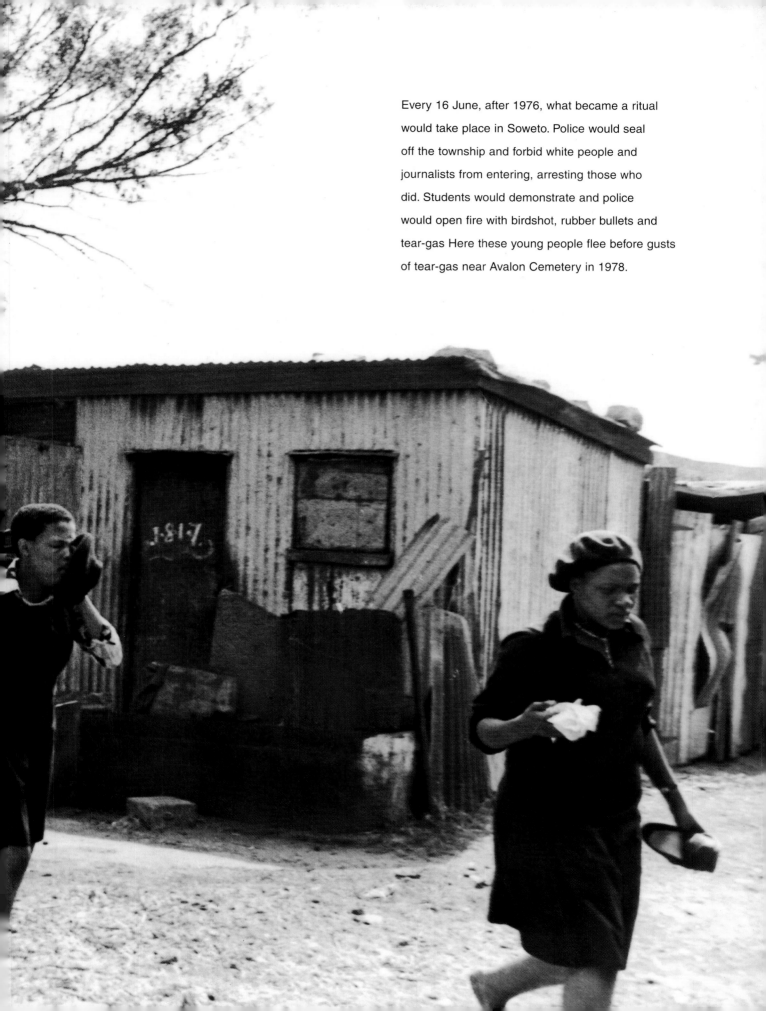

Every 16 June, after 1976, what became a ritual would take place in Soweto. Police would seal off the township and forbid white people and journalists from entering, arresting those who did. Students would demonstrate and police would open fire with birdshot, rubber bullets and tear-gas Here these young people flee before gusts of tear-gas near Avalon Cemetery in 1978.

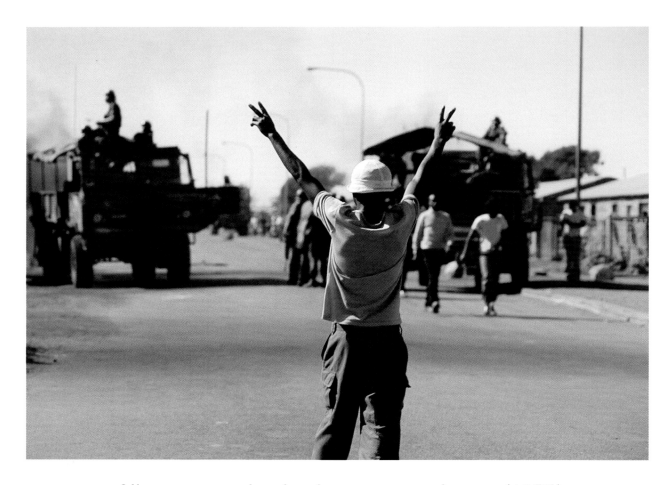

All we are saying is give peace a chance (1978)

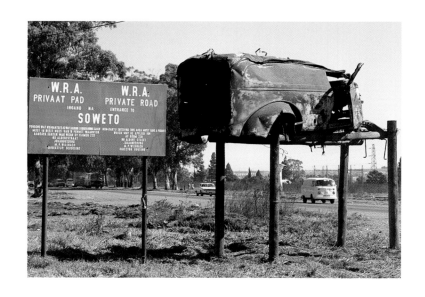

Signs like this one served to warn of restrictions on white access to black areas, and vice versa.

Between 1976 and 1994, one of the easiest targets for demonstrators was delivery vehicles: they were stoned, hijacked and burnt. At times deliveries into Soweto would stop for days, or consignments would be taken in vehicles that had heavy mesh across windows and radio contact with the police. Some were even landmine-proof, although landmines were never used in South Africa's urban warfare.

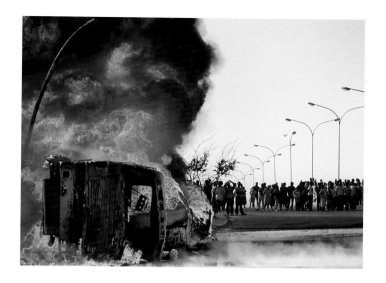

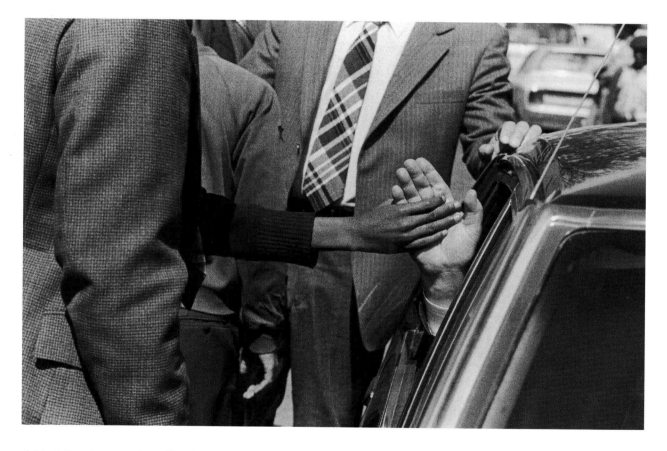

A black hand grasps the stiff, raised hand of State President Pieter Willem Botha who came to power a few years after the Soweto uprising. Botha was more inclined to drive past the people he governed, and to wag a pointed finger at them, than to grasp the hand of a fellow citizen, especially that of a black person in friendship. Under his rule apartheid was militarised and death squads proliferated.

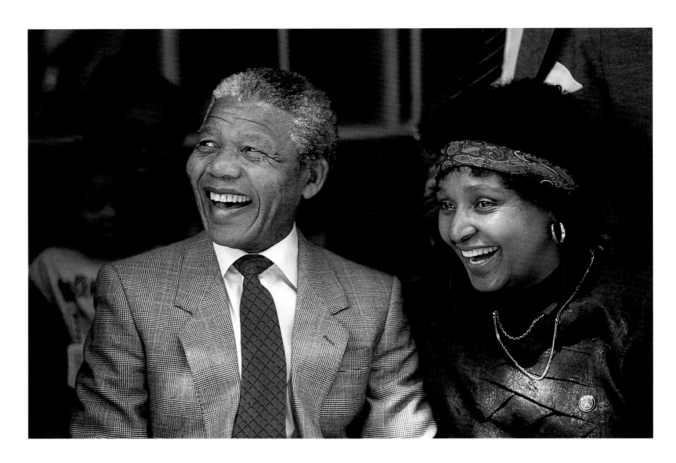

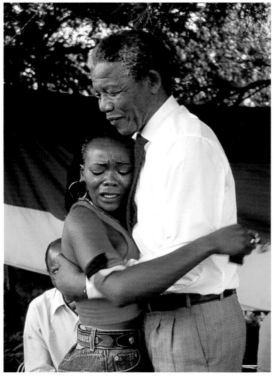

Joyful scenes following Nelson Mandela's 1990 release from 27 years in prison: during happier times with his ex-wife Winnie Madikizela-Mandela (*above*); well-known singer Brenda Fassie tearfully welcomes her long-lost relative (*left*); the late Oliver Tambo and Mandela share a joke (*opposite top*); and Mandela marching between Cyril Ramaphosa and the late Joe Slovo (*opposite bottom*).

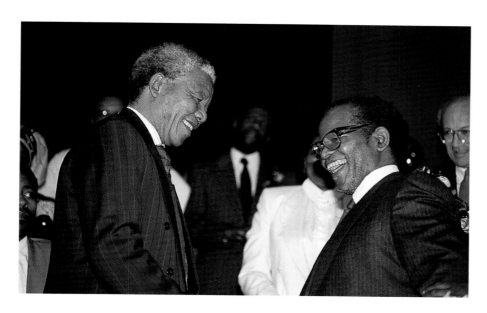

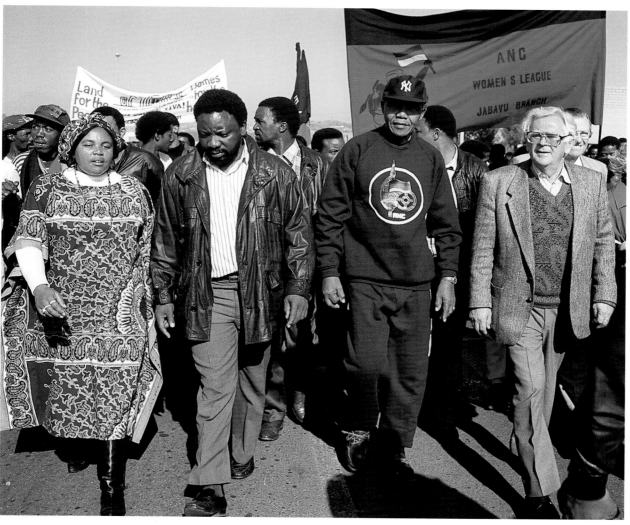

The most loved man in South Africa:
Nelson Mandela walking with his
bodyguards and youth leaders
through Soweto shortly after his release
from prison in 1990. A leader of the
African National Congress for most of his
life, he was elected as South
Africa's first democratic president in
1994. He governed the country until
1999, and has since then been an
international ambassador for peace. One
of Mandela's most endearing attributes
is his unqualified love of children.

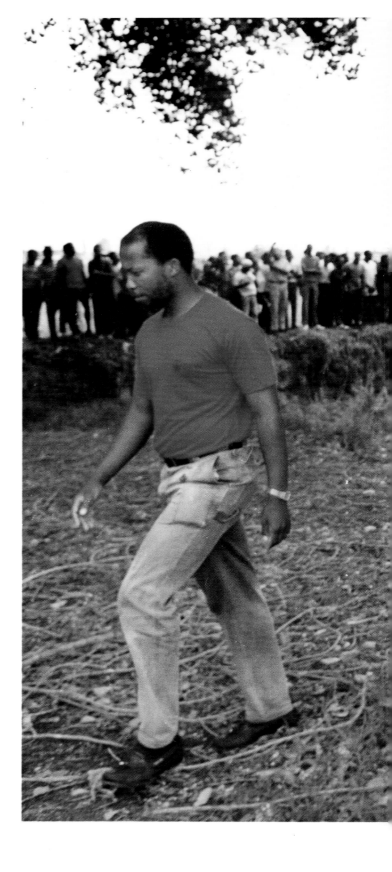

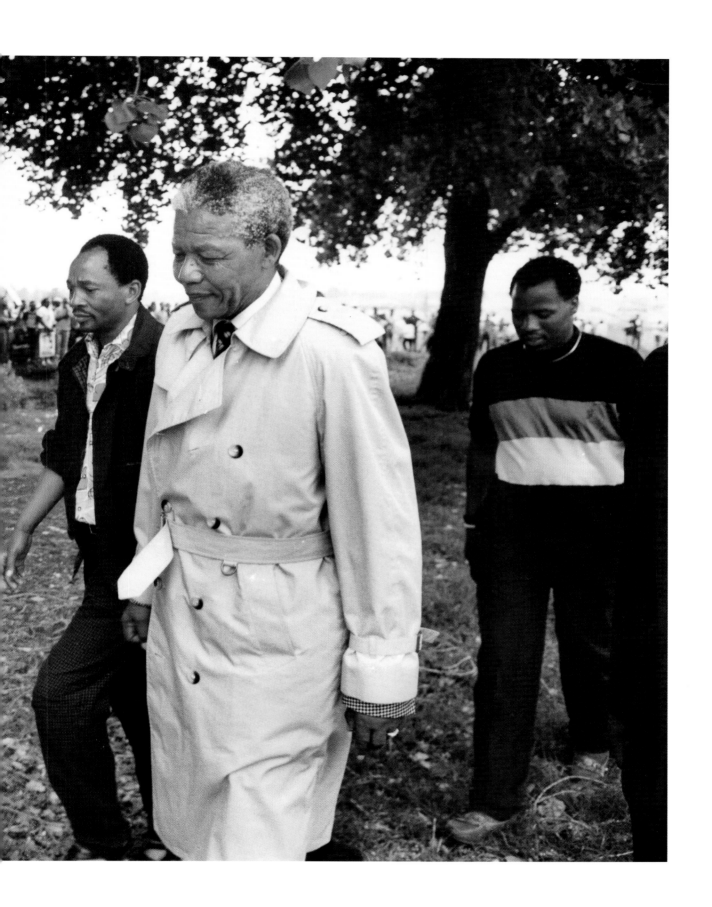

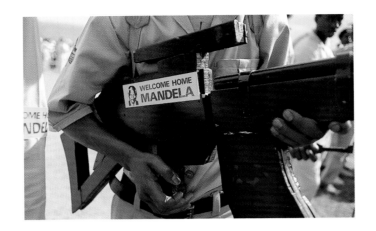

On the day Nelson Mandela came home to Soweto an unprecedented tidal wave of people filled the streets: people left their homes and walked to his home in Orlando West. The release of Mandela symbolically released every South African from the prison of apartheid. And in the end freedom came through negotiation and not the barrel of a gun.

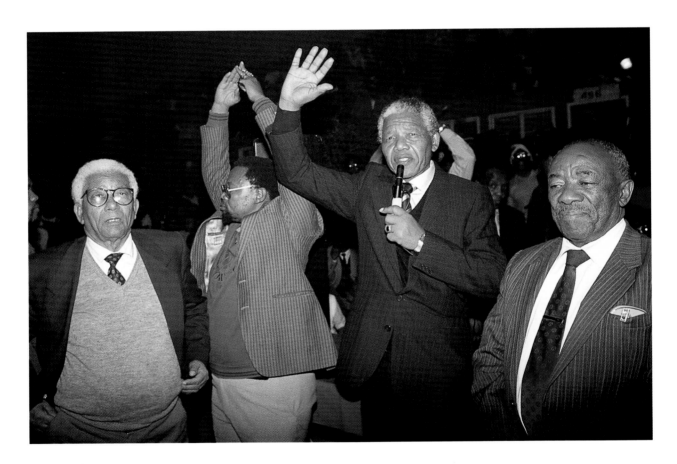

We are one people

Nelson Mandela greets crowds soon after being released from prison on 11 February 1990; with him are (*from left*) fellow Rivonia Trialist Walter Sisulu; Popo Molefe, a leader of the United Democratic Front, which waged the struggle against apartheid within South Africa on behalf of the African National Congress (ANC); and-long time secretary general of the ANC, the late Alfred Nzo.

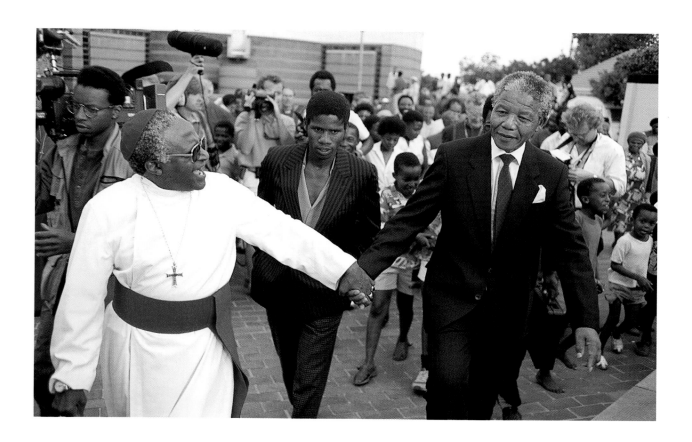

Come, my brother, let's celebrate our rainbow nation

An exuberant Archbishop Desmond Tutu with Nelson Mandela

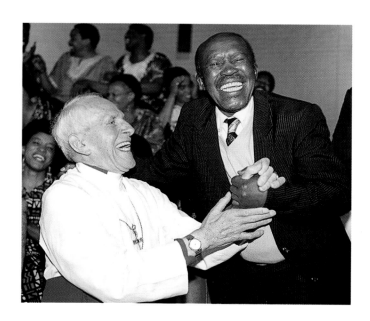

A great champion of the liberation struggle, and a priest in Sophiatown when black residents were forcibly removed to Soweto, Bishop Trevor Huddleston of the Anglican church returns to South Africa after being deported almost 30 years before. Clasping his hand is George 'Kortboy' Mpalweni, a former member of the Americans, a Sophiatown gang. As a young man he was sentenced to death for murdering a school principal. His sentence was reduced to life through Bishop Huddleston's intercessions.

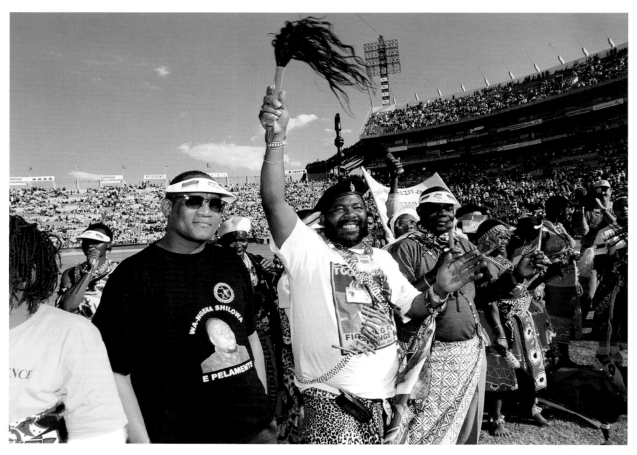

During the build up to the 1999 elections, supporters of former Congress of South African Trade Unions leader Mbhazima Sam Shilowa wear t-shirts and caps calling for his election to the Gauteng parliament at a political rally at FNB Stadium on the outskirts of Soweto. Shilowa was elected premier of the province.

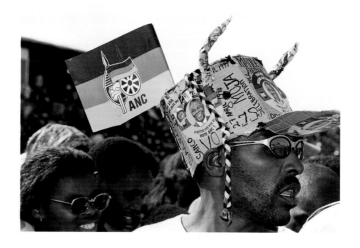

At a political rally at Orlando Stadium a supporter of successful presidential candidate Thabo Mbeki wears a cardboard hat of the sort made to show support for soccer teams; its *equtu* 'cattle horns' denote strength.

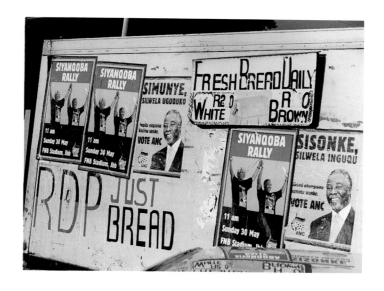

Political activism is the soul food of Soweto. This bread shop, announcing 'RDP Just Bread', refers to the ANC's Reconstruction and Development Programme, that was designed to uplift communities. The DDP was abandoned a few years into democracy.

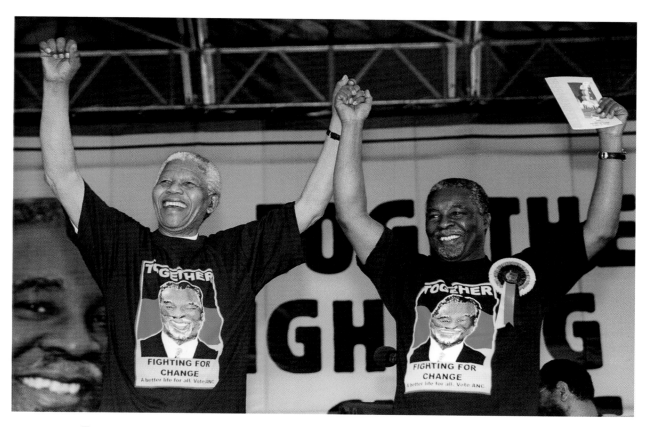

Together fighting for change: outgoing president Nelson Mandela introduces his successor Thabo Mbeki to crowds at Orlando Stadium during the run-up to the 1999 elections.

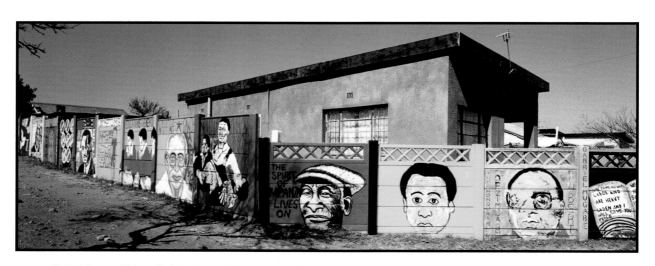

Wall of Heroes. This wall of freedom, painted by young Soweto residents, salutes those who helped bring about democracy in

South Africa. It also emphasises some of the needs of a new society, most importantly respect for knowledge and education. Heroes

depicted include (*from right*): Alan Boesak, a churchman and leader of the anti-apartheid United Democratic Front; Chris Hani,

chief of staff of the ANC's armed wing Umkhonto we Sizwe, who was assassinated in 1994, shortly before the first democratic elections;

James 'Sofasonke' Mpanza ('Housing and Shelter for all', *see* page 12); Hector Petersen, the first child to die in the 1976 Soweto uprising;

Mohandas Gandhi, who advocated active non-violence; and Walter Sisulu, a leader of the African National Congress (ANC).

Today my return to Soweto

fills my heart with joy

Nelson Mandela, on his return to his home in Soweto

on 13 February 1999 after 27 years in prison

(*Long Walk to Freedom*, Macdonald Purnell, 1994)

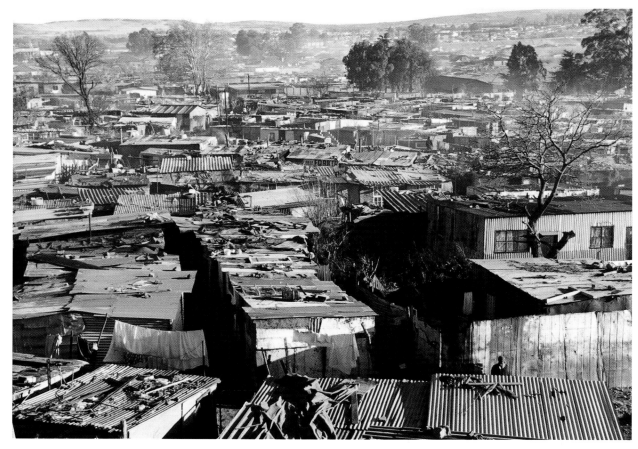

One of the squatter camps scattered around Soweto, where people live in overcrowded shacks, with no electricity and limited access to fresh water. The relaxation of influx controls in the 1980s, followed by democratisation and the opening of the country's borders to fellow Africans, has resulted in an influx of people from across southern Africa, and indeed the continent. They come to Soweto in the hopes of finding work in nearby Johannesburg.

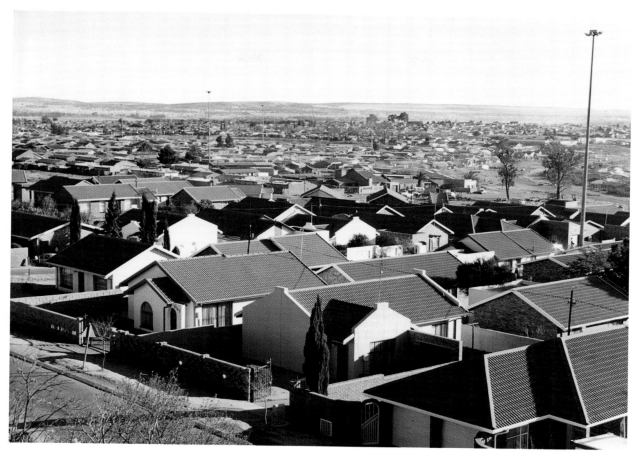

Black suburbs began being constructed during the late 1970s. Following the Soweto uprising, the apartheid government hoped that an emergent black middle class would quell revolutionary desires. They were wrong.

South Africa generates over 80% of the electricity used in Africa, but it was only in the 1980s that government began in earnest to distribute electricity to black areas, among them Soweto. In some informal settlements today, prepaid electricity meters bring light to many humble homes. In newer shack locations, however, candles and gas still provide the only light.

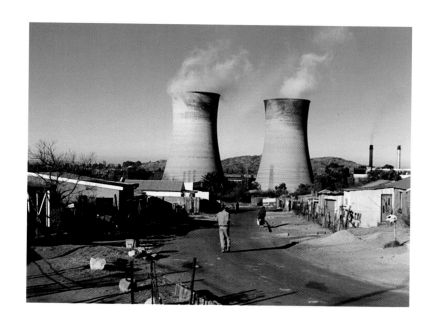

Although black people are now free to live wherever they wish in South Africa, not all of the rich have left the townships for tree-lined suburbs. Many families prefer the sense of community found in old townships like Soweto, where walls are lower than in prison-like suburbs, and neighbours still wander over for a chat and communal gripes. The plush new houses depicted on these pages are in Soweto's Diepkloof Extension Phase 3 (*below*) and Phase 2 (*bottom*), Dube Village (*right*), and Orlando West Extension (*opposite bottom*), not far from the residence of Mrs Winnie Madikizela-Mandela.

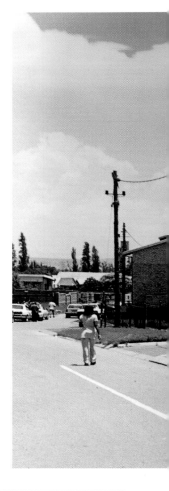

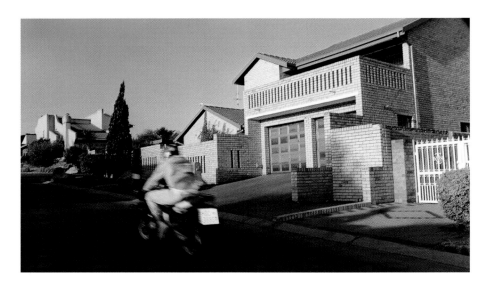

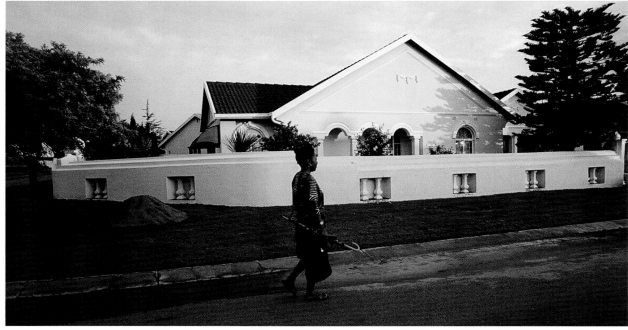

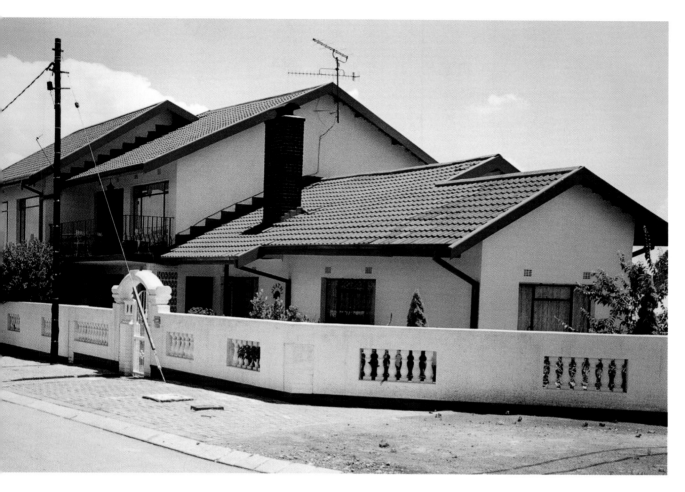

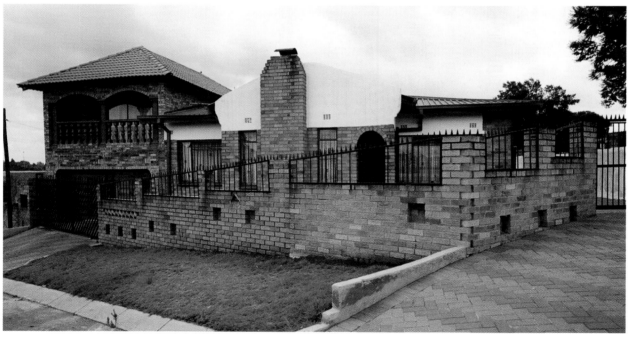

Poverty is a game of chance, the capacity to

manipulate the odds against a cruel world,

and the ability to take the risks that survival often

necessitates. These women gamble in the hopes

of augmenting their housekeeping money.

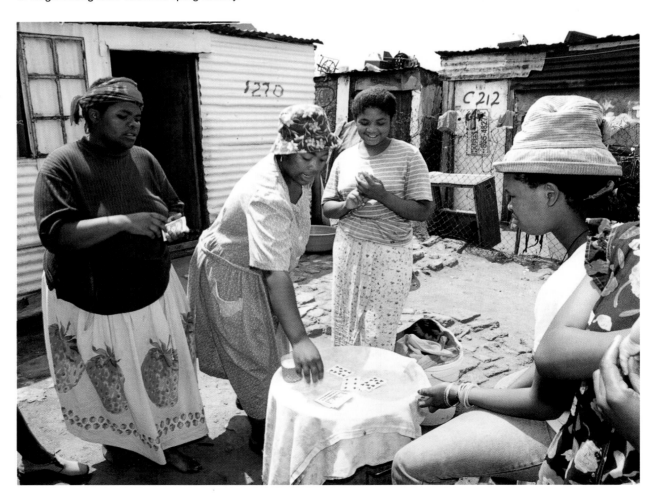

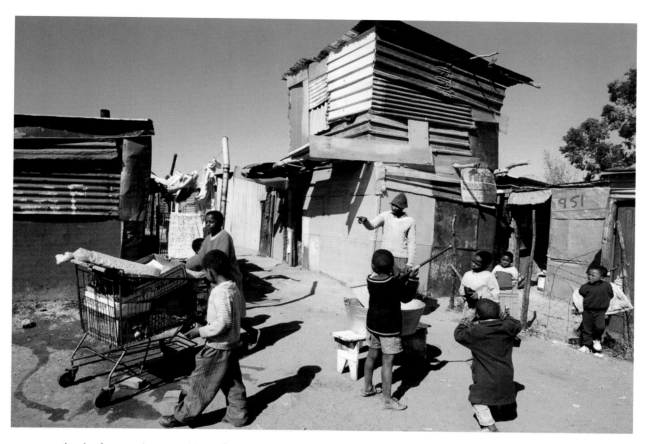

Lack of space is no problem if you are inventive: a second storey balances precariously on top of
a shack (*mkhukhu*) in Mandelaville Squatter Camp.

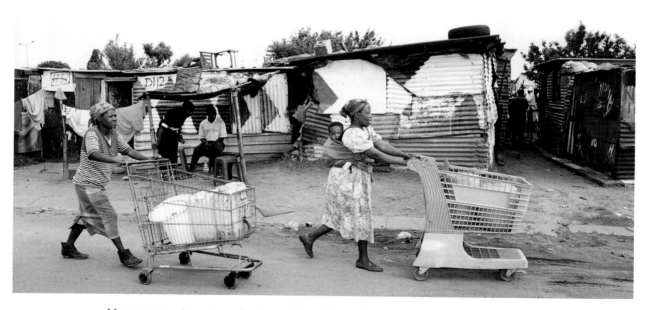

Many women have to make long daily walks to fetch clean water for their families.

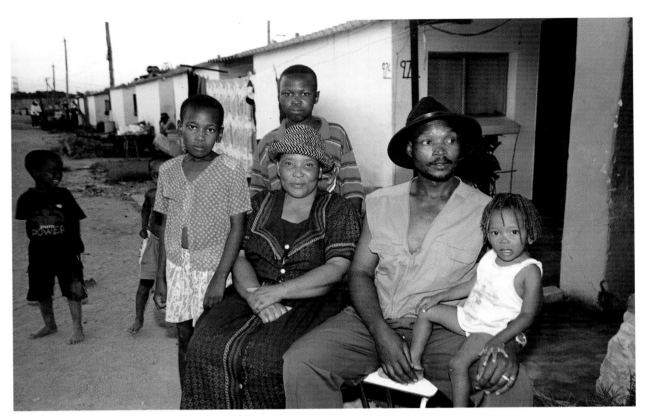

Single-sex hostels in Soweto, especially Mzimhlope, were the site of violent war-mongering in the 1980s and early 1990s. When the new democratic government came into power in 1994, they immediately set about transforming these male-only bastions into family housing. These hostels are now places where traditional African culture, in particular Zulu culture, is kept alive. In this picture, the Mtshali family are sitting outside their home, a renovated family unit at Mzimhlope hostel, into which they moved in the mid-1990s. Photographer Peter Magubane spotted Mrs Mtshali sweeping outside her home with her family around her, and thought they might be candidates for a good family portrait. And they were. Says Magubane: 'What I believe needs to happen now is that those communities need to be further improved. At present a family is living in only two rooms. I hope with time there will be ongoing development.'

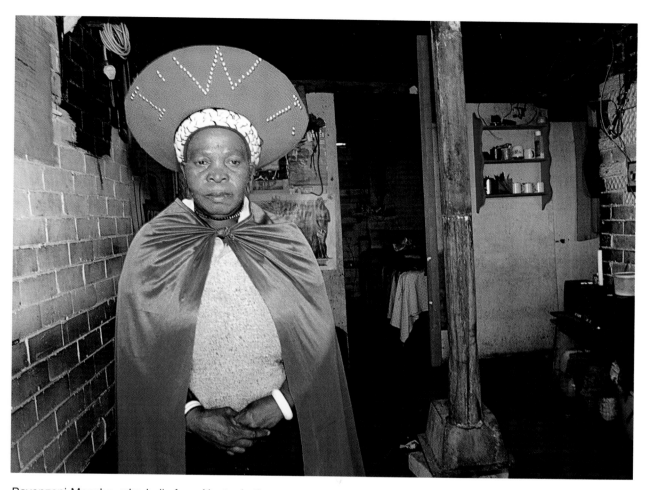

Bayenzeni Mncube, who hails from Nqutu, in the communal cooking area of one of Soweto's converted hostels. She is wearing an ochre-coloured headdress with a white woven wool border and silver studs. Travel in tightly-packed buses and taxis makes large headdresses impractical, and as a result urban women tend to adopt smaller head coverings. The woven wool border has replaced the beads that are traditionally a mark of respect to a married woman's parents in-law. A black greased leather skirt is another token of her married status.

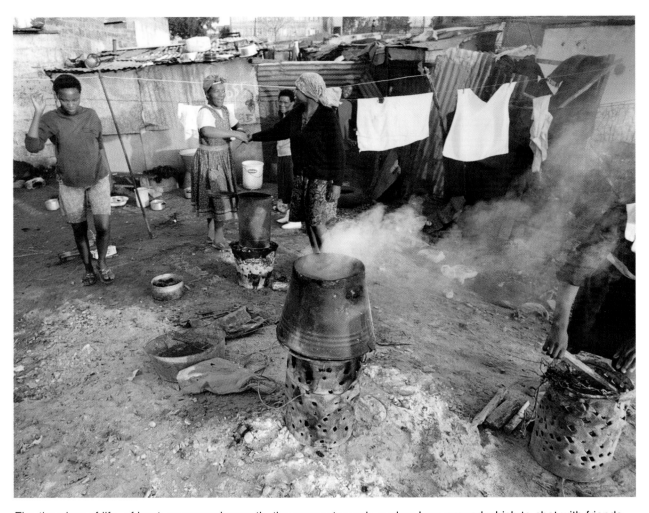

Fire the giver of life, of heat, communal warmth, the means to cook, and embers around which to chat with friends.

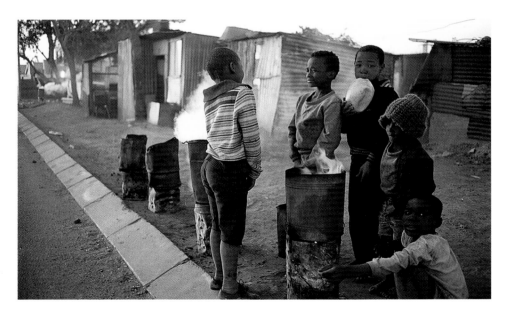

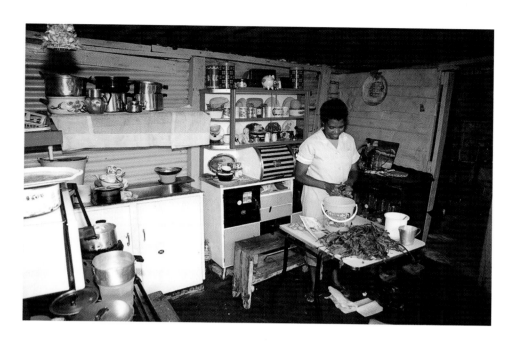

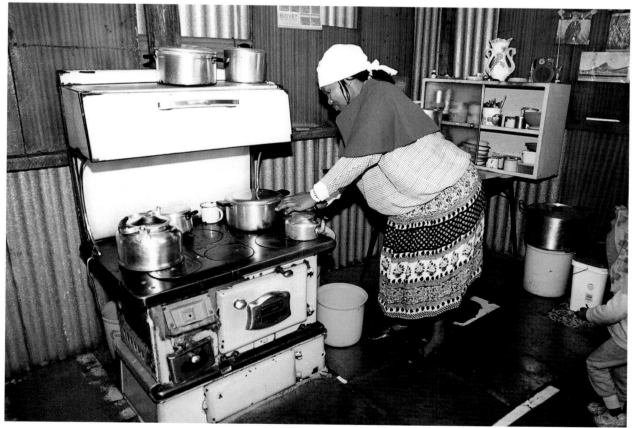

The kitchen is the heart of the home, where food is prepared (*top* and *above*) and family members congregate. Coal stoves may be chic in some communities, but in Soweto the old coal stoves in shacks often belch out thick smoke, burn women's skirts if they stand too close, and can make homes uncomfortably hot, especially in summer.

Beautiful genes: international star of cabaret and theatre Mara Louw with her daughter Lerato who was born in Mzimhlope, Soweto. Mara Louw, whose professional career spans some 25 years, became a solo artist after she returned home from an overseas tour with the musical *Meropa* in 1976. She has performed for many African presidents and other dignitaries.

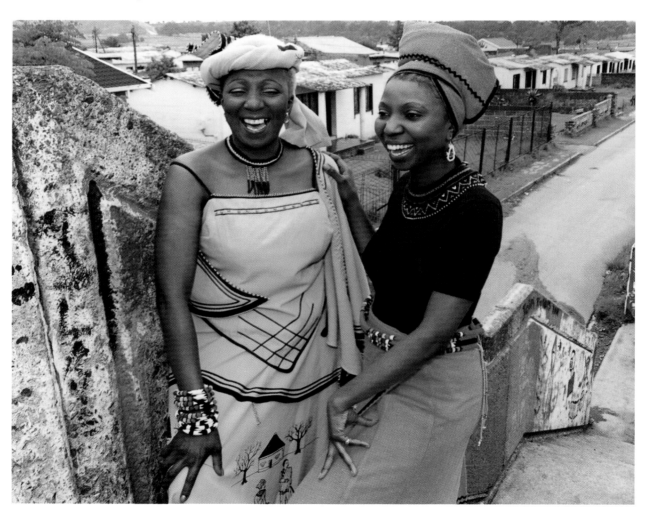

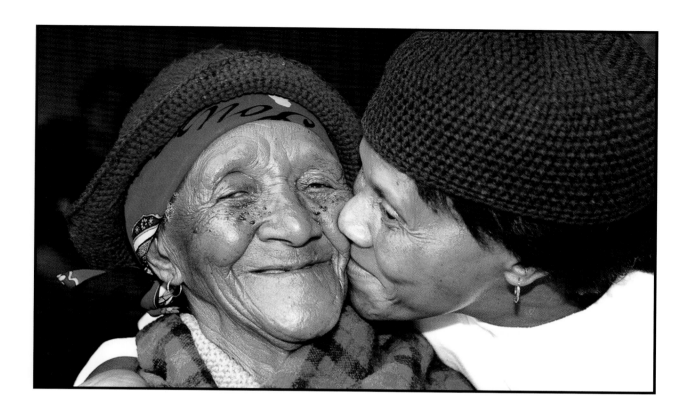

A kiss for *gogo* (grandmother), Mrs Maliwase Manonyane Asinata Kolisang, who celebrated her 100th birthday on 18 November 2000 in Dube. She was born at Qwacha's Nek in Lesotho, where her father was a court guard, but her family was originally from Matatiele in the former Transkei. The youngest of three boys and two girls, she recalls her childhood with happiness: 'We used to play with a skipping rope or hide and seek, the usual children's games.' In 1910, when she was nine, she was privileged to witness an event that shook the entire world: *Mochochonono*, as the Sotho people call Halley's Comet.

She was a sickly child when she was growing up, 'but the doctor said I would get over it, and maybe even live to be a hundred.' She recalls: 'My sister and I ... took pride in our clothing and home duties, and my father sent us to a college to learn domestic science so that we would be good wives.' In 1918, she and her family survived an influenza outbreak that killed thousands of people in southern Africa: 'You would come home from burying one and find another dead.' She lived through another devastating event between the two world wars, the so-called 'red dust' of 1933: 'People were very poor, and then we had drought. It was terrible.'

A highlight of her life was the visit of the British royal family in 1947, when she found herself among hundreds of spectators welcoming the royal couple and the two princesses. By that stage she was a married woman and the mother of eight children – four boys and four girls. She has outlived three of her boys.

She first went to Soweto in 1970 for an eye operation, and returned to visit her daughter, Mapaseka Alice Lekaba (*above*), who lives in Soweto, in 1995 and again in 2000. 'I don't like Soweto. There are a lot of people and a lot of killings. I can't move freely in that place.' She lives in Bloemfontein with her granddaughter Tiny Kolisang. 'I am happy there.'

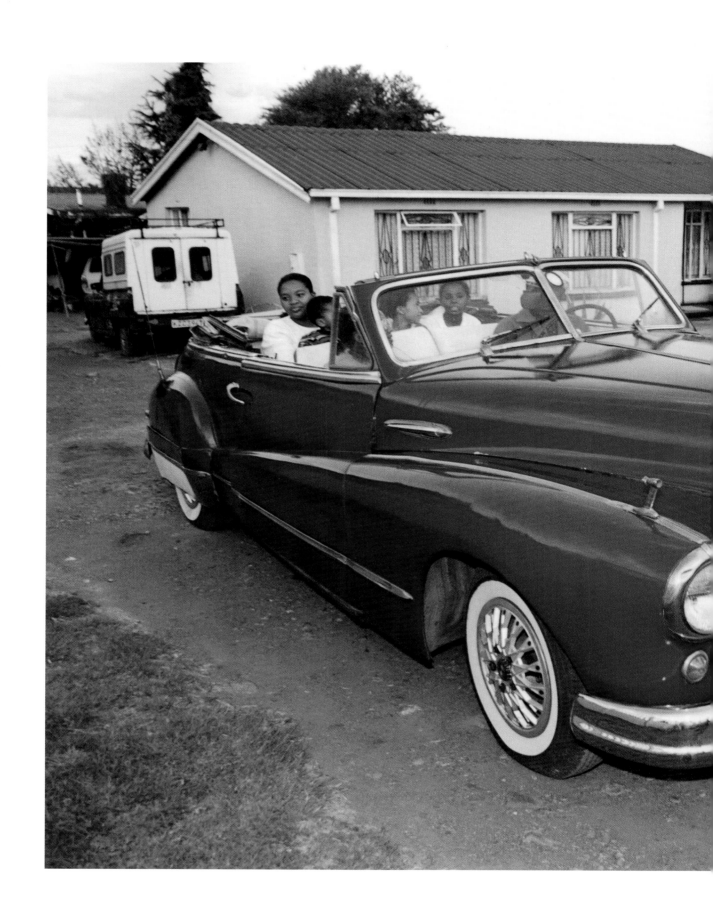

58

SOWETO
PETER MAGUBANE

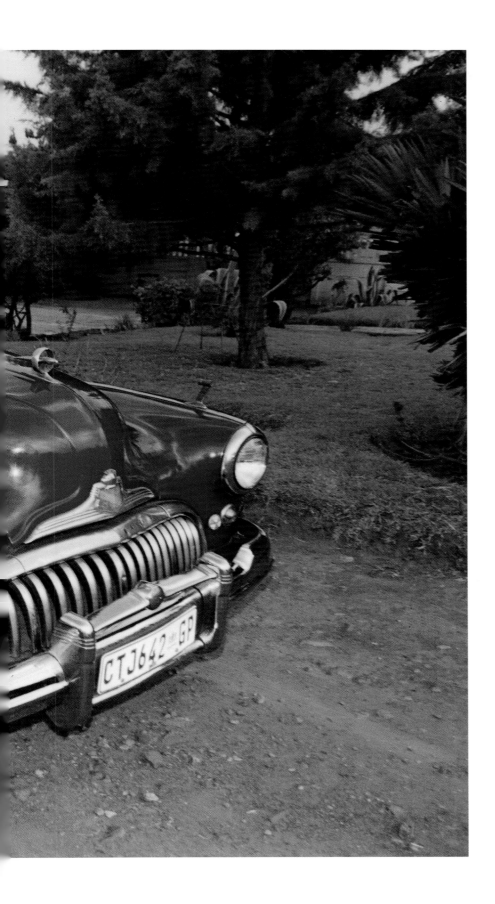

A mirror shine for a gem. Mr Kubheka takes his family for a spin in the 1948 Buick that he bought in 1958 and has treasured ever since.

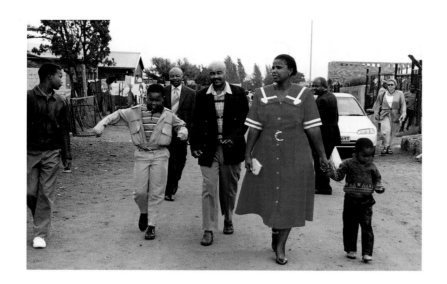

The Ntuli family of Zone 1
Diepkloof walk to church:
(*from left*) Doctor, Derek,
Ivan (the father), Thandi
(the mother) and little Arnold.

It can be hard for a small
boy to concentrate during
a long sermon. Arnold tries
to attract Thandi's attention.

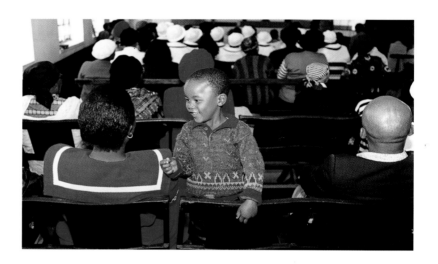

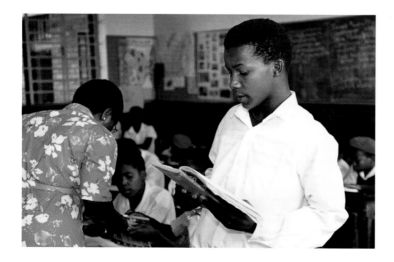

Doctor (21) reads from a manual
at the technical school where he
is studying to become a vehicle
mechanic.

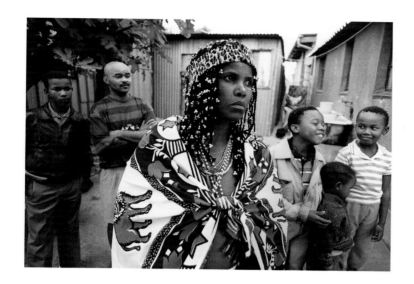

In 1992, Thandi graduated as a *sangoma*, a traditional African spiritualist. Here she wears her robes of office with her family looking on: Doctor, Ivan (her husband), Derek smiling with a friend, and a disconsolate Arnold.

A young man needs his space: Doctor has his own room in a backyard shack at his parents' home. Here he is chatting to his dad and younger brother Derek, whose eye was injured when a scrap of metal flew off a toy into his eye.

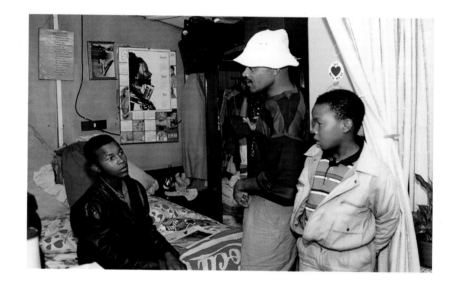

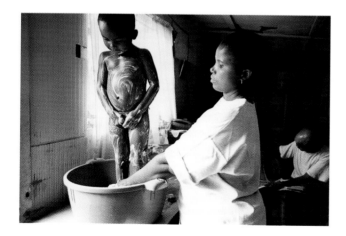

Bathtime in the Ntuli household: Arnold gets a good soaping down from Thandi.

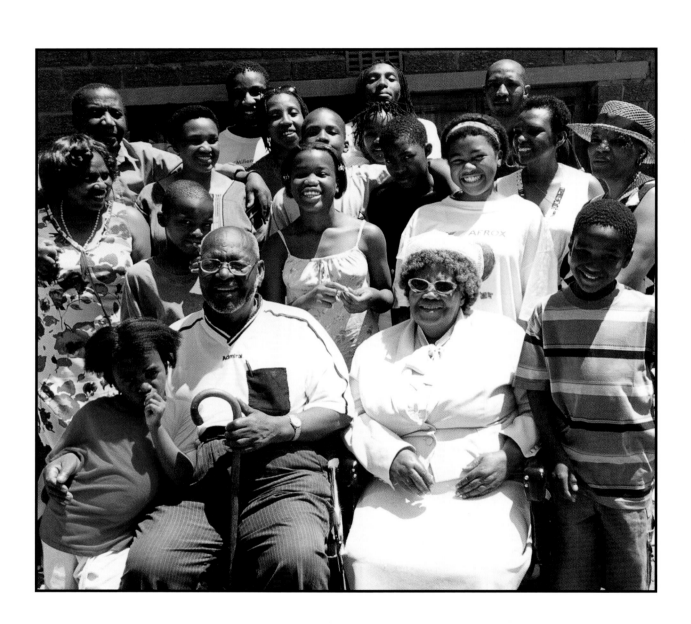

Reverend Benjamin Rajuili with his wife Ellen and some of their seven children and 18 grandchildren in Soweto. Reverend Rajuili, who was ordained a minister of the African Methodist Episcopalian Church in 1952, retired from pastoral work in 1981. Before retiring, he oversaw a huge area of Gauteng and parts of Mpumalanga (in the former Transvaal province), with 14 ministers under his leadership. Reverend Rajuili was also a member of the opposition party, the Transkei Democratic Party, in the Transkei 'bantustan' (homeland) on the east coast of South Africa. 'In parliament I was the first to stand up and condemn apartheid.' He laughs when asked what sort of effect that had on the apartheid government. 'They swallowed it. Before they had taken away my travelling document to travel to America, and then I contested a parliamentary seat. I was told I could say anything I liked, as long as I said it in the House.'

Reverend Rajuili quickly rose to become Chief Whip of the opposition party in Umtata, Transkei. His constituency was the Maluti region, comprising the Mount Frere magisterial district and Matatiele, the region in which he was born. Reverend Rajuili came to Johannesburg as a young man in 1944. 'When I contested the Transkei seat I was already a Johannesburger, but in those days you could contest a seat anywhere. I never saw the voters' roll until the morning of the voting day when they called out my name. I was a thorn in the side of the government, who did not know what to do with me. They made sure I never got back to parliament. My mother was a princess in the Moshoeshoe family, and at the next election some of my family, who were involved in counting ballots, came and told me that ballots were being deliberately spoilt to ensure I could not get voted in. The mode of counting in those days was that there would be 28 people on the list and you had to place your tick next to four names. The government had engaged people to put extra ticks on the ballots to spoil papers that would have voted me in.'

Revered Rajuili is not content to sit back and watch life pass by. 'I've resigned from politics but not from civic duties. I am part of a village forum where we we are opposing ever-escalating service charges. People just get billed amounts that are beyond their ability to meet. We have just briefed an attorney and advocate to bring an action against local government to reduce service charges. We have collected all the necessary money to fight this, because some people have been told if they cannot pay service charges they will lose their homes.'

And so the spirit of civil resistance lives on among the people of Soweto.

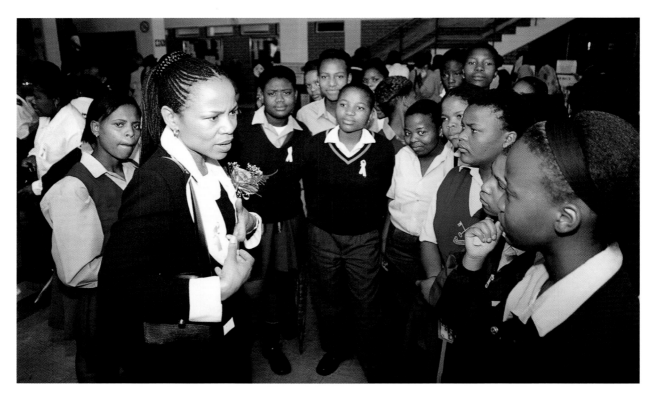

Dr Precious Moloi discusses breast cancer with school pupils visiting Chris Hani-Baragwanath Hospital.

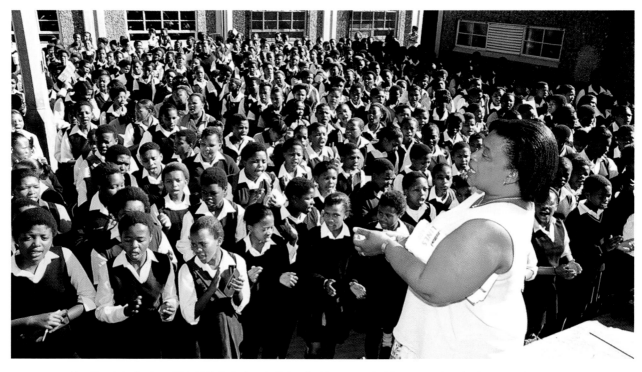

Pupils at Lofentse Girls' High School, Orlando East, are led by a teacher in the morning prayer.

The denial of adequate education was a keystone of apartheid policy. As a result, decent education became critical to anti-apartheid resistance. The 1976 Soweto student rebellion against Afrikaans as a medium of instruction saw the beginning of the end of apartheid. Despite the demise of apartheid, there is still a way to go before all children have access to good education. Racial inequality has been replaced by class and wealth divisions as the democratic government battles to extend decent education to all.

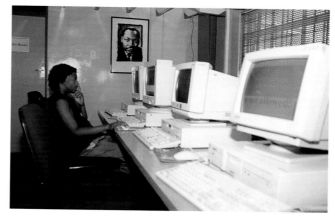

This state-of-the-art library in Soweto is funded by the government of the United States of America and run by the US Information Service.

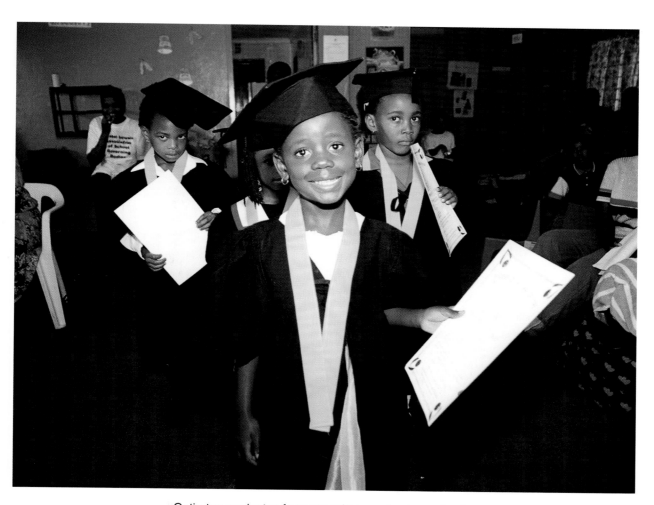

Ontiretse graduates from pre-primary school *cum laude*.

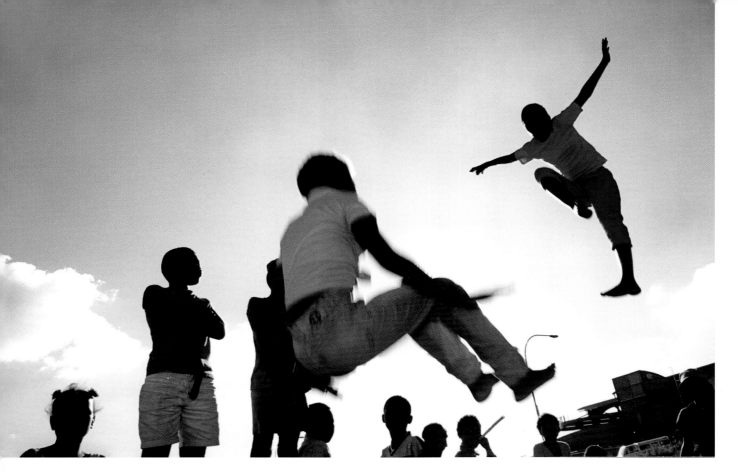

*The aim of education
shall be to teach the youth
to love their people and
their culture, to honour
human brotherhood,
liberty and peace*

(extract from the Freedom Charter, adopted
at the Congress of the People, Kliptown,
Soweto, 26 June 1955)

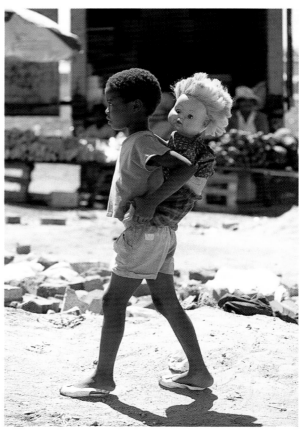

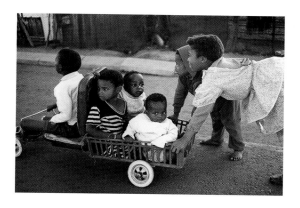

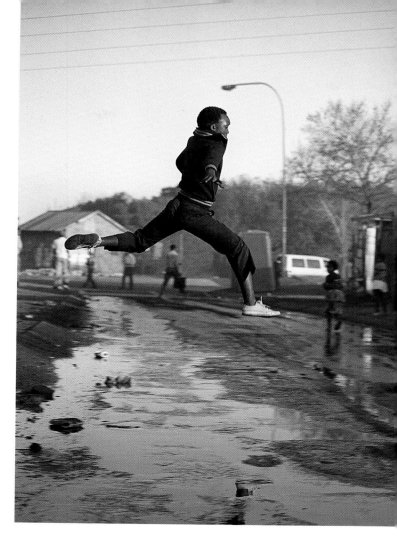

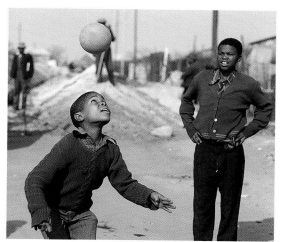

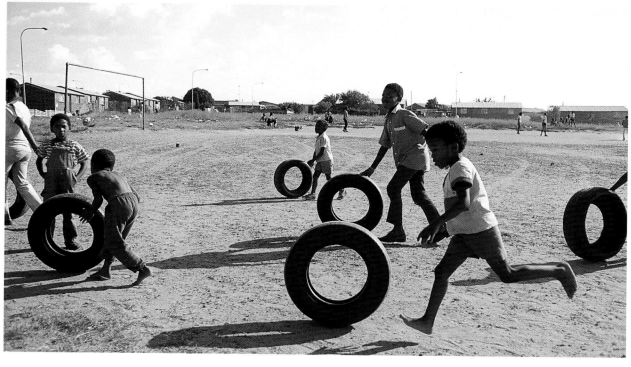

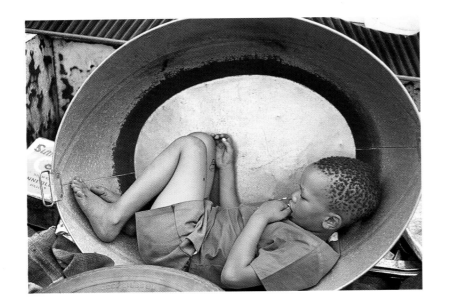

*It takes a village
to raise a child.*

African proverb

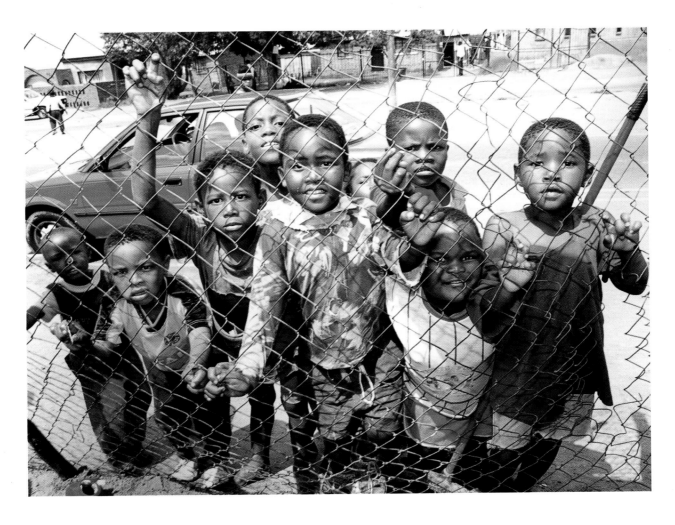

SOWETO
PETER MAGUBANE

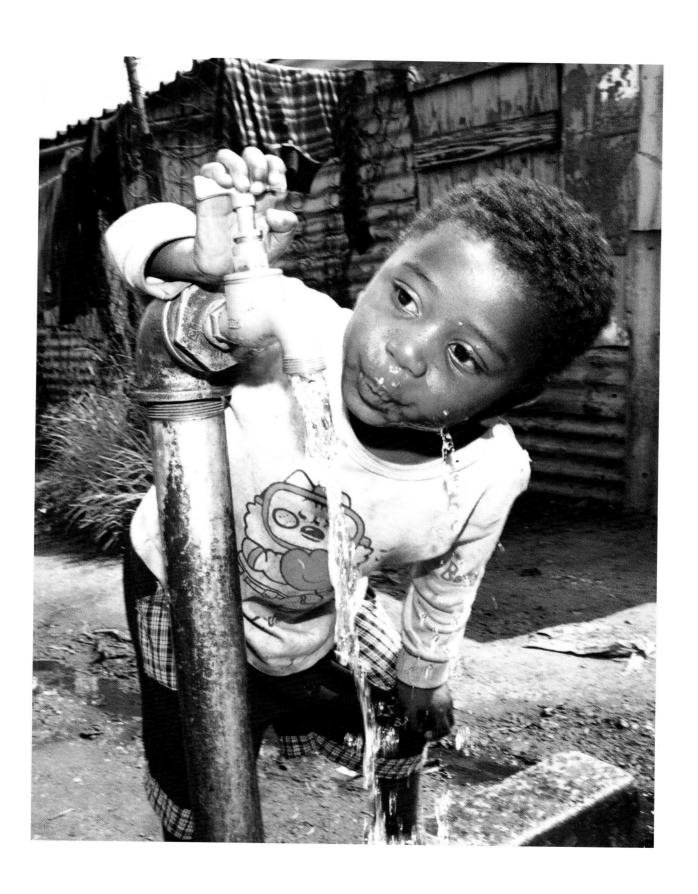

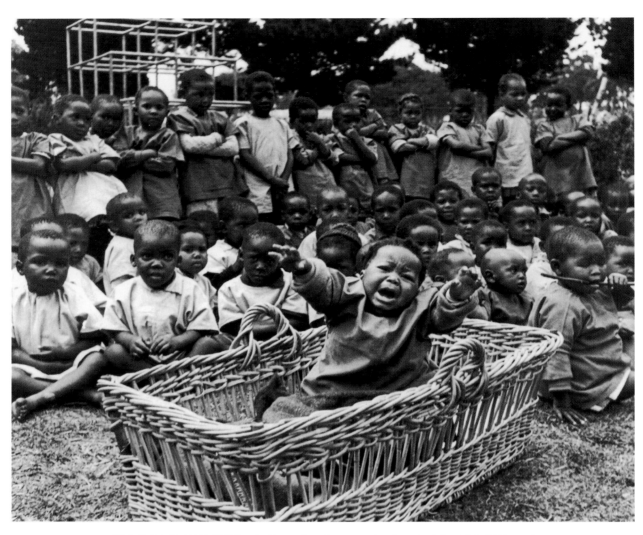

The Orlando East Children's Home has been caring for abandoned babies and children for decades, as this picture, taken in 1957, shows.

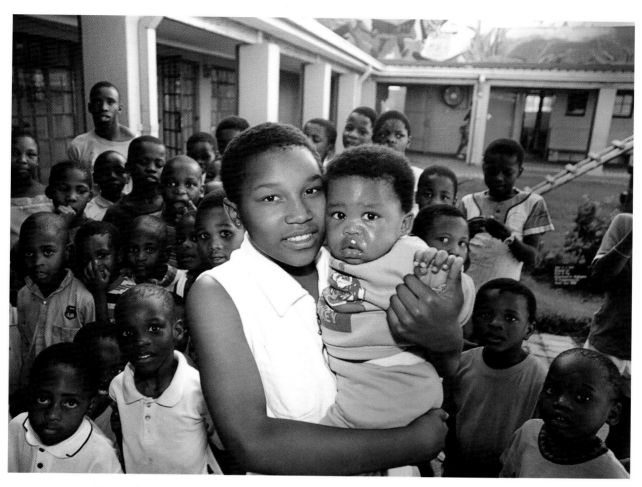

Many of the abandoned babies in Orlando East Children's Home today are orphans.
This baby was orphaned when both his parents were killed in a car accident.
AIDS is ensuring that the numbers of parentless children in South Africa's hospitals
and orphanages are soaring, straining already limited resources.

During the apartheid years, many employers exploited workers who were not in possession of the correct papers (*see* pages 14–15), paying them low wages. The workers in turn eked out an existence on the fringes of society. This family (*below*) followed a migrant labourer to the city, where he lives in a hostel. The family are living in a squalid disused truck in Soweto, far from the mountainous villages of the childhood of the *gogo* (grandmother). Today the numbers of homeless in South Africa have been augmented by refugees, asylum seekers and illegal immigrants from as far away as Senegal, Somalia, Ghana, Kosovo, Poland, Bulgaria, Ethiopia and Rwanda.

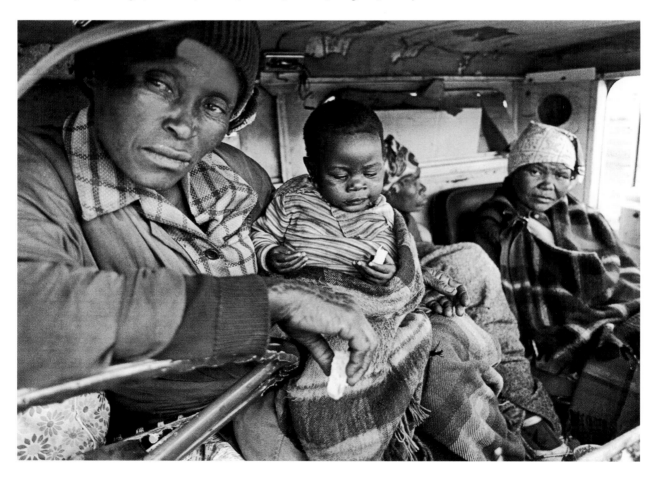

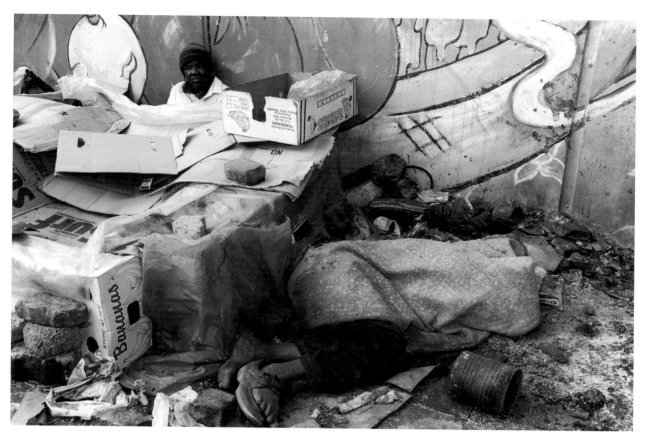

Chris Hani-Baragwanath Hospital is the largest hospital in the southern hemisphere. Among the tens of thousands of patients it treats each year are people who come from right across Africa. Others are abandoned at the hospital by their families: babies with AIDS, mentally ill adults, the crippled and the aged. The hospital places some in institutions, but others leave the gates only to hug its walls as homeless people. They live close to garbage bins, rummaging through them for food by day and using them as braziers during the cold winter nights. They may hawk traditional medicines (*muti*) outside the hospital, or sell fruit to commuters and soft drinks to the families of the ill. 'In rural areas the poor simply starve,' one doctor observed, 'but in Soweto even the poorest can usually find a slice of discarded bread in a bin or earn a few cents helping someone. Survival becomes possible.'

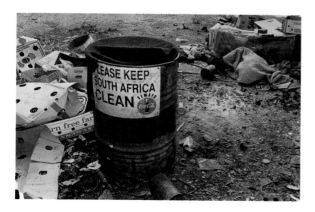

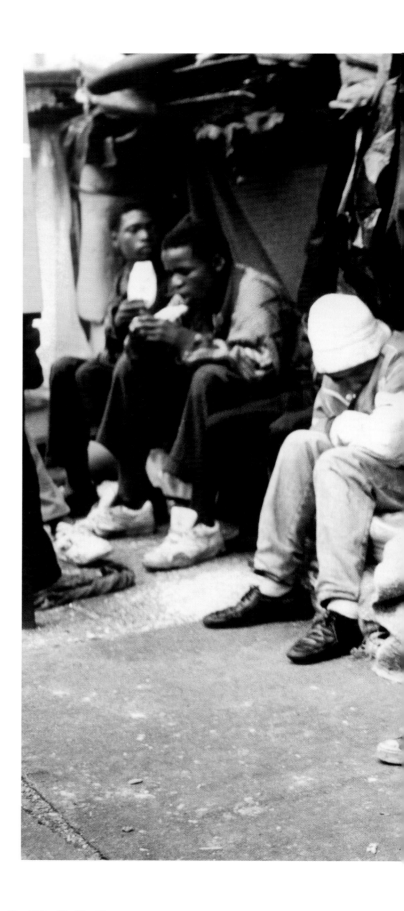

Fourteen-year-old Oscar Makhubo (*extreme right*), who originally comes from Emdeni in deep Soweto, sits outside his makeshift shelter in Hillbrow with some of his friends.

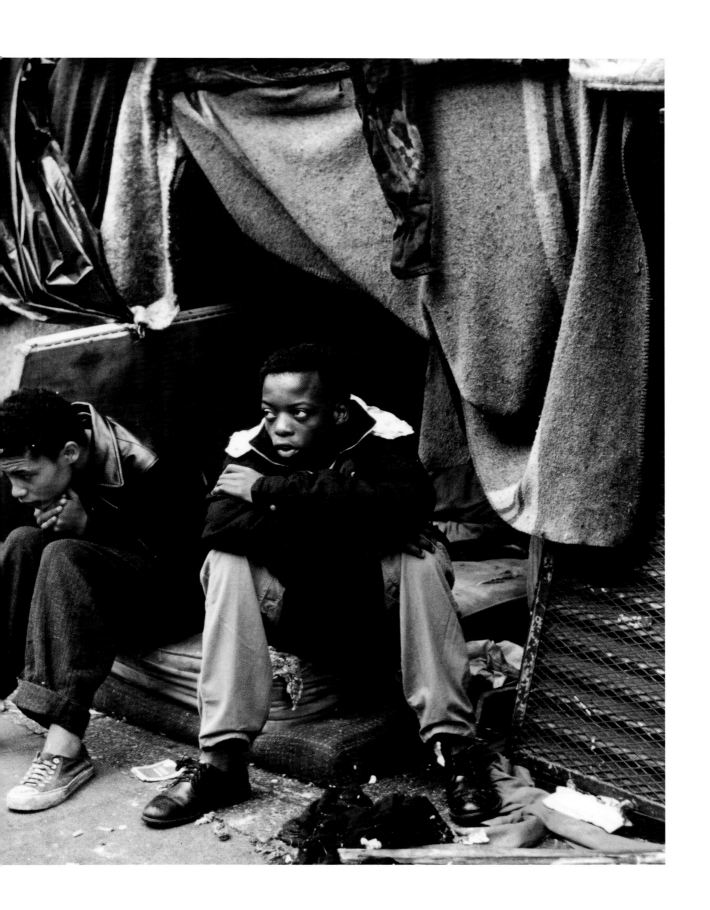

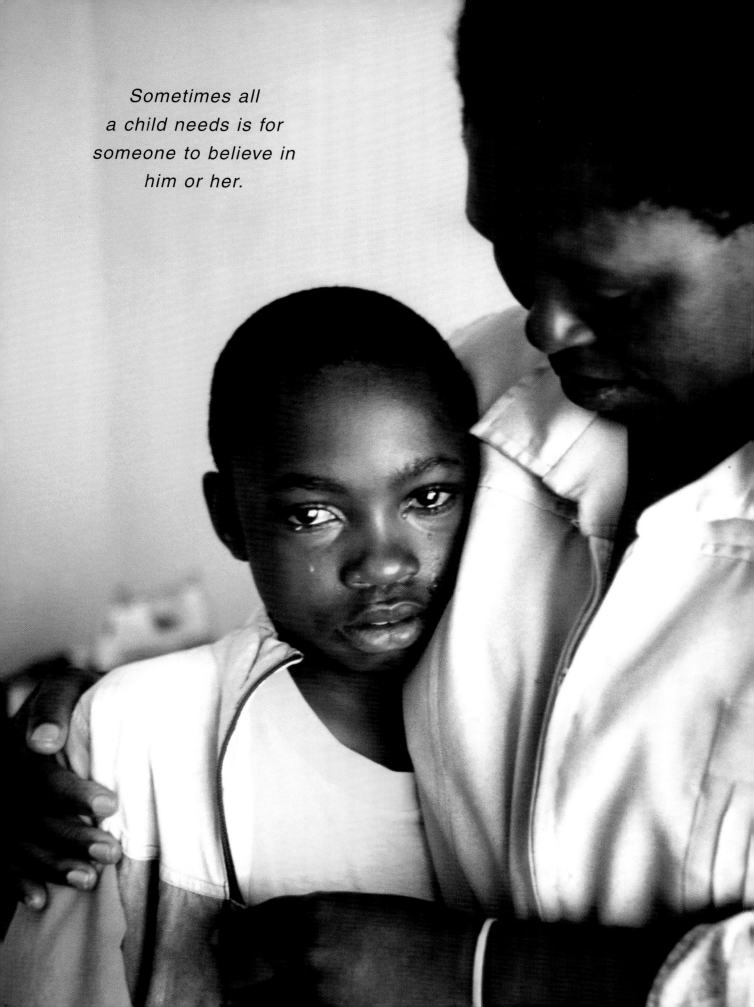

Sometimes all a child needs is for someone to believe in him or her.

Across the world, particularly in developing countries, children who are forced out of their homes through poverty, AIDS or other causes may be found living on the street: begging, sniffing glue or engaged in prostitution. It is rare for these children to be reintroduced into society once they have been on the streets for some time, and few are successfully reunited with their parents. One of the reasons for this is that the social ills that put them on the streets still prevail. Children who have lived on the street also find it difficult to conform to routine and discipline. Nonetheless the ideal is to reunite children with their families where possible, as this picture essay displays.

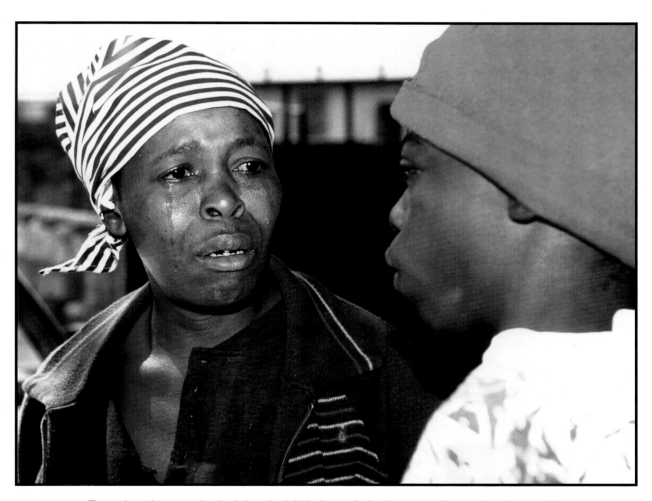

Tears, happiness and pain (*above*). A little boy safe in the arms of his mother (*opposite*).

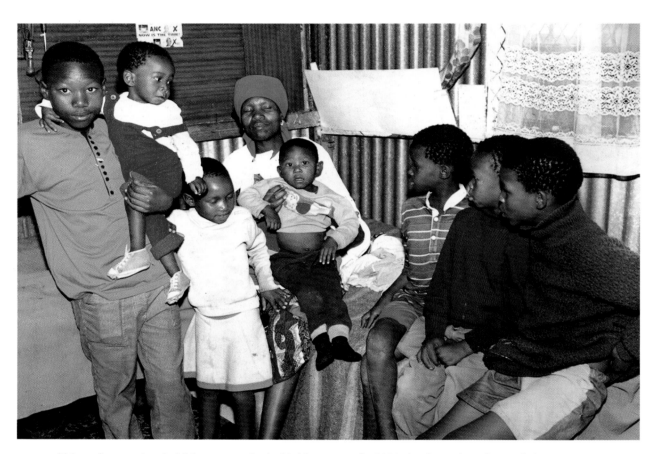

Mdu, a former street child, was reunited with his parents in 1992 thanks to the efforts of photographer Peter Magubane. He is pictured with his family on the day he returned home (*above, extreme left*), and in 2000 with his parents while he was in Grade 12 (*opposite, centre*).

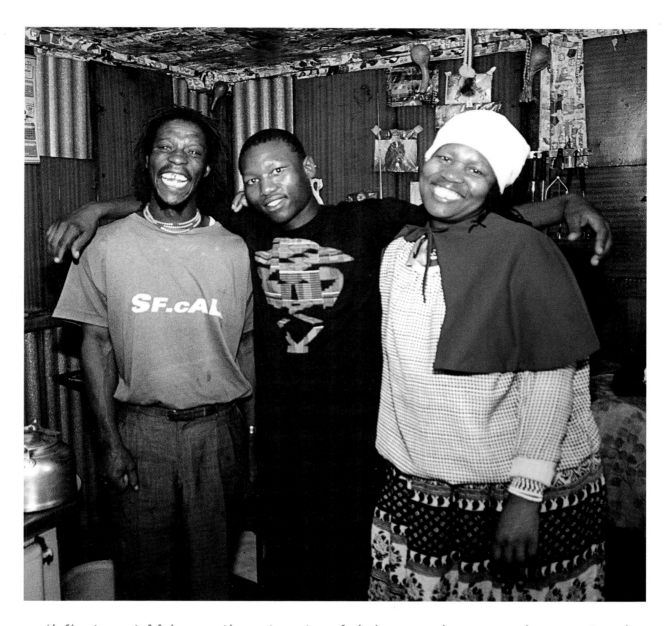

'I first met Mdu on the streets of Johannesburg, and was struck by the youthful intelligence of this young man. I struck up a relationship with him, counselling him and later helping him to find his family and return home to them. This is one of the things I have done that have given me a sense of great joy, to see this fine young man today living up to his potential.'

Peter Magubane

Electricity began being introduced to Soweto when the Orlando power station was established in the late 1940s, but the major electrification drive came in the mid-1980s. In the days before most of Soweto had electricity, coal yards abounded. Despite being owned by Soweto residents, the yards exploited homeless children, children who had run away from home (*below* and *opposite*, taken during the 1980s), or the children of the very poor. Child labour was illegal then, as it is now, yet it persists. Peter Magubane took an intense interest in the hardship experienced by these coalyard boys, and maintained contact with them over many years. He went so far as to reunite three of the coalyard boys with their families, one of whom has since completed his school education and is studying further.

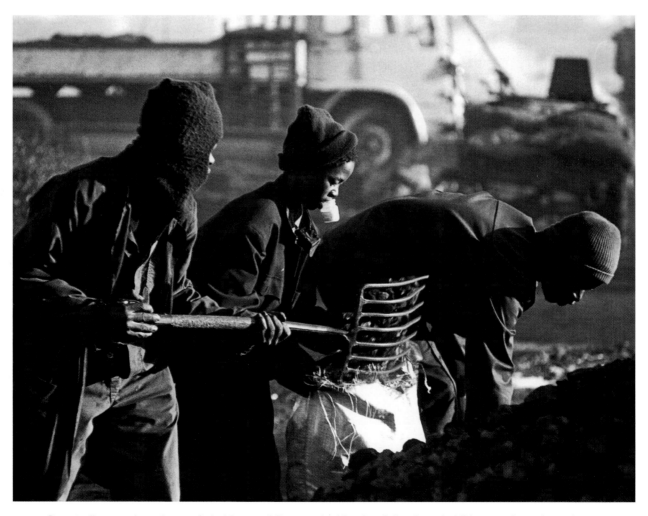

Soweto lives under a haze of choking coal fires, stoked by the deliveries of children such as these boys.

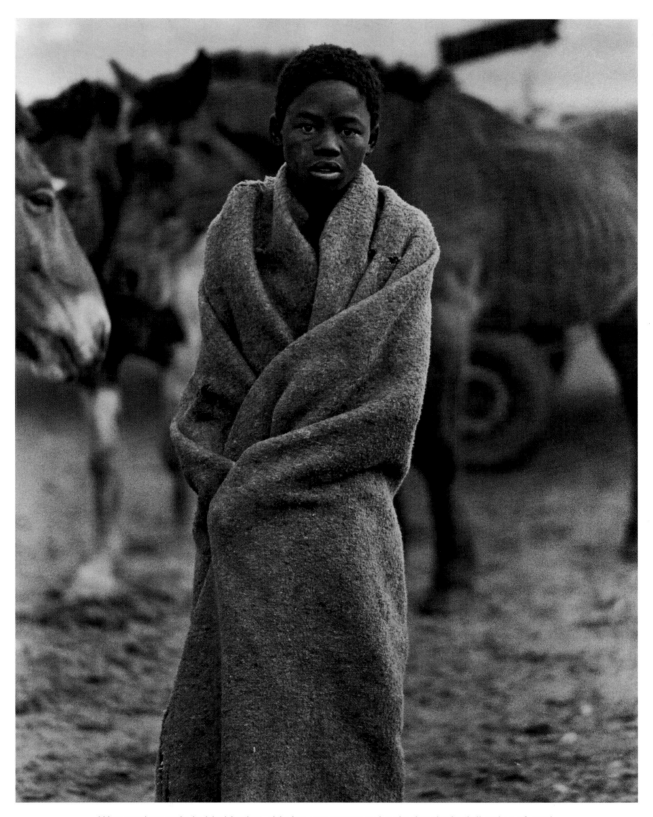

Wrapped warmly in his blanket, this boy prepares to begin the day's deliveries of coal.

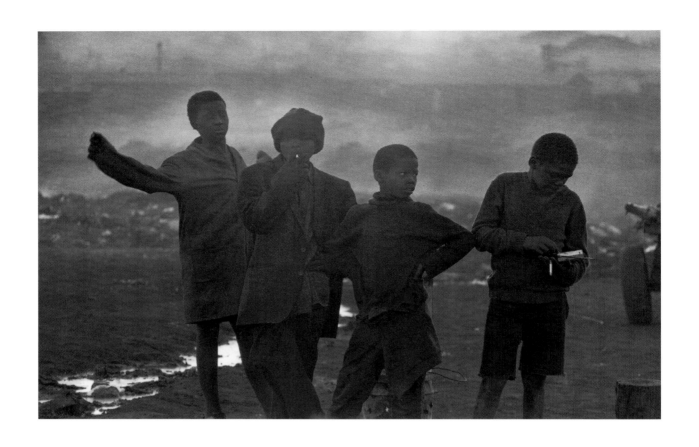

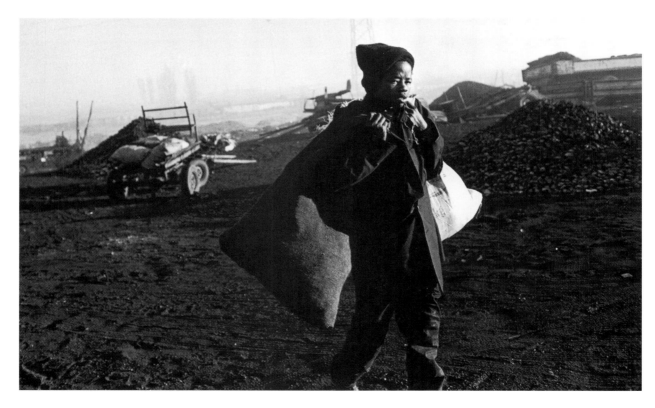

S O W E T O
PETER MAGUBANE

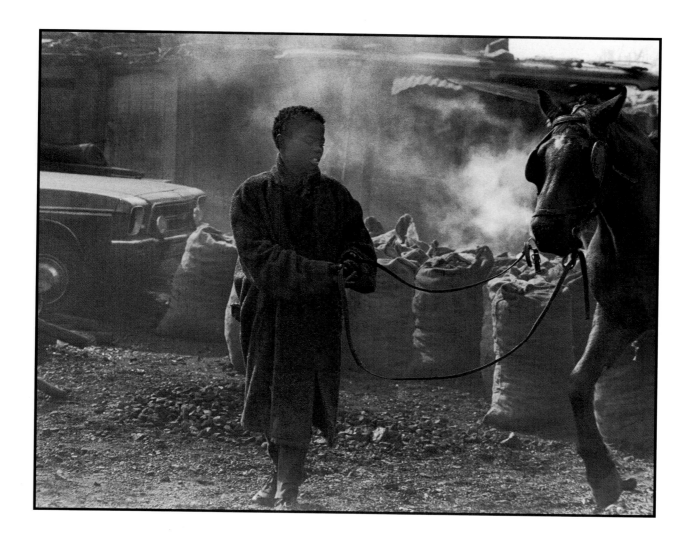

The Universal Declaration of the Rights of the Child, to which South Africa, as a founding member of the United Nations, has long been a signatory, expressly forbids child labour. In the past in South Africa children could frequently be found at work. Even today, in a democratic state in which every child has the right to free education, and where child labour is outlawed, this is sometimes still the case. Poverty speaks louder than noble declarations, even in a country that is sensitive to the rights of its children. Says Peter Magubane: 'These boys I photographed over a period of time, under the gloom of the apartheid years. They touched me with their childlike vulnerability, their adult meanness, and the desperation of their lives. They were up early, worked long, muscle-building, soul-destroying hours, and had their rights to a childhood removed.'

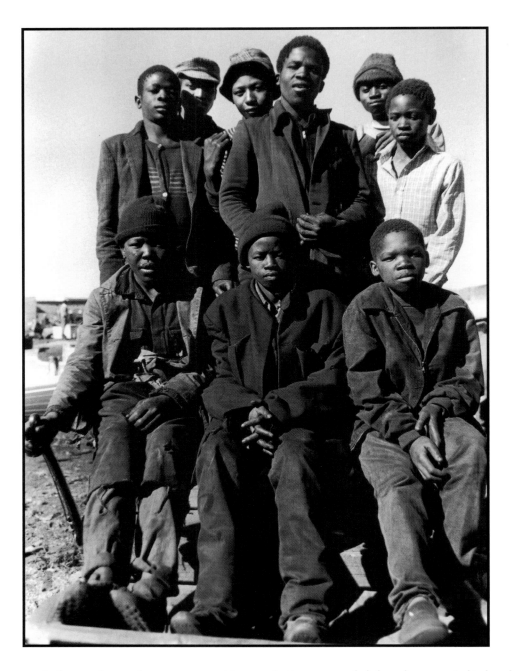

We want freedom because the whites and blacks got it in USA.
White's get more money at work, here in South Africa.
If they have standard ten cetificates both of them,
the white one is going to earn more money than the
black one who is more educated than the white.

Dexter, 13 years (*Two Dogs and Freedom*, a compilation of writing by township children, Ravan Press, 1986)

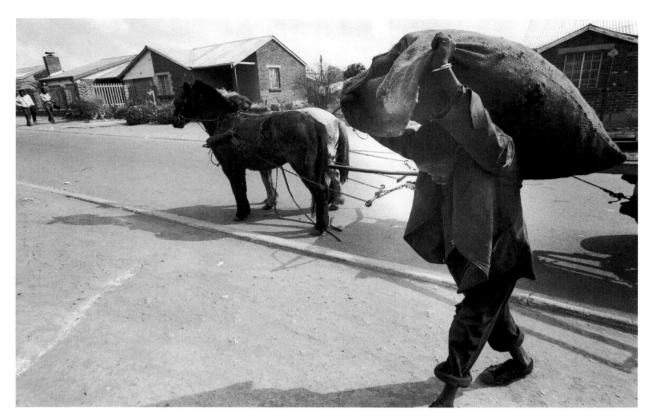

Nkwana (14) hauls a bag of coal almost as big as himself to the home of a Soweto householder.

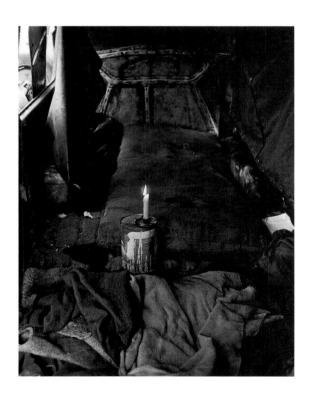

A solitary candle brings a tiny spark of light into the gloomy, dusty quarters of children who work for Soweto coal merchants. But candles like this, and the paraffin stoves used in humble shacks, are a dire fire hazard in South Africa. Every year, particularly in winter, dozens of people die and hundreds of shacks are destroyed – and with them everything the poor own – when a single unattended candle falls.

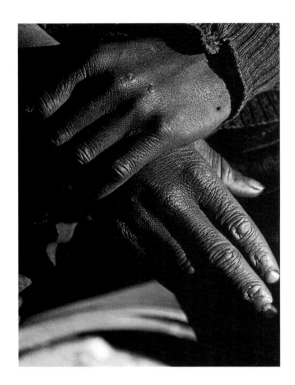

The hands of a 14-year-old boy
who has worked as a manual
labourer in Soweto for much
of his short life.

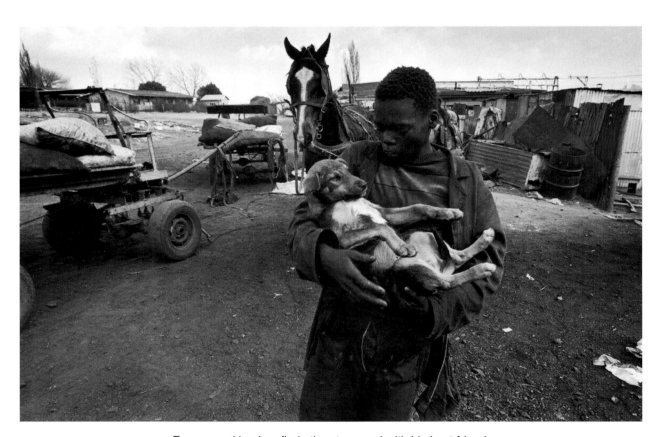

Even a working boy finds time to spend with his best friend.

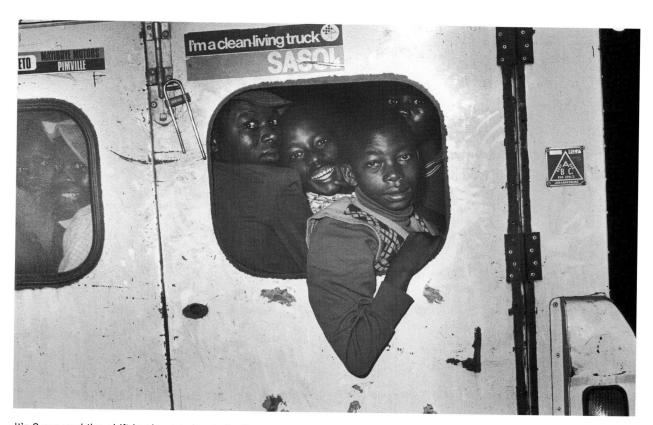

It's 3 am and the shift is about to begin for these young newspaper sellers. Locked into this truck, they are on their way to pick up bales of today's newspapers to sell to morning commuters around Soweto and Johannesburg.

This little boy selling newspapers in Africa Road, Soweto, should be in school, but he is playing truant to earn some extra money. Today child labour is illegal, but, as in most developing nations of the world, it persists in some areas.

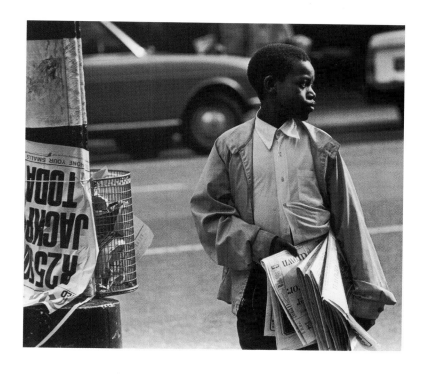

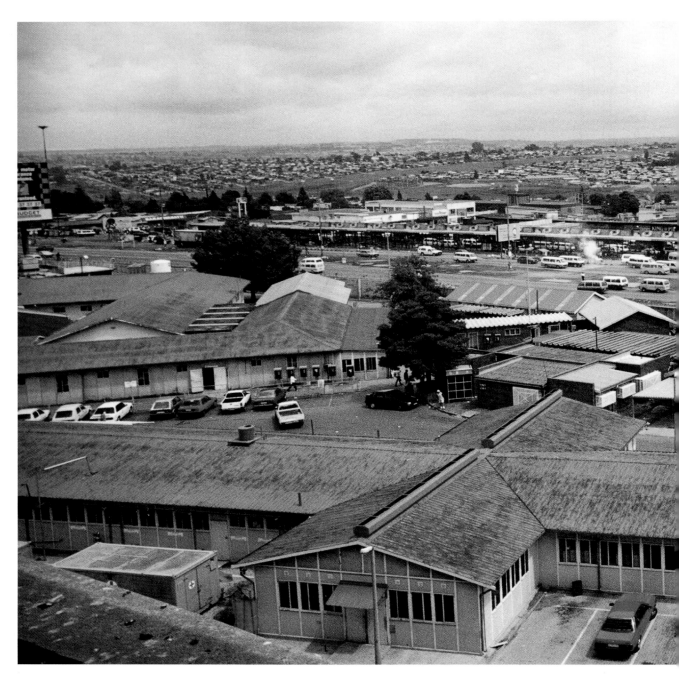

Chris Hani-Baragwanath Hospital is the largest hospital in the southern hemisphere, with some of the world's finest specialists working in its overcrowded wards. This view, taken from its high administrative block, shows only a small part of the hospital, with some of the many prefabricated buildings that comprise its sprawl. In the foreground in the left of the photograph is the pedestrian bridge that connects the hospital to a small shopping area and one of the busiest taxi ranks in South Africa. Beyond that stretches the suburb of Diepkloof.

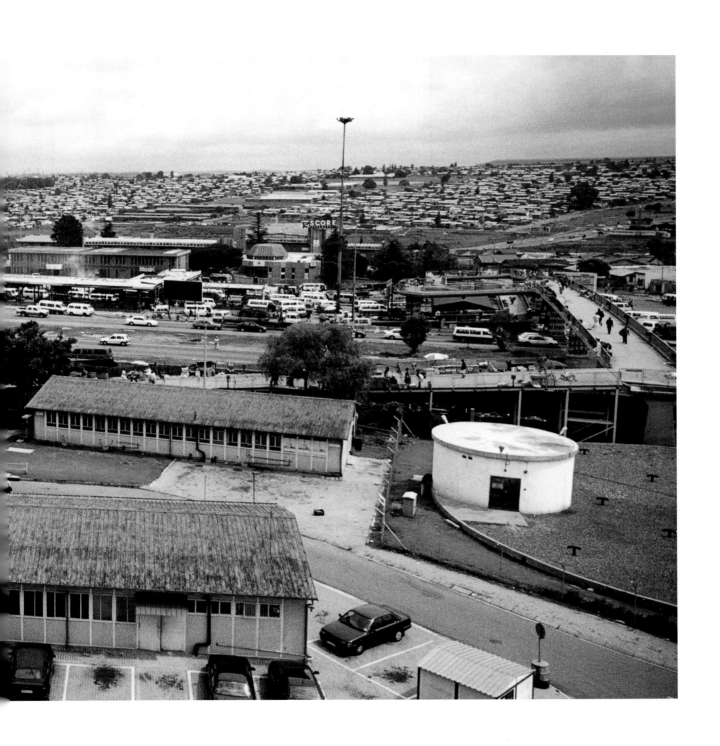

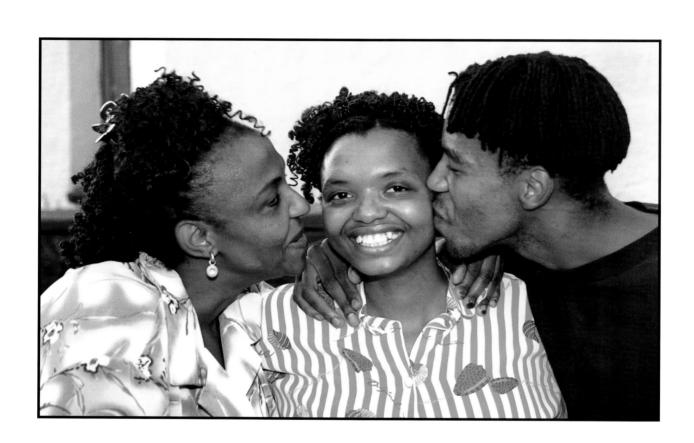

During the 1950s black people were denied access to alcohol, which led to the proliferation of speakeasies, better known as shebeens, that were run from people's homes. Ironically, the crumbling of apartheid in 1990 and the lifting of restrictions on the sale of liquor destroyed an industry that had provided many people with a good livelihood. One of those who sold liquor from her home was Tselane Mohasoane, who as a teacher and a single parent was battling to make ends meet. Her gentle, convivial nature ensured the success of her outlet. This allowed her to send her three children to school and her daughter, Katleho Mohasoane, (pictured here with her mother and brother in Dube Village), studied medicine at the University of Natal. 'It was difficult to pay and Katleho also had to take out a small loan, but I wanted her to have a bright future, so she can look after herself. A shebeen ensured a better income than teaching during those times, but now it is better to be a teacher than sell liquor. Now there are many liquor outlets; during that time I could still make money.'

She is still putting her two boys through school and technical college. 'It was sometimes very hard, but as a single mother you have to be focused and determined and do the right thing. Success is tied up with the way you think. I used to plan on Sunday what I would do for the whole week. I have found that most single mothers raise their children with a far greater commitment to education and self-betterment than children in families with both parents. With single parents there is no fighting, so the children listen to you better and they do well. As a single mother your children are closer to you. They can see you are working and struggling. They say, I wish I could be educated so I can help you.'

Katleho is working at Chris Hani-Baragwanath Hospital and plans to specialise in neuro-surgery.

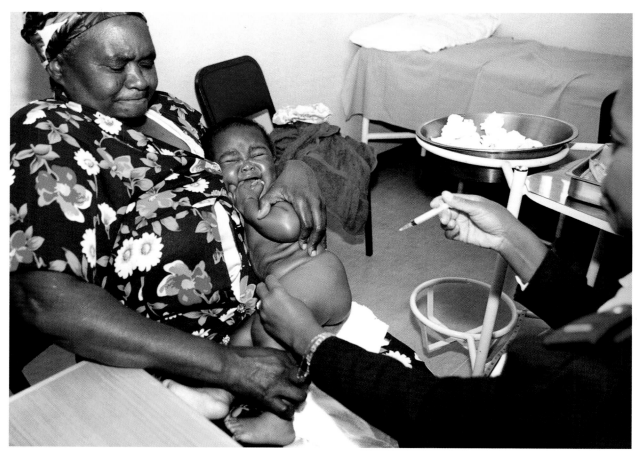

Sometimes anticipation is worse than reality. At Diepkloof Clinic, a mother grimaces and her baby wails, as a nurse pauses with the instrument of medicine every child dreads.

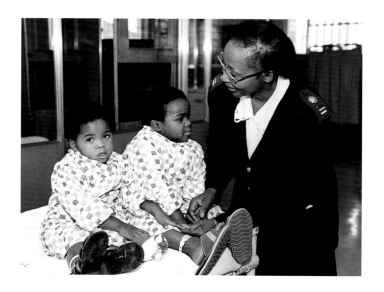

Kind nurses make hospital stays easier. Sister Serobatse chats with two small patients at Chris Hani-Baragwanath Hospital.

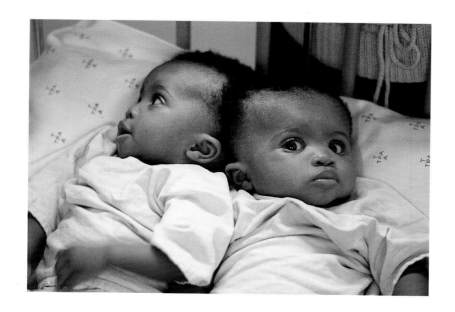

Chris Hani-Baragwanath Hospital is one of the best centres in Africa specialising in operations to separate conjoined (Siamese) twins. Mpho and Mphonyane Mathibela, who were joined at the back, made world news in 1987, when they were separated at the hospital. Sadly one of these twins did not survive the operation.

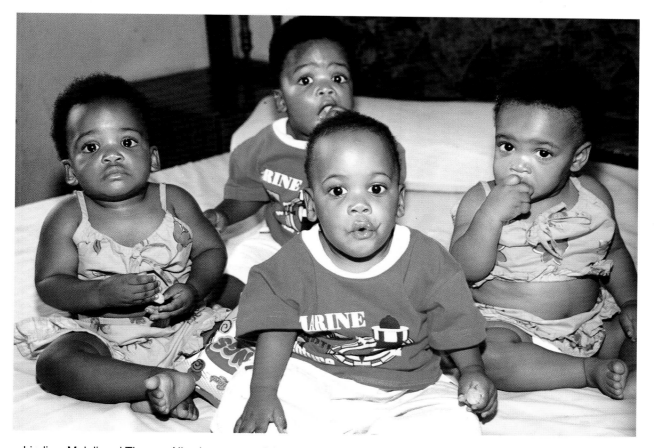

Lindiwe Meluli and Thomas Nkosi were astonished to learn they were expecting not one, not two, but four babies! Sipho and Simphiwe (the boys) and Jabu and Jabulile (the girls) celebrated their first birthday on 28 January 2001.

During the apartheid years, an entire subculture sprang up around public transport in Soweto. Train carriages would be separated according to preference. In some carriages there would be preachers conducting church services or Bible readings. In others political discussions would take place, with activists hotly debating black consciousness and congress politics. In other carriages musicians would practise the saxophone or discuss the relative merits of the harmonica versus the penny whistle. Commuting was more than just a tedious part of the day's work: it was an essential element of community life.

The advent of minibus taxis in the early 1980s, which the apartheid government tried unsuccessfully to squash, merely perpetuated what was happening in trains. In taxis today, commuters grapple with religion and politics, and talk about the last football match. Taxis make their own tapes, and they also sell advertising space on their exterior. Trade unions or political parties frequently use a taxi ride to try to recruit new members.

Commuters in Soweto live with the ongoing possibility of being robbed or raped, or caught in crossfire between rival taxi organisations at taxi ranks. Later during the apartheid years, in the early 1990s, death squad assassins went onto trains and opened fire on commuters, killing dozens.

The taxi industry is a billion rand industry, but it is hard work. The already narrow profit margins are always under siege from escalating fuel prices, maintenance costs and relatively poor passengers who quibble about every price increase. As a result, most taxis operate on turnover, speeding from place to place, with as many passengers as possible crammed into poorly maintained vehicles.

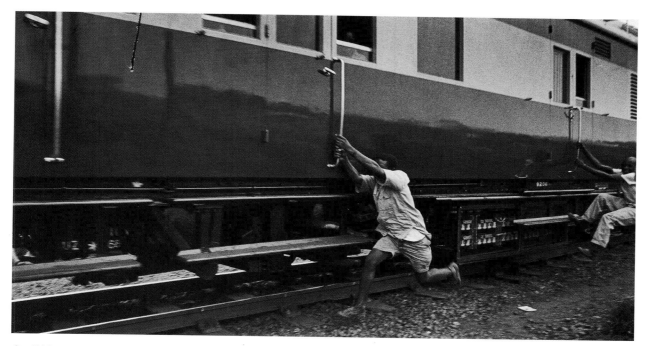

Staffriders are one of the classic symbols of Soweto train journeys. They are usually young men who, to avoid paying the fare, run alongside trains, and then grab onto outside bars for dear life to get a free – and dangerous – ride into and out of Johannesburg. These staffriders were photographed near Pimville in 1962. Today this is an unusual sight, as modern trains are designed without convenient rails.

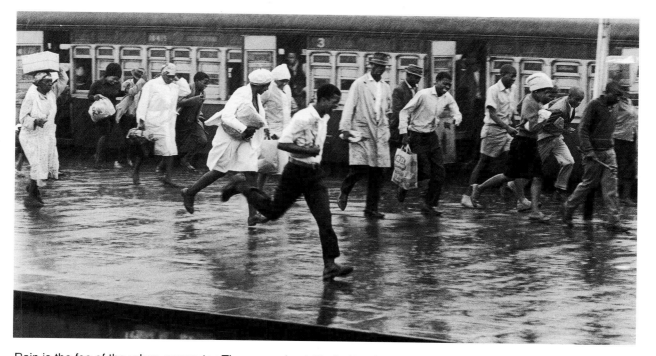

Rain is the foe of the urban commuter. These people at Phefeni station in Orlando West dash for cover (1978).

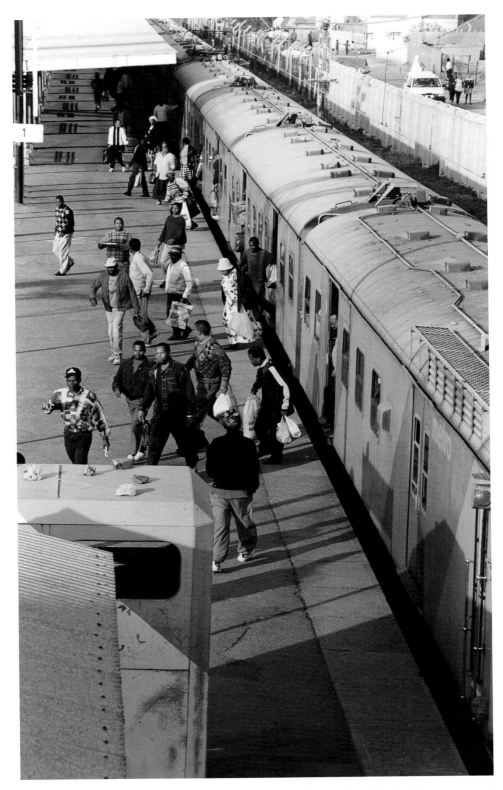

Mzimhlope station is one of the busiest stops on the Soweto line. Most of those who get off or board at this station are migrant workers from nearby Mzimhlope hostel.

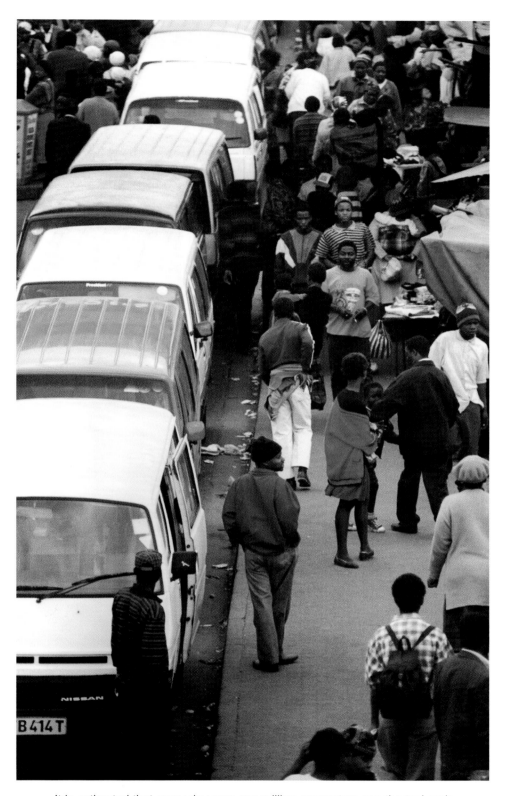

It is estimated that every day over one million commuters use the taxi rank situated opposite Chris Hani-Baragwanath Hospital.

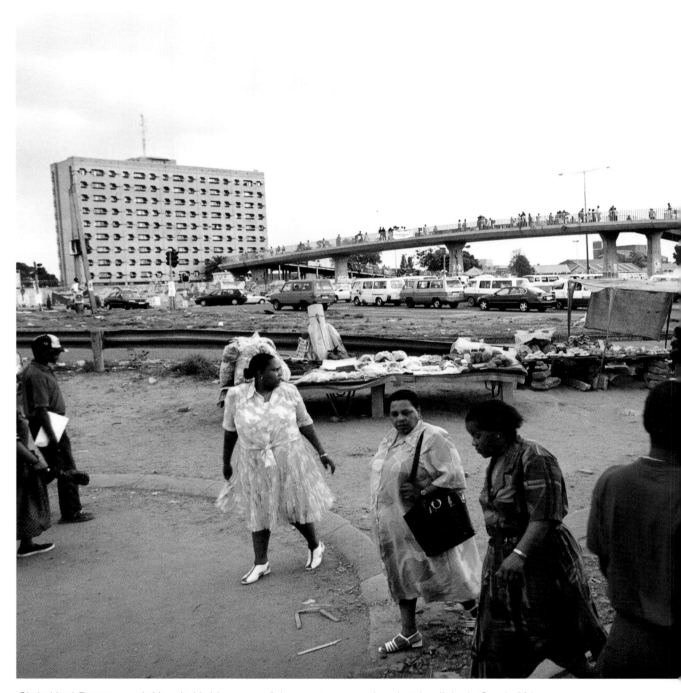

Chris Hani-Baragwanath Hospital bridge, one of the most traversed pedestrian links in South Africa.

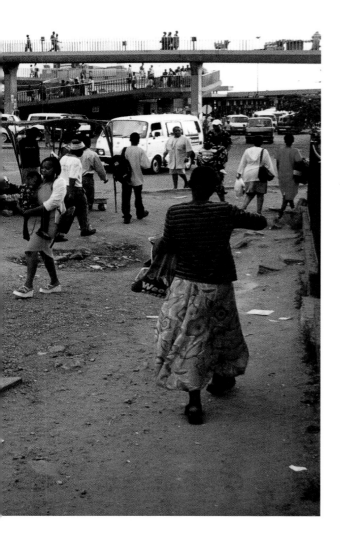

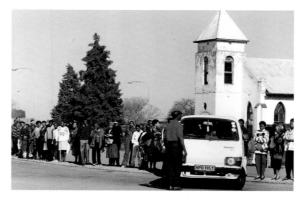

Commuters queue outside a traditional church in Orlando East. During the apartheid era it was used as a place for the local community to meet and discuss grievances about township administration, schooling or political issues.

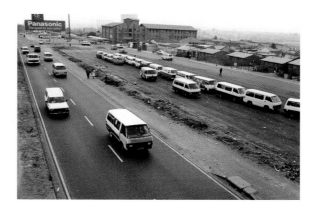

Potchefstroom Road is one of the primary access routes into Soweto, leading past Chris Hani-Baragwanath Hospital. Opposite the hospital gates are one of the main taxi ranks serving Johannesburg and surrounding towns.

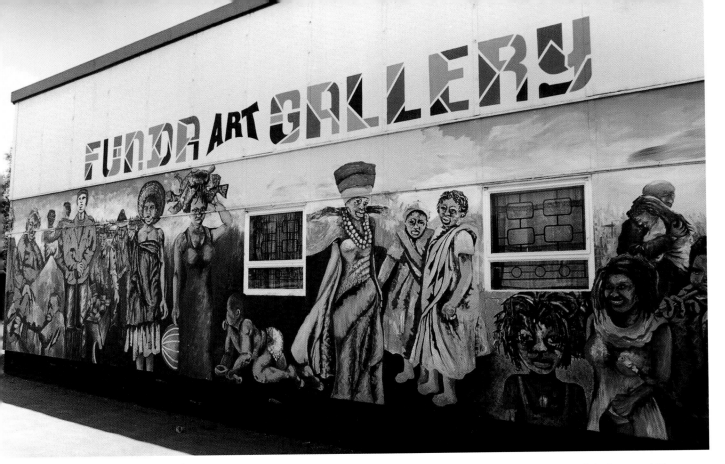

The murals on the outside of Funda Art Gallery in Diepkloof, depicting people's struggles and their way of life, serve to attract visitors to the gallery. However, in traditional African culture, particularly among the Pedi, Zulu and Ndebele, wall painting is an important activity carried out by women. In the past, pigments obtained from the soil and plants were daubed onto walls. Even the colours used carry meaning: red ochre facilitates communication with the spirits of ancestors, white guards against bad spirits, and blue is the colour of the sky and good spirits.

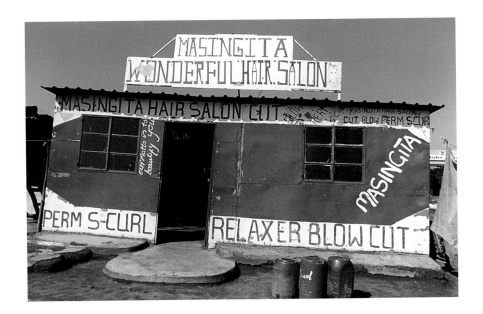

Masingita's Wonderful Hair Salon lures its clientele across Freedom Square with its enticing offers.

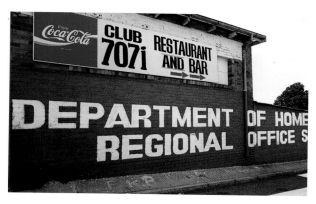

A Department of Home Affairs office is a new addition to Soweto. Throughout the apartheid years it was extremely difficult for black people to obtain passports or documents to travel abroad. All of that has changed in the past decade. Offices such as these also strike fear into the hearts of the many illegal immigrants from across Africa who live in Soweto. South Africa's tough immigration laws are perceived to be in place in order to keep out as many *kwere-kwere* (a derogatory term for foreigners) as possible.

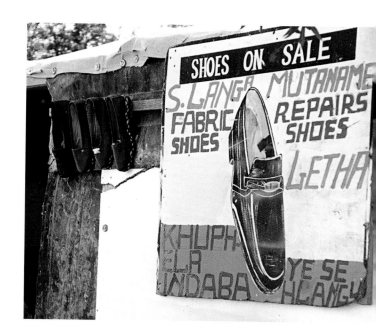

He wears
the latest Levison's suits
'Made in America';
from Cuthbert's
a pair of Florscheim shoes
'America's finest shoes',
He pays cash
that's why
he's called Mister.

He goes for quality, man,
not quantity, never –
the price is no obstacle.

Good shoes are a national obsession, as Oswald Mtshali captures in this excerpt from his poem, 'The Detribalised' (*Black Poetry from Southern Africa*, 1982).

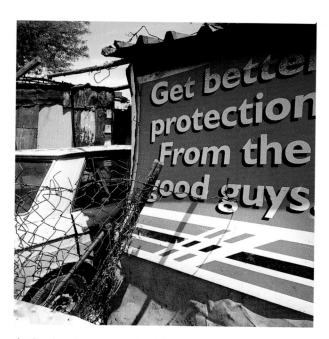

An ironic advertisement advises people to 'Get better protection. From the good guys.'

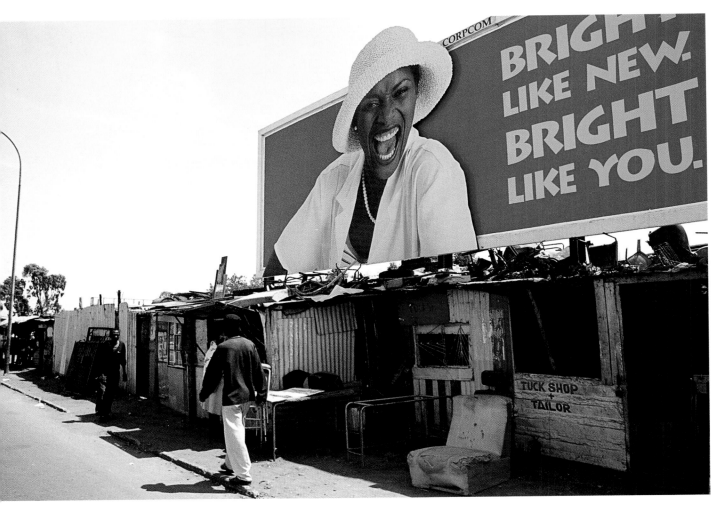

Despite its dilapidated air, Mandelaville Squatter Camp in Diepkloof is relatively new. The vibrant washing powder advertisement above these shacks reflects the optimism of Africa's youngest democracy.

Rhee's Place in Zone 2 Diepkloof is one of the many taverns where tired workers go to relax after work or during the weekend.

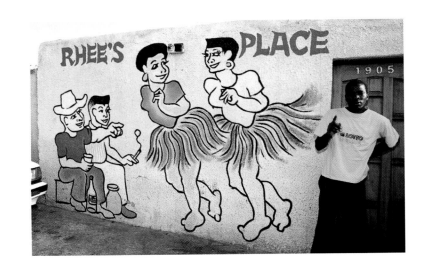

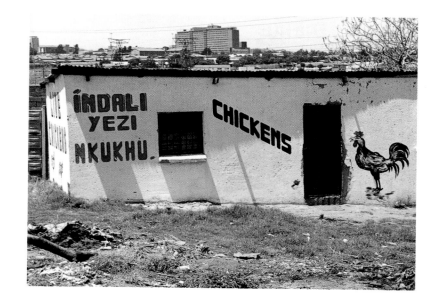

During the struggle, the cock crow was an African symbol of freedom, the awakening of a new dawn. This cock is merely inviting buyers to select a chicken for the cooking pot.

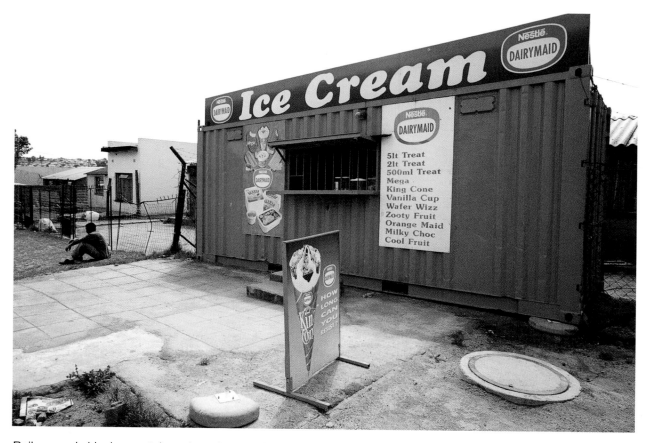

Railway and shipping containers have been artfully used in Soweto and other townships in South Africa as premises for businesses. They serve as anything from offices to voting centres, to phone shops, spaza stores, or, in this instance, an ice cream bar in Zone 6 Diepkloof.

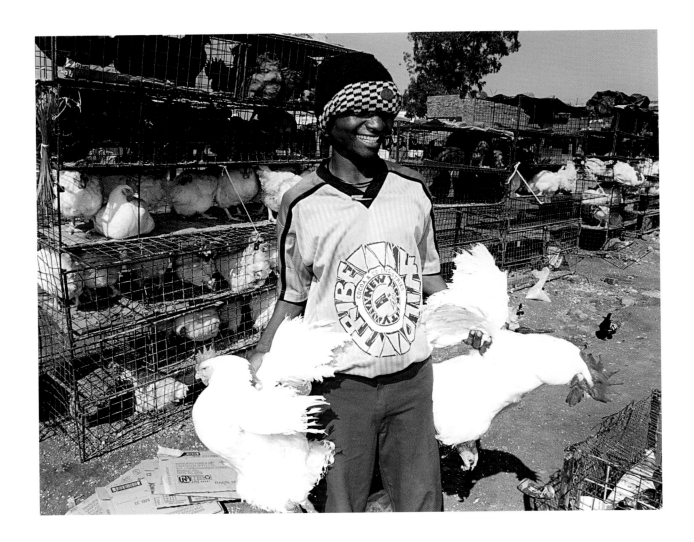

On 26 June 1955, some 5,000 people gathered at a square in Kliptown, now known as Freedom Square, to ratify the Freedom Charter of the African National Congress. The Freedom Charter begins: 'We, the people of South Africa, declare for all our country and the world to know that South Africa belongs to all who live in it, black and white, and that no government can justly claim authority unless it is based on the will of the people ...' The young chicken seller (*above*), vegetable hawker (*opposite top*) and second hand clothes retailer (*opposite bottom*) pictured here at Freedom Square are exercising their rights in terms of section three of the Charter: 'The people shall share in the country's wealthy'. Among other points the Charter notes that 'all people shall have equal rights to trade where they choose, to manufacture and to enter all trades, crafts and professions.'

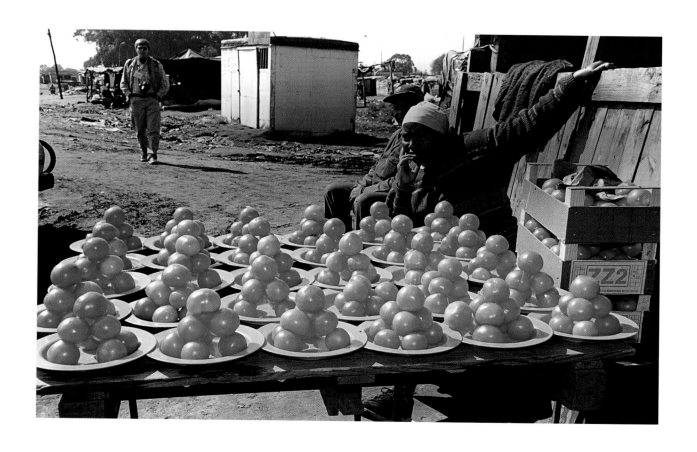

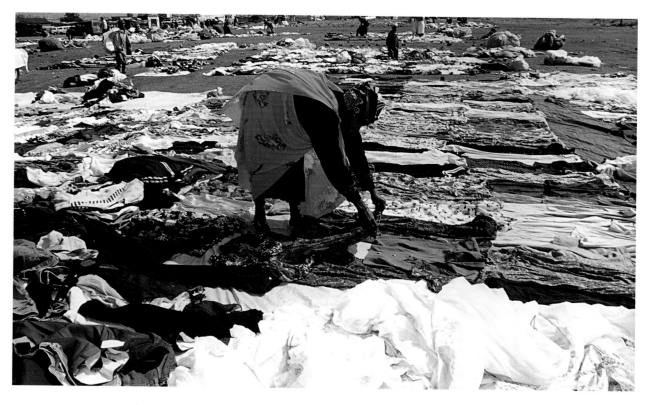

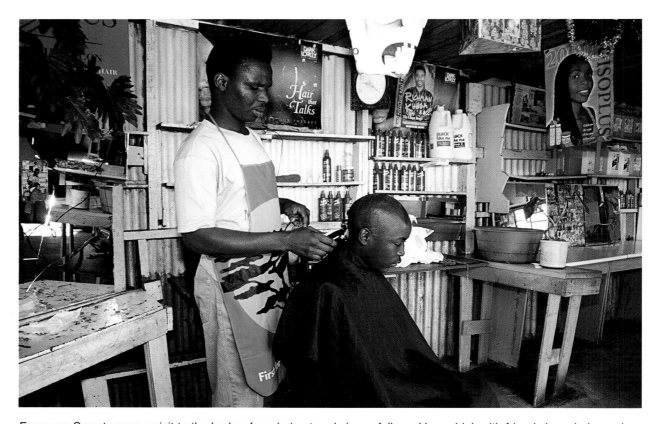

For many Soweto men a visit to the barber for a haircut and shave, followed by a drink with friends in a shebeen, is a ritual of manhood they refuse to give up. This man goes for the shorn look at a Freedom Square barber.

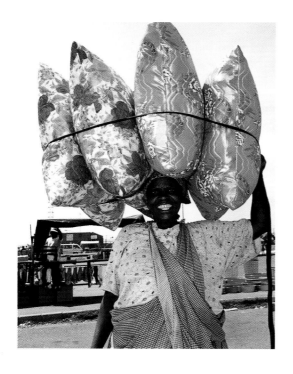

One of the most coveted and rare items for collectors of African art and artefacts is a traditional carved wooden headrest. These beautifully wrought objects began disappearing rapidly as migrant labourers came to the cities at the turn of the 20th century seeking work. They would return home proudly bearing a soft white pillow or a colourful cushion like those sold by this woman.

Bright plastic plates and
basins are a feature
of street sellers on the
Chris Hani-Baragwanath
Hospital walkway, helping
to keep goods clean
and quickly transportable.

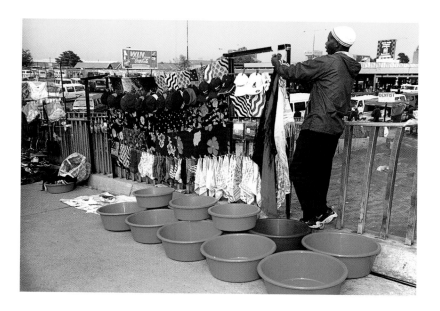

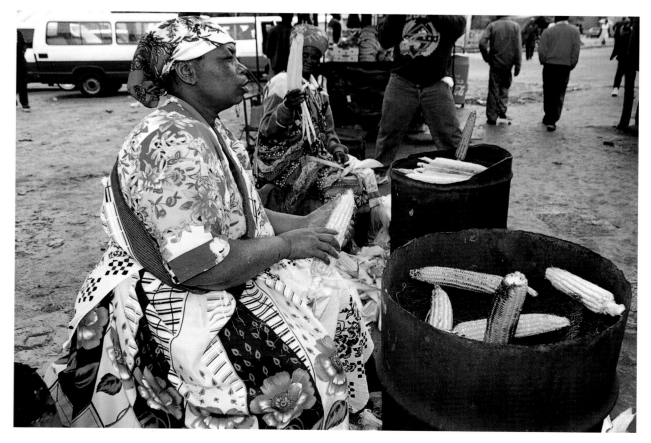

One of the most evocative sights in the northern parts of South Africa is that of women sitting at braziers. Frequently dressed in Shangaan robes like the women above, they grill fresh mealies (corn on the cob) until they are blackened and delicious, for sale to commuters.

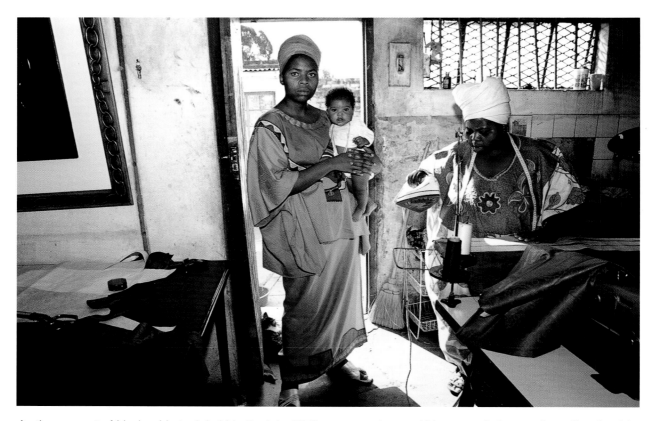

As the concept of black pride took hold in the late 1970s, more and more African people began discarding the tight collars and cuffs of Western dress in favour of traditional African garb, which draws primarily on West African styles. Bheki Gumbi is a popular clothing and furniture manufacturer in Orlando East who typifies the new fashion consciousness of the Sowetan.

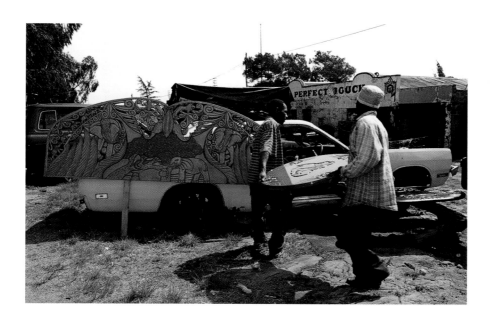

These beautifully carved headboards and table tops come from Bheki Gumbi's Perfect Touch furniture factory in Orlando East.

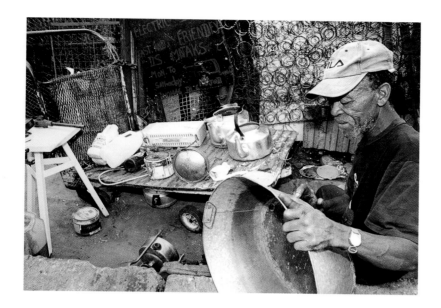

Little gets goes to waste in Soweto. This craftsman makes tin baths, kettles, mugs and plates from recycled metal at his workshop in the township.

Soweto is home to numerous artists, sculptors and craftspeople who make everything from traditional clay pots to silkscreen prints and delicately woven baskets. There is not a single outlet for art in Soweto. Instead, many artists, such as sculptor Grant Sihlahla (*below*), have had their works exhibited abroad and bought by international museums.

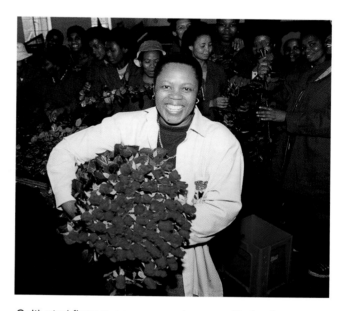

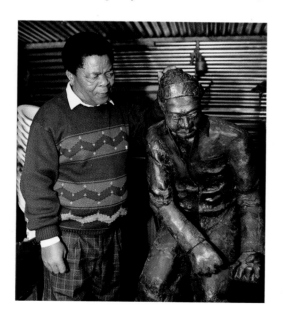

Cultivated flowers are an export commodity for the countries of the southern hemisphere to the wealthier northern countries. Soweto-born Jean Davidson began growing roses at the farm she now lives on at Tarlton, an hour to the west of Johannesburg. Each year Caroza Farm exports three and a half million long-stemmed roses to the markets of Europe, Saudi Arabia and Scandinavia.

Etchings in despair: an exhausted coal worker rests his head in his hand at Nancefield railway station (1978). South Africa has the most extensive rail network in Africa, and loans or rents rolling stock to nations across the continent. These wagons at Nancefield might later find themselves in the Democratic Republic of Congo, Namibia, Botswana or Mozambique.

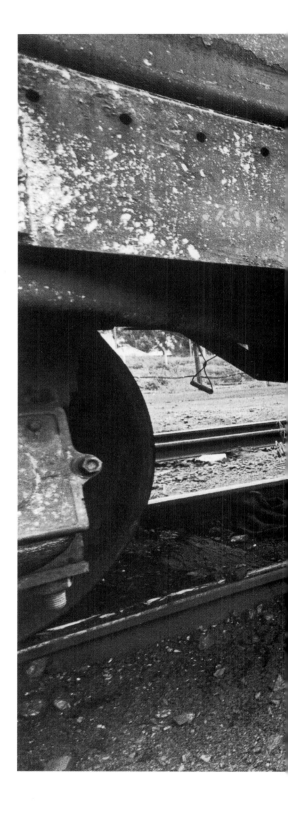

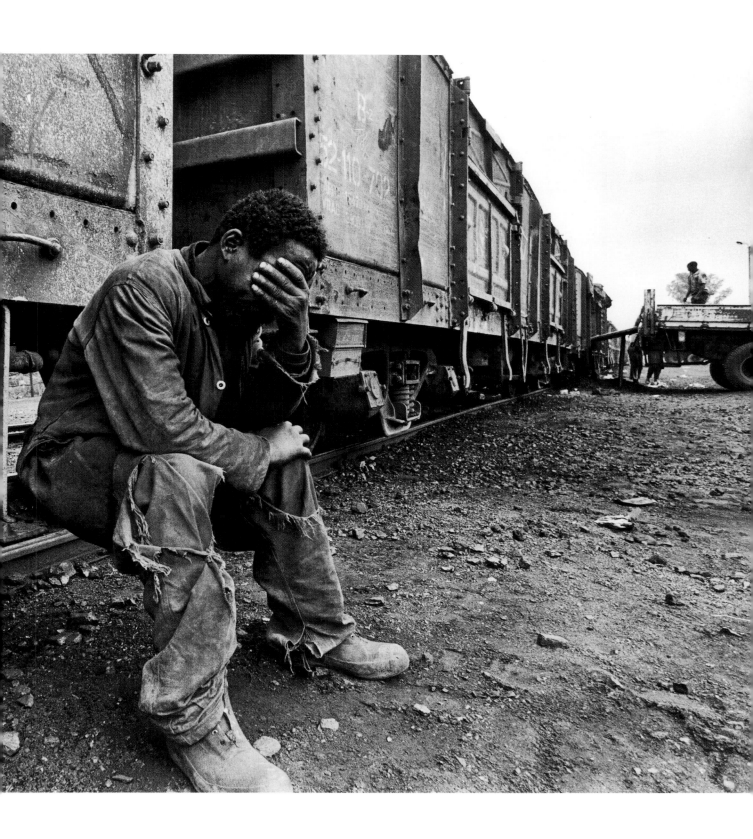

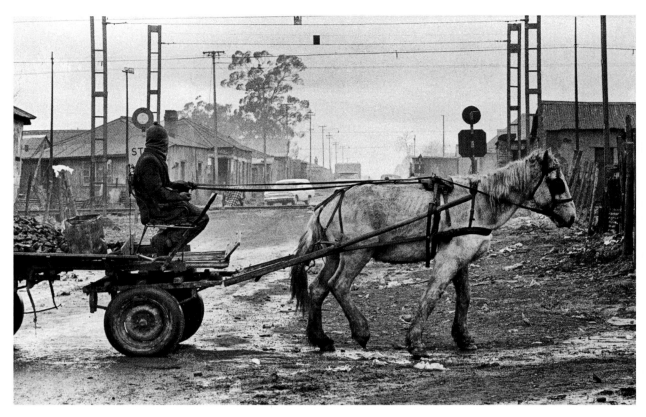

A coal merchant and his mangy horse drive through the streets of Pimville in 1962. Coal merchants were the backbone of Soweto life and industry until an electrification drive took place in Soweto in the 1980s.

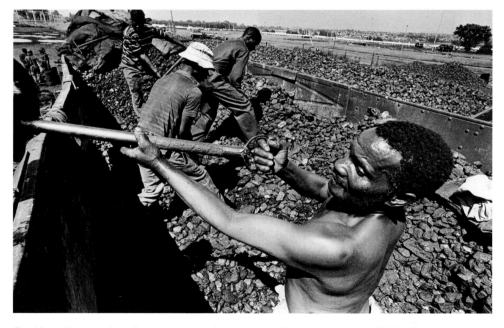

Backbreaking work: railway workers shovel coal off a truck at Nancefield railway station.

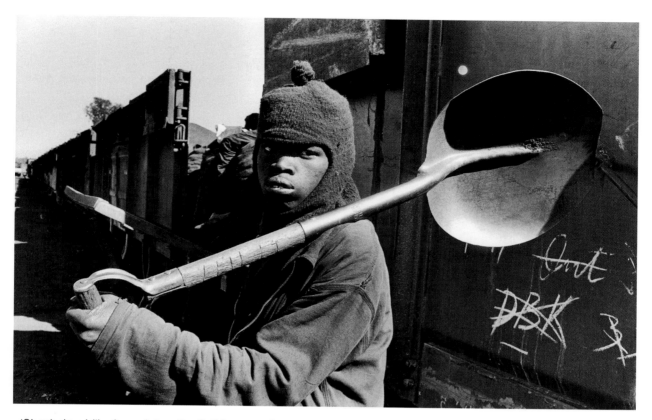

'Shosholoza' ('Let's work together'): this song, that originated with spade-wielding workers on the roads, farms and railways, became an unofficial national anthem during South Africa's transition to democracy in 1994.

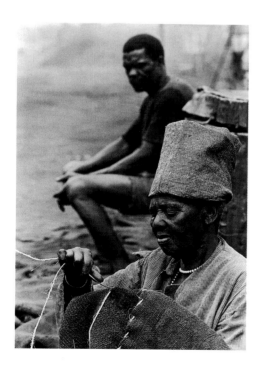

Sackcloth is commonly worn by haulers of coal and railway labourers. This woman stitches together a sackcloth garment.

Cattle play an important role in the life, customs and wealth of African people (*below* and *bottom*). Even among city families, cattle are exchanged as *lobola* (payment by the groom to the family of a bride). The number of head of cattle a man owns signifies his wealth and status in his community, and wealthy men loan out cattle as a form of currency. Villagers and city dwellers alike use the dung of cattle to make beautiful floors with a high gloss, or to bind the daub in walls. Historically, cattle were sacrificed to the ancestors, and today a cow is still slaughtered at great festivities, such as weddings and funerals, or to commemorate a new house or enterprise.

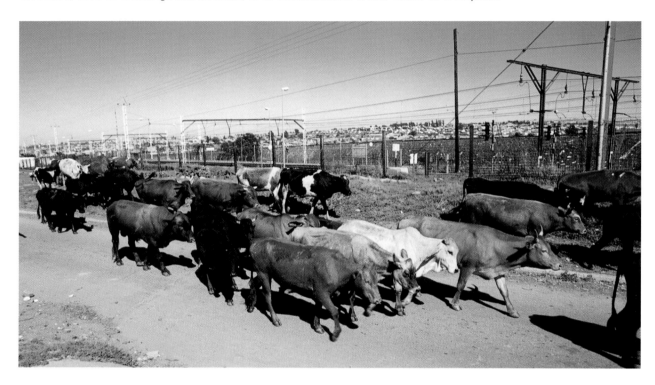

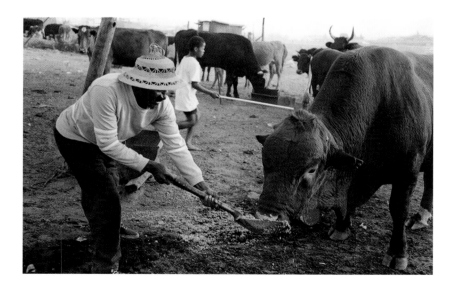

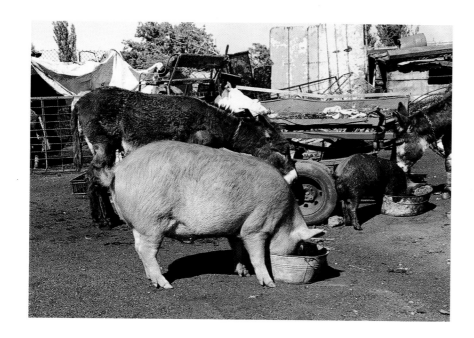

Pigs are not eaten by some African ethnic and religious groups, but in Soweto it is not uncommon to see a sow and piglets foraging for food on the sides of roads and the banks of streams.

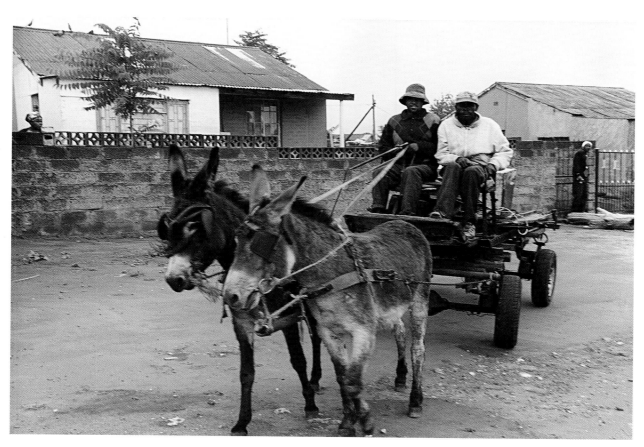

The donkey is an essential means of transport for poor people and their goods. Scrap collectors drive around Soweto in their donkey carts, collecting glass, metal, paper or other discarded goods for resale to merchants.

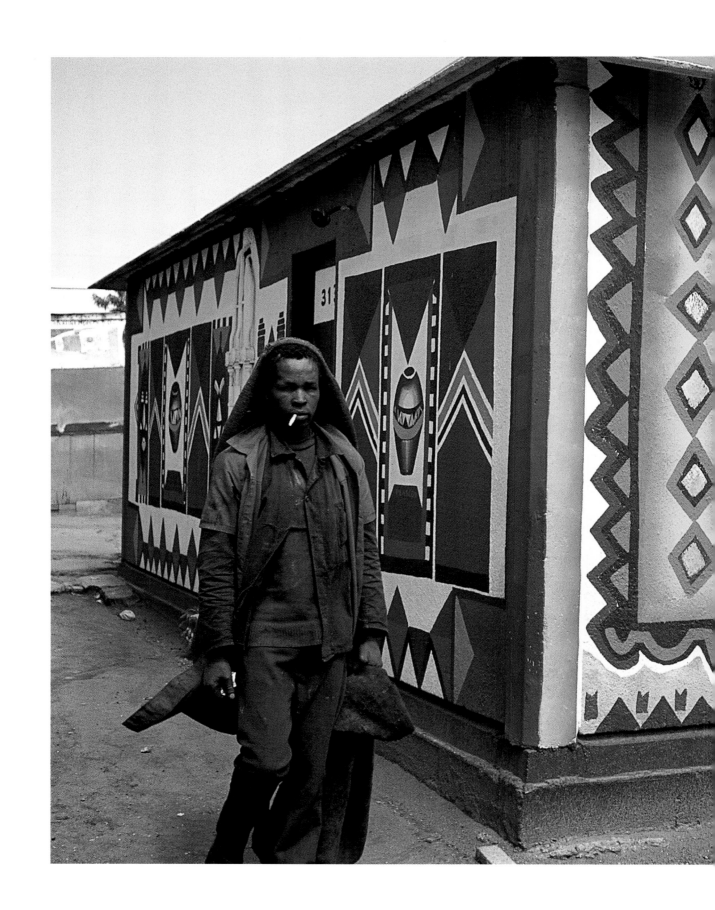

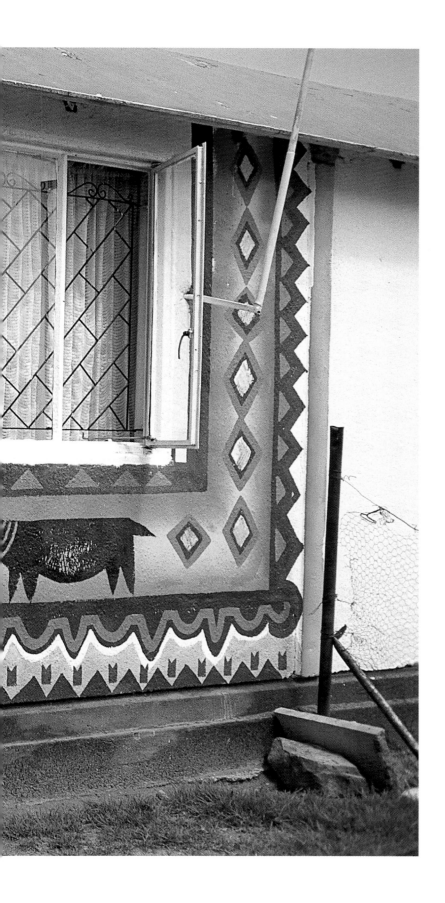

House painting, which holds an important place in African culture, is always the preserve of women. Murals have been modified over the years to incorporate new themes and new colours, some devoid of the meaning of the past. They are no less evocative in their impact, as this house in White City Jabavu shows (1980).

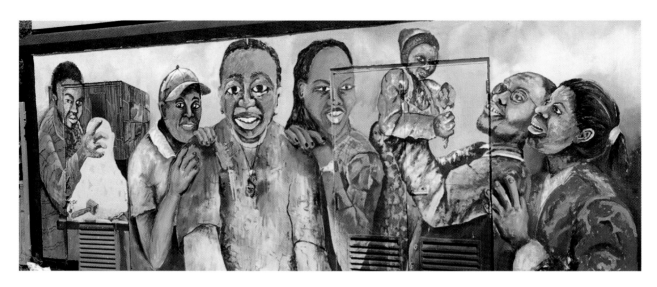

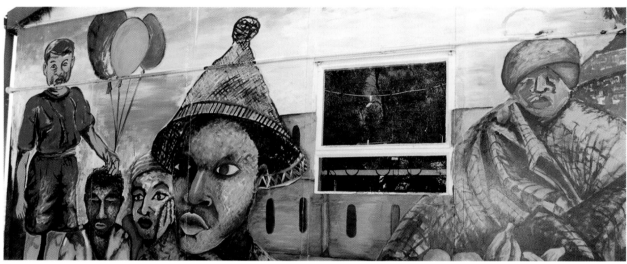

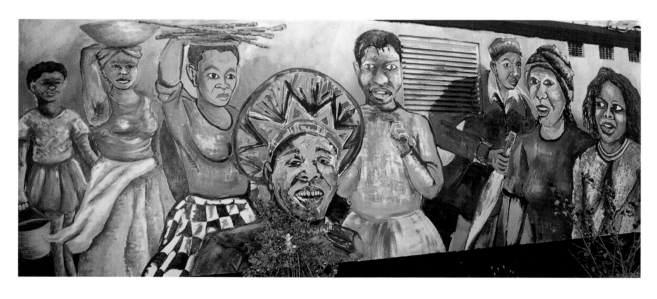

In 1986, 40% of the 40,000 people in political detention in South Africa were children. Township residents should have been emotionally crushed, but instead they created 'peace parks': they cleared open spaces and painted rocks and walls; they planted flowers, made little benches, and constructed fishponds out of old tyres. The apartheid police retaliated by destroying these simple symbols of the determination of people not to allow their spirits to be crushed. The destruction of these parks led to the emergence of mural artists whose work can be seen across Soweto. The greatest challenge facing black artists today is persuading foreign buyers to accept them as artists.

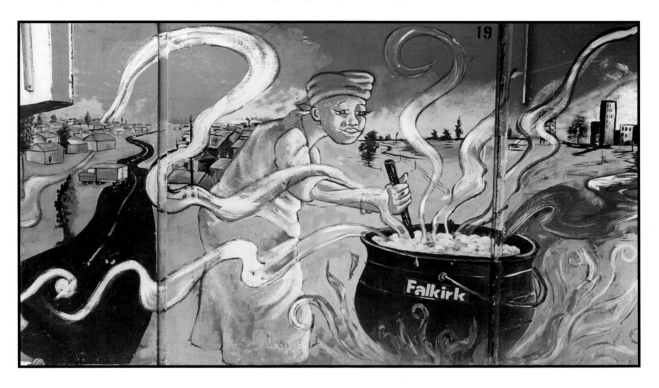

The art of Africa has changed. The tribal past, glorified in the glossy pages of African art magazines, presents a view of African art as European collectors would like to see it ... The curator of the Federated Union of Black Artists Gallery, David Koloane, has complained that the art market has prevented artists from experimenting: 'The more naïve the artist, the more they want him to remain that way.' Cut off from their buyers by language and the Group Areas legislation, black artists have had scant chance of assessing if their work is communicating.

Gavin Younge, artist (*Art of the South African Townships*, Rizzoli, 1988)

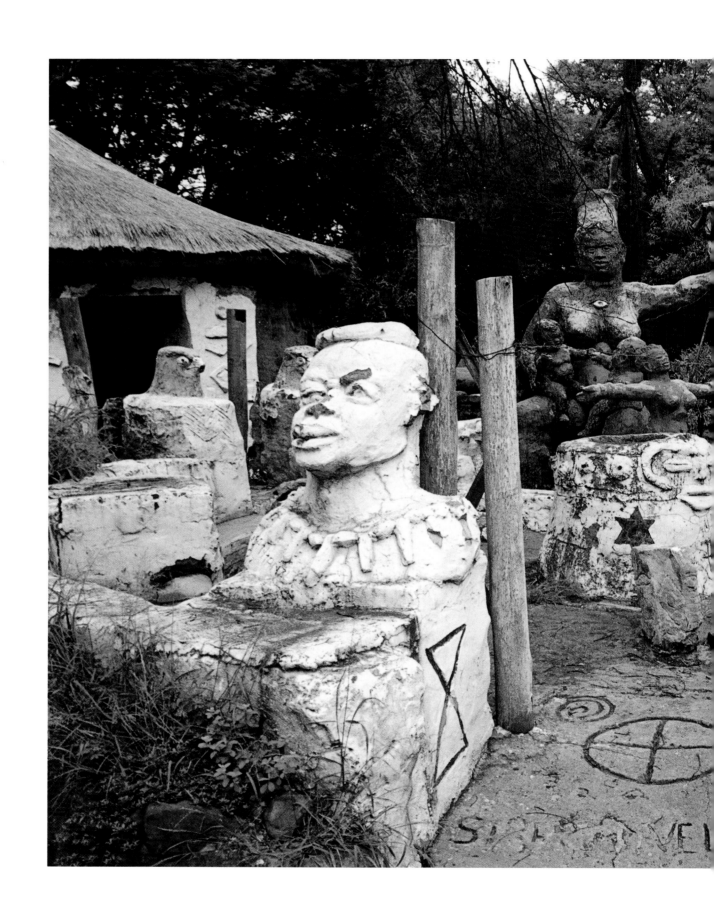

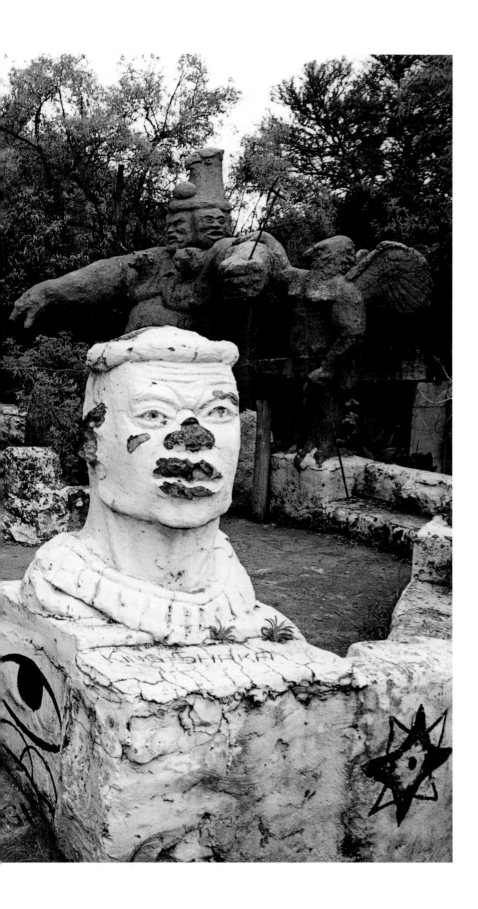

'These are the stories that old men and old women tell to boys and girls seated with open mouths around the spark-wreathed fire in the centre of the villages in the dark forests and on the aloe-scented plains of Africa.' So begins *Indaba my Children*, the seminal book on African history, legends, customs and religious beliefs, written in 1966 by South Africa's sage mystic and *sangoma* Vusamazulu Credo Mutwa. A few years later the Johannesburg City Council gave Mutwa funds to build a village filled with the figures of African mythology. Mutwa, with the help of other *sangomas*, spent years constructing this village in Oppenheimer Park. Student activists partially destroyed it during the 1976 student uprising, which began a stone's throw away. Today, despite its dilapidated air, this national cultural treasure is still a place of magic and mystery.

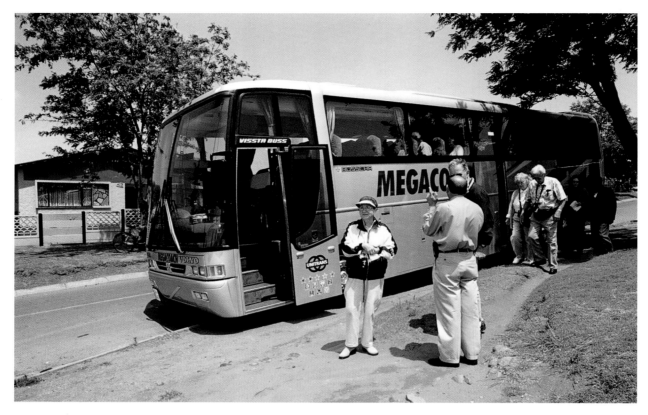

More than 1,000 tourists visit Soweto each day in luxury, airconditioned coaches that take them in comfort from one venue to the next. Here tourists take a breather in Orlando West, one of Soweto's oldest suburbs and at times home to Nelson Mandela, Winnie Madikizela-Mandela, Archbishop Desmond Tutu, and Walter and Adelaide Sisulu.

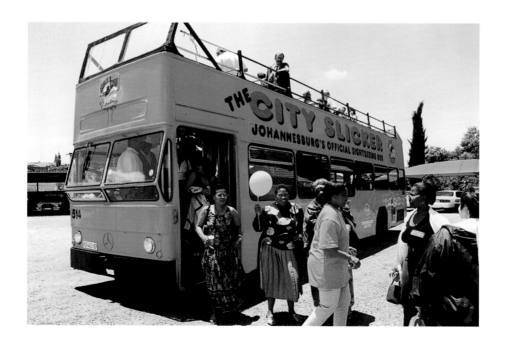

The 'topless' bus runs daily shuttles between central Johannesburg and Soweto. The region's fine, dry and mild weather allows passengers a comfortable ride with excellent views.

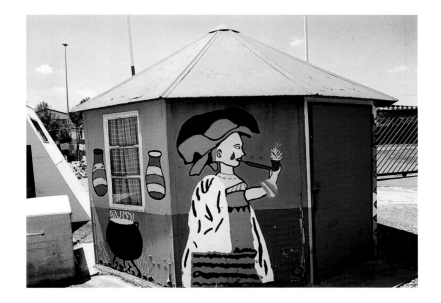

A painting of a Pondo woman smoking a traditional clay pipe does little to disguise the temporary nature of this prefabricated building at Ubuntu Kraal.

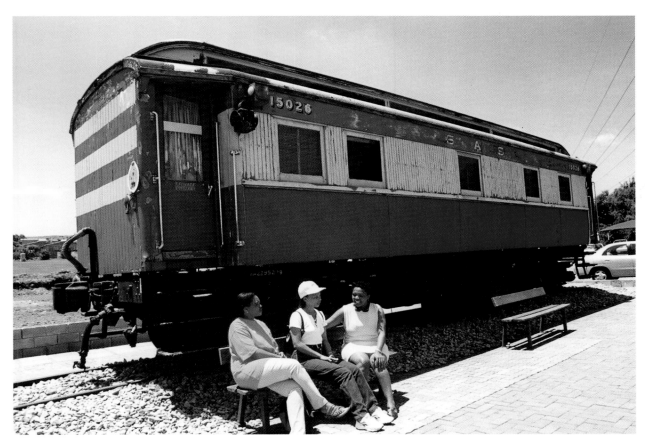

Ubuntu Kraal is a primary attraction for tourists to Soweto and is a favoured recreational spot for Soweto residents. Many wedding receptions are held here, and its old mainline railway coaches are going to be converted into honeymoon suites for bridal couples.

Jimmy Ntintili of Soweto's best known and oldest travel agency, Jimmy's Face to Face Tours, began his business in 1985 after showing friends and visitors around for years before. He developed a fascination for Soweto at the knee of his grandmother, with whom he lived in Orlando East. 'My grandmother used to work at the Donaldson Community Hall [now the YMCA] in Orlando East. From the age of six I would go with her to listen to stars like Miriam Makeba. Ah, those were wonderful years.' He says tour operators now crowd Soweto, but when he began he was the only one. 'Most people come expecting to see poverty – they want to see poverty – and they get the shock of their lives when they see it is a place like any other. Most people like to feel they can help. When Mandela came out [of prison] everyone wanted to see his house. Winnie's house is not so important. Although lots of people lay flowers on the grave of Hector Petersen, few know anything about him.' Jimmy Ntintili gives intensely personal tours, speaking rapidly in a slightly mid-Atlantic accent. 'Reading about a beautiful country doesn't tell you anything about it. I say, when you come with us, I don't care about what you've read, we want you to live the experience. You can read anywhere ... you are getting to see it face to face.' He explains the origin of the name 'Face to Face': 'South Africans never used to look at each other as people, and this is why we were in such a mess. Only when we know each other can we understand and respect each other. Take for example the African male tradition of going through doorways first ... many Western women are offended. But we do this because in the old days an African man would go ahead in case there was danger. He would have to fight, to protect the woman. In Western society, men open doors for women, but we as Africans see that as exposing women to possible danger ahead. If we don't have respect for each other then we have nothing.'

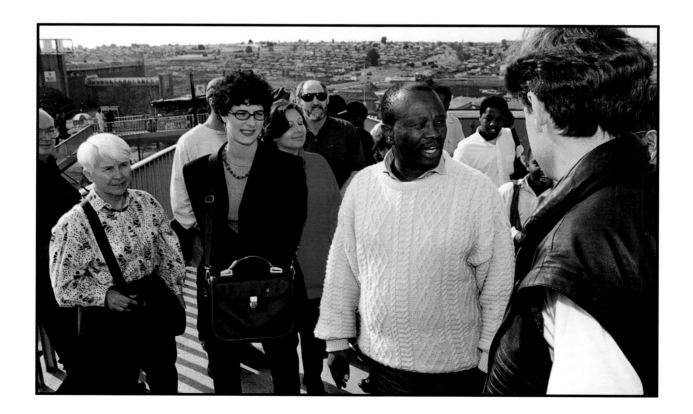

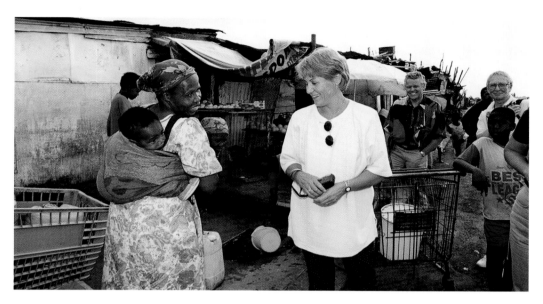

A mother about to purchase vegetables, with her day's supply of water in a big plastic container in a supermarket trolley, stops to exchange pleasantries with a visitor.

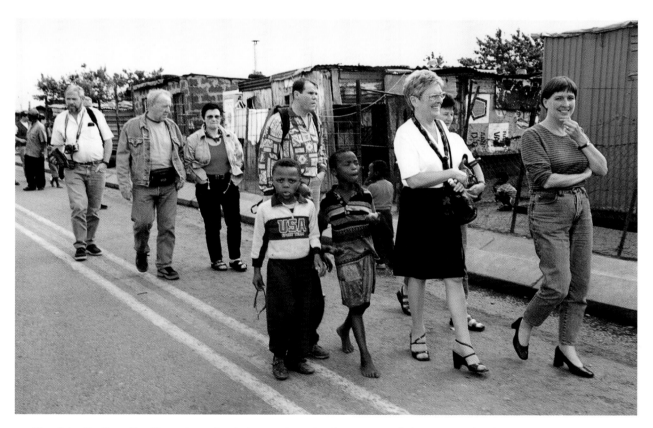

Mandelaville Squatter Camp is a shanty town where tourists can stroll the streets chatting to locals. They often find themselves followed by crowds of curious children listening to the different languages being spoken.

The two faces of Soweto

A child in a tattered shirt stands next to his better
dressed friend, while well-to-do tourists
chat with Soweto residents.

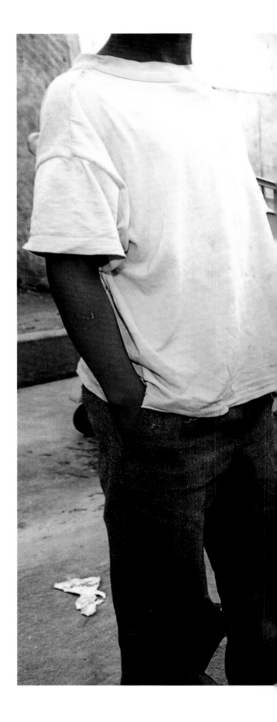

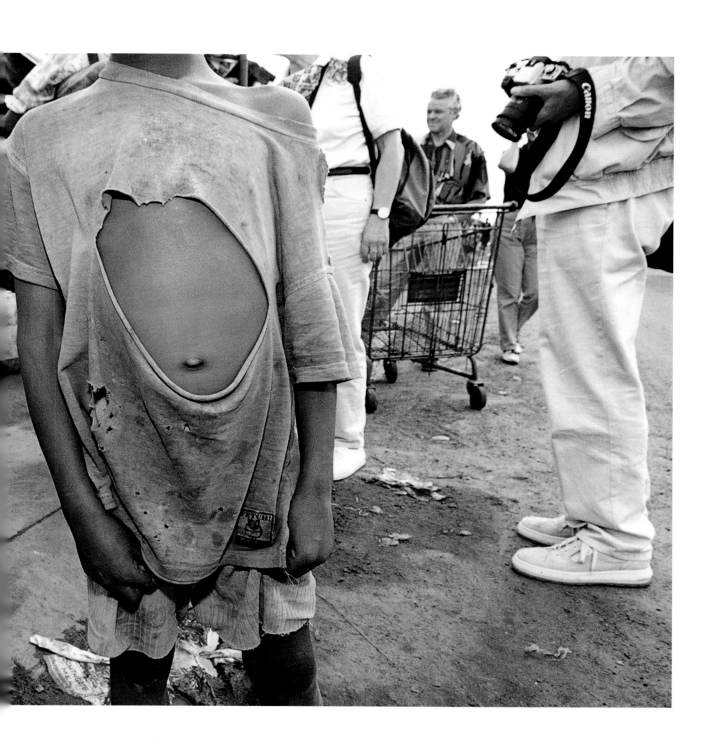

SOWETO
PETER MAGUBANE

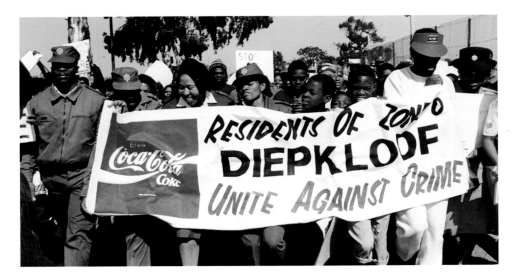

South Africa has the world's highest incidence of reported violent crime, with 65 murders per day, one rape every 26 seconds, and a high rate of violent hijackings. Residents of Diepkloof demonstrate their anger at the ongoing crime in their area. In many areas, community policing forums, in which residents and police unite to fight crime, have proved effective in lowering the criminal activity.

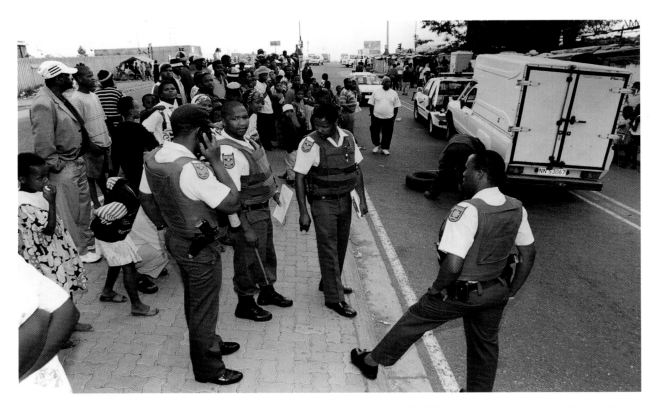

These officers have just apprehended the driver of a stolen vehicle; some 90,000 are stolen each year in South Africa.

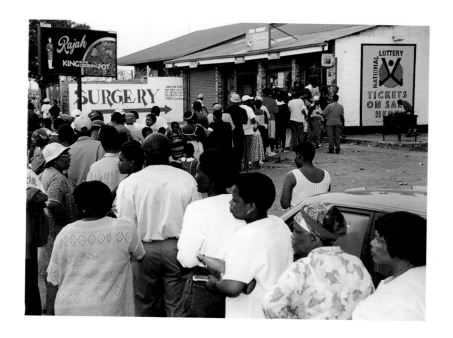

The national lottery, the Lotto, was introduced to South Africa in 2000. It has proved so popular that, according to commentators, some people are neglecting to pay their hire purchase instalments, instead using the money to buy lottery tickets.

At the end of each month, post offices, welfare bureaux and hospitals see old people patiently sitting on benches, leaning on their canes, or standing in line, as they wait to collect their pension payouts.

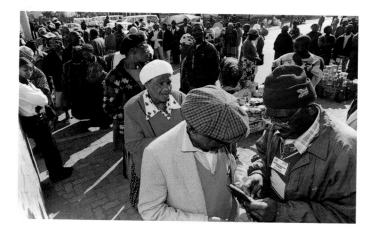

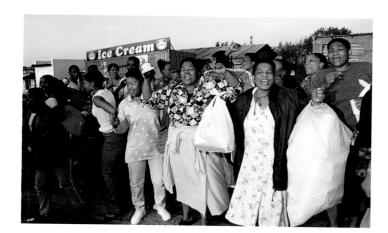

Choral singing is a passion among the people of Soweto. Competitions between choirs from Soweto and other parts of southern Africa attract huge crowds of spectators. They are also broadcast to a wide audience on both television and radio. These jubilant Soweto choristers are returning from one of these competitions.

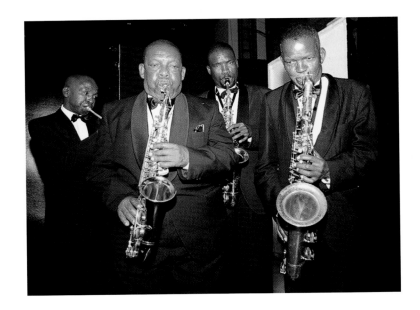

Some of the best saxophone cheeks in South Africa come from Soweto. This is also the home of township jazz, *kwaito*, *mbaqanga*, soul, and the penny whistle.

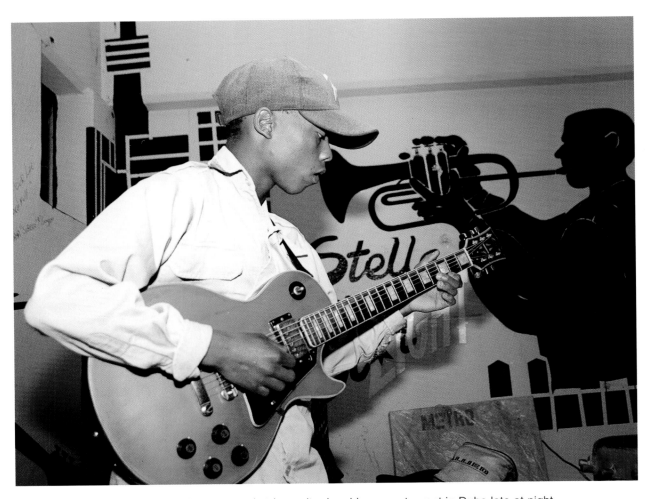

A young man picks on a steel-string guitar in a bluesy restaurant in Dube late at night.

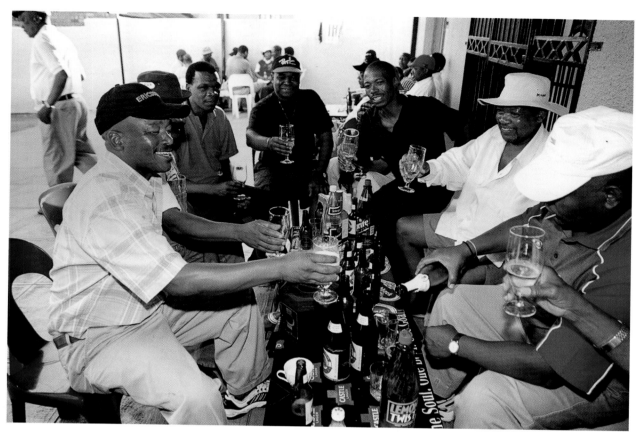

It's Saturday afternoon ... Soccer will be on the box soon, and the men get together
to shoot the breeze at Mathabo's Shebeen in Orlando West.

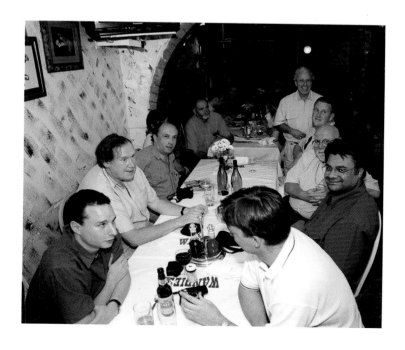

By the early 1990s, Soweto had
become one of South Africa's top
tourist attractions. At the end of
a long dusty tour most visitors would
retire to up-market shebeens like
Wandie's Place in Dube, which
is still popular today.

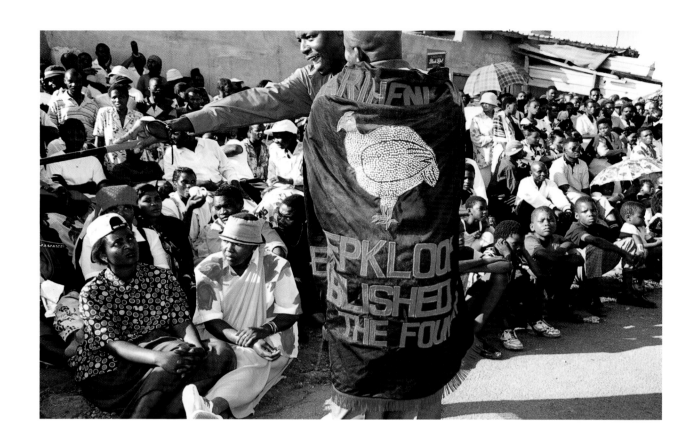

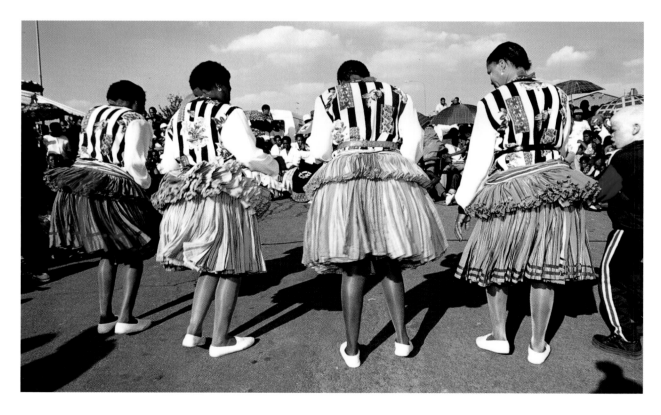

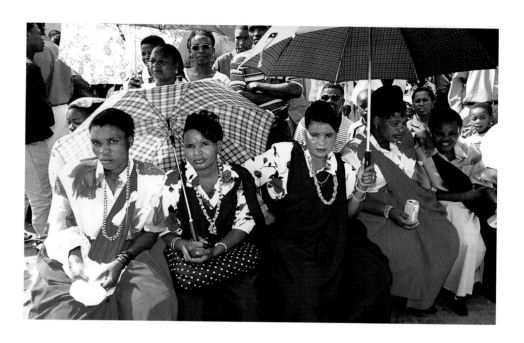

Under the apartheid government, people in Soweto had to live in areas according to their ethnicity. This promoted separateness, as was the intention, but it also had the effect of encouraging the preservation of traditional values and practices. These pages depict a Tsonga dance contest, during which xylophones or a tambourine-like drum may be played; the latter, which is struck with a stick and played by men, is most often used in rituals to exorcise spirits. A flute is also played to drive away thunderstorms. It is made of a hollow bone covered with leguaan skin and stopped at one end with a black substance, said to be the flesh of the lightning bird (*ndlati*), and three seeds of the lucky bean. Onlookers accompany the dancing with chanting and clapping. Children are initiated and welcomed into dancing groups from a very early age, so that they may learn tradition and in turn teach their children the ways of an ancient and noble people. In traditional African culture, a woman with broad child-rearing hips is admired, and skirts often accentuate that feature. Although now made of fabric, in they past they would have been made of grasses or leaves, or even thin pleated animal hide. Some of the participants also wear elaborately embroidered cloaks.

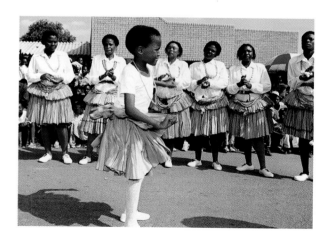

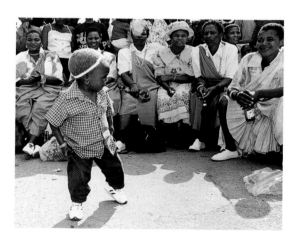

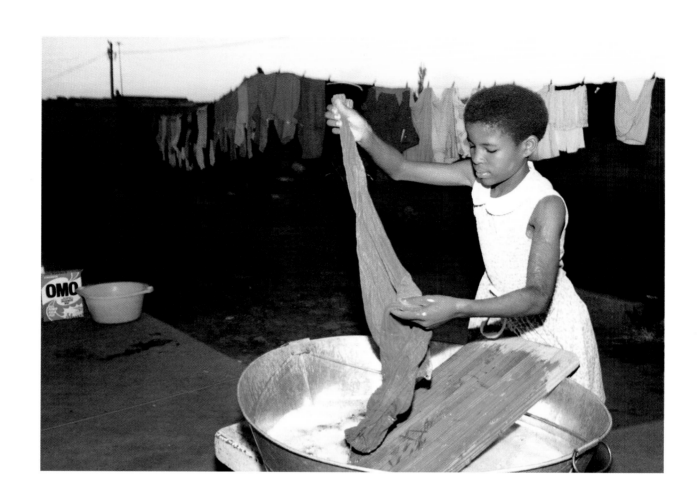

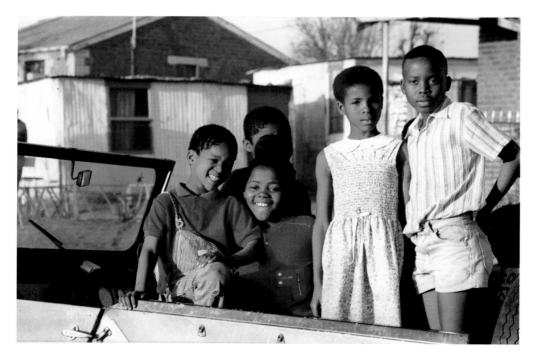

S O W E T O
PETER MAGUBANE

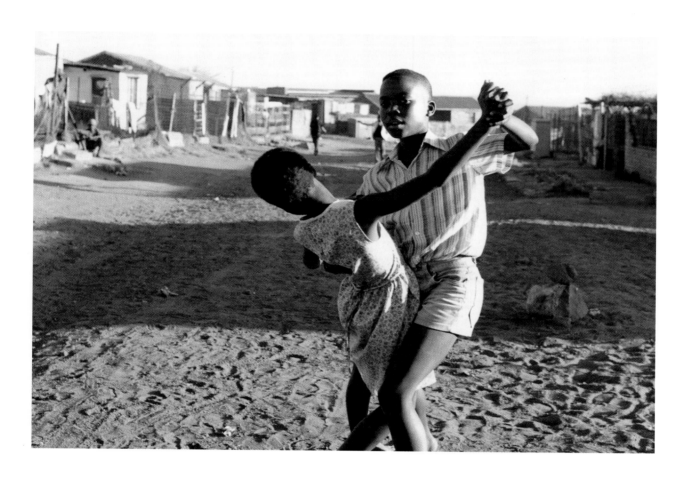

A picture that made dreams come true (*above*). In 1994 Peter Magubane took this photograph of talented Gugulethu Nkosi and Molaodi Machitse (who were both 13 at the time) practising ballroom dancing in the streets of Orlando East. He sent it, with an article, to the *Los Angeles Times* and as a result they were invited to the United States of America to dance in events across that nation. 'It was,' Gugulethu breathes, 'just beautiful. It was the best thing that has ever happened.' The two children have dreams of one day being world champion ballroom dancers. But even ballroom dancers find time to help out with chores around the house and to play with their friends (*opposite*).

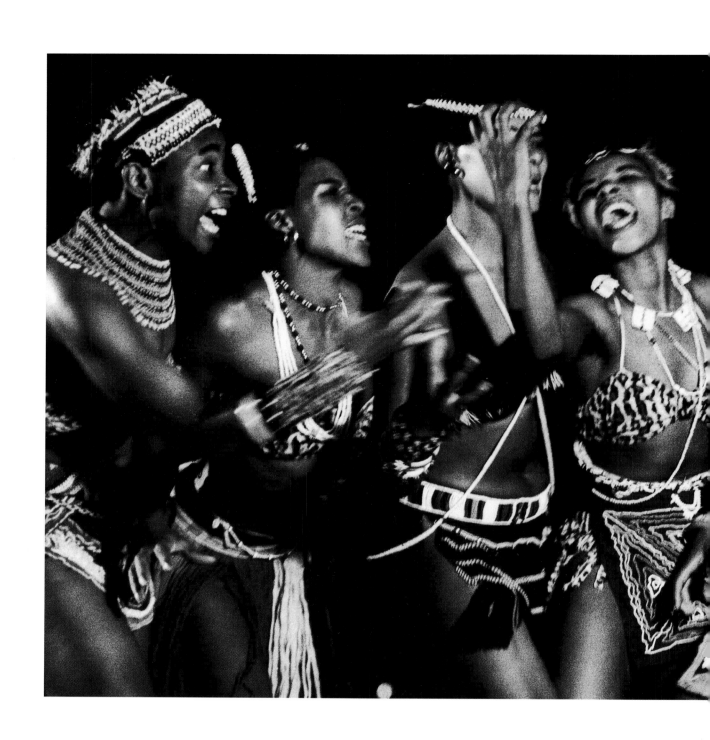

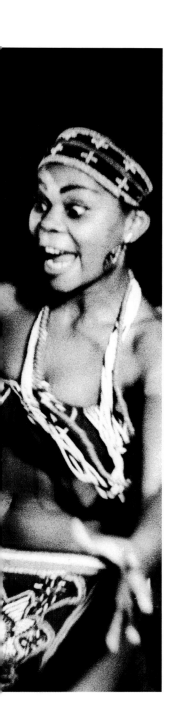

The song 'Meadowlands', named after a Soweto
suburb, is redolent of the 1950s when Miriam
Makeba, Dollar Brand (now known as Abdullah
Ibrahim), Todd Matshikiza and Hugh Masekela
were taking the sounds of South Africa to foreign
markets. Here the Mzumba group rehearse the
song during the 1970s.

Music is one of the defining features of Africa. While South Africa's white musicians have tended to imitate American and British performers, with little success, South Africa's black musicians continue to develop some of the most original sounds in the world. Among the many well-known musicians who were born in Soweto, or who lived there for a time, are jazz supremo Hugh Masekela, Ray Phiri, leader of the band Stimela that provided instrumental backup for Paul Simon's *Graceland*, and Sipho 'Hotstix' Mabuse.

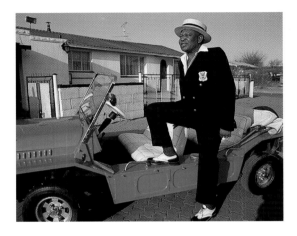

No one told better stories about Soweto of the 1950s to the late 1990s (when he died) than husky-voiced Godfrey Moloi, a sometime smuggler, shebeen king and occasional gangster. One of the most colourful people in a rainbow city, Moloi entertains the crowds at his Flamingo nightclub in Mapetla, Soweto (*below*). Moloi, ever the dandy when he had a chance, poses next to a township runaround, dressed to the nines (*right*).

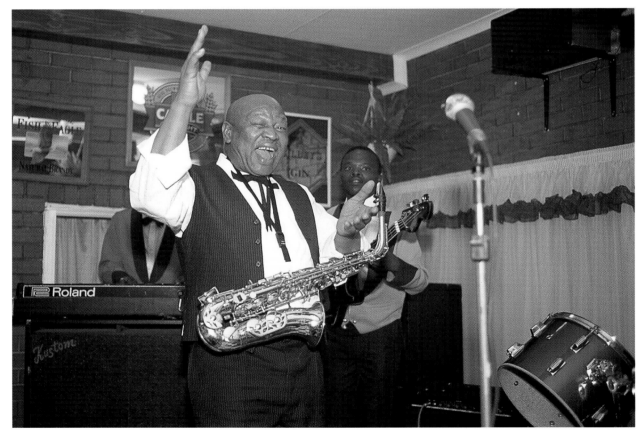

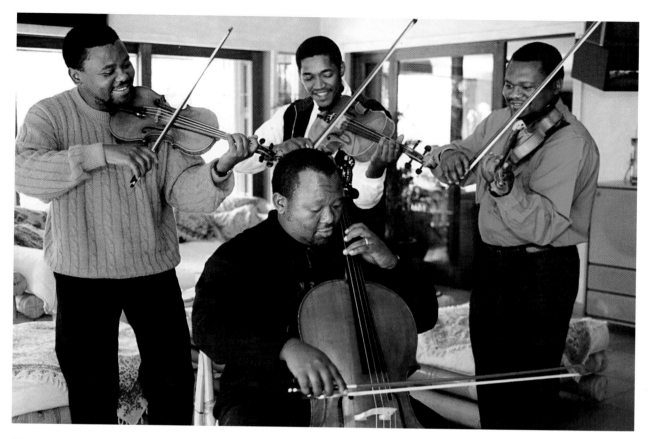

The Soweto String Quartet – brothers Reuben (cello, *front*), Sandile (violin, *left*) and Thami (violin, *right*) Khemese and their friend Makhosini Mnguni (viola, *centre*) – had humble origins. Initially they played in shopping malls and at garden parties before their vibrant sound captured the interest of record producers. Today the quartet has played in most of the world's major centres, has produced a number of compact discs and won numerous awards.

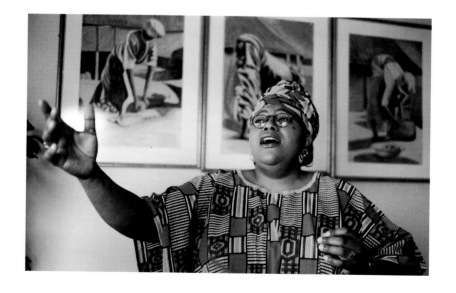

Sibongile Khumalo, Soweto's opera diva , is one of the most beloved songstresses in South Africa. She has sung for Nelson Mandela, and queens and foreign rulers around the world, bringing the rich tones of Africa to resonate in opera halls and concert venues across the globe.

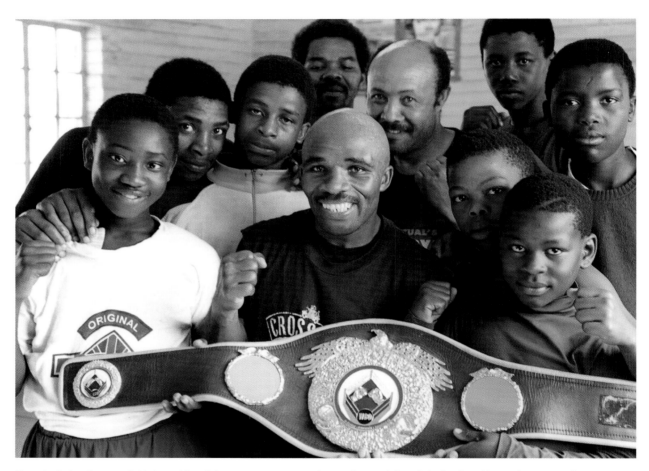

Soweto is boxing mad. Nelson Mandela was an amateur boxer for a while when he lived here. In gymnasiums around Soweto young boys dream of one day fighting in an international ring, watched by a world television audience. Baby Jake Matlala, now at the end of his professional boxing career, has achieved that goal.

In addition to a strong following of fans, he endorses consumer goods ranging from clothes to softdrinks.

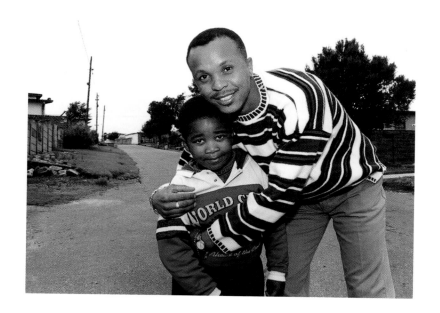

Doc Khumalo, a child of Soweto, is one of South Africa's star soccer players. A role model for thousands of young people, he dedicates a considerable amount of his free time to charity work.

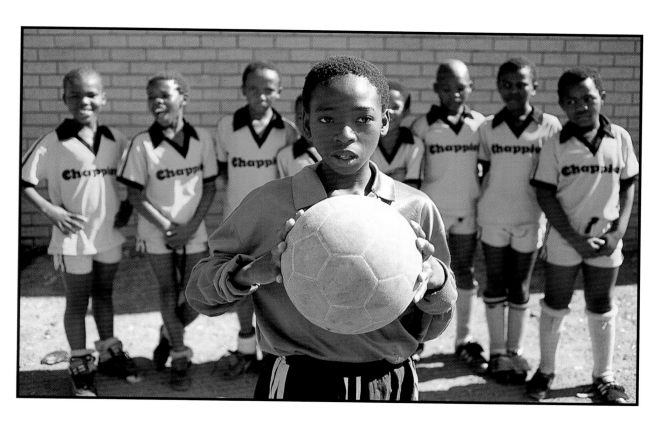

*Every Soweto boy's dream
is to be a Pele, Jomo Sono, Doc Khumalo
– a great soccer player.*

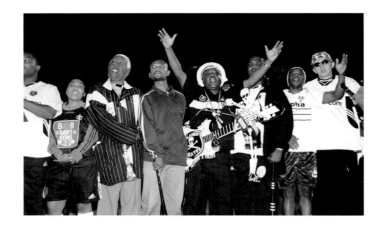

Extravagant clothes and antics are the trade mark of South African soccer fans. Supporters at the Orlando Pirates–Ajax Cape Town match of the Rothmans Cup get up to high jinks at the FNB Stadium (*left* and *below*).

Soccer is not just a sport in Soweto. It is an unbridled passion. Before a match, cars, buses and taxis full of fans sweep through the streets of Johannesburg and Soweto, with flags, balloons and scarves in team colours being waved from windows. Faces are painted, and some fans spend weeks making ornate helmets, hats and outfits to wear to matches. During the games, fans sing and dance in the stands, wave banners, and blow whistles, horns and sirens when their team scores a goal. If Bafana Bafana, the national team, wins against a foreign team, then the whole township celebrates. Soccer fanaticism is so intense some homes are painted in the colours of different teams: maroon and white for Moroka Swallows, black and yellow for Kaiser Chiefs, and black and white for Orlando Pirates.

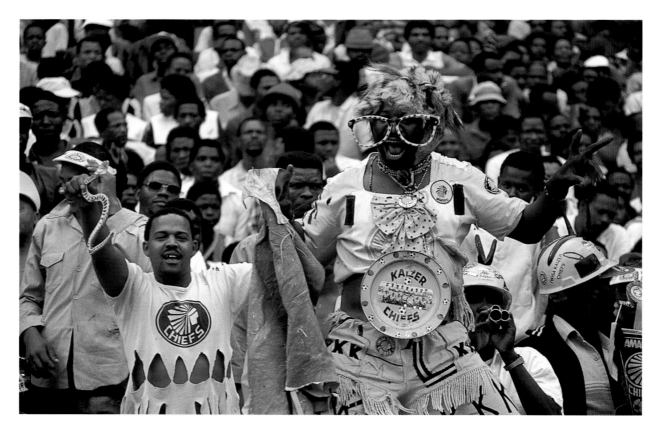

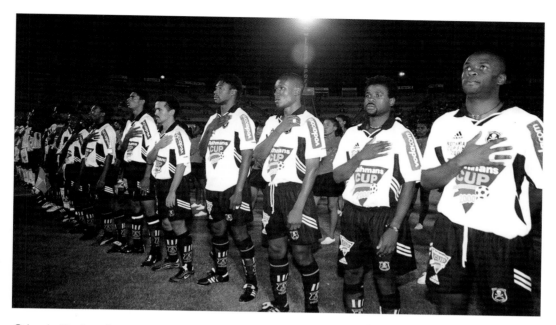

Orlando Pirates players sing the national anthem at the start of the Pirates–Ajax game

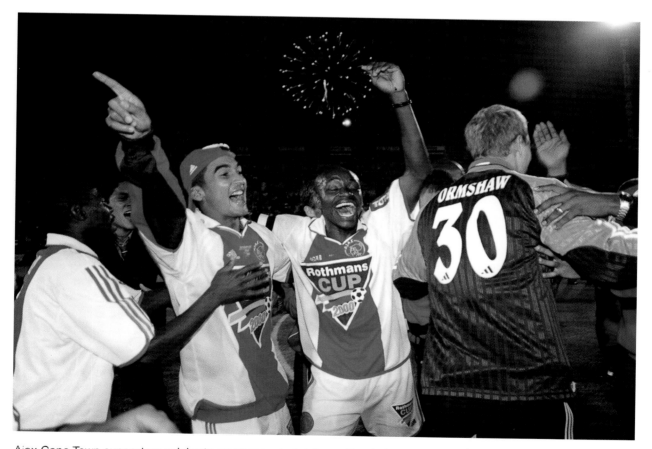

Ajax Cape Town supporters celebrate an unexpected victory, after their team beat Pirates 4–1.

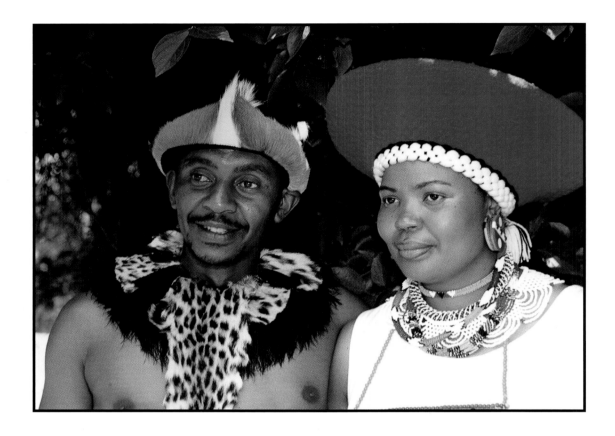

While it was fashionable in the past to wear whatever was on the catwalks at Paris or Milan to Soweto weddings, many couples increasingly prefer to add a traditional sense to their nuptials. Bride Thulile Tholo and groom Mphindiselwa Nkomonde (*above*) are attired in traditional Zulu garb at their wedding celebration held at Ubuntu Kraal. The groom wears the leopard and cheetah skin regalia of a high-ranking Zulu warrior, while the bride wears increasingly rare Zulu beadwork and the red cone hat of women of the Tugela Ferry area. Her hat is made of wool rather than the traditional red clay of days gone by. The Tholo women, Mumsie and Nomsa (*opposite top*, *left* and *right* of picture), have headdresses and facial markings of the Xhosa. Completing this picture of African fusion couture are the female relatives of the groom (*opposite bottom*), dressed in contemporary West African-inspired garb (*extreme left*), a traditional Swazi sarong (*second from left*), a Pedi-inspired outfit (*second from right*), and a more contemporary African-inspired frock and headdress (*extreme right*).

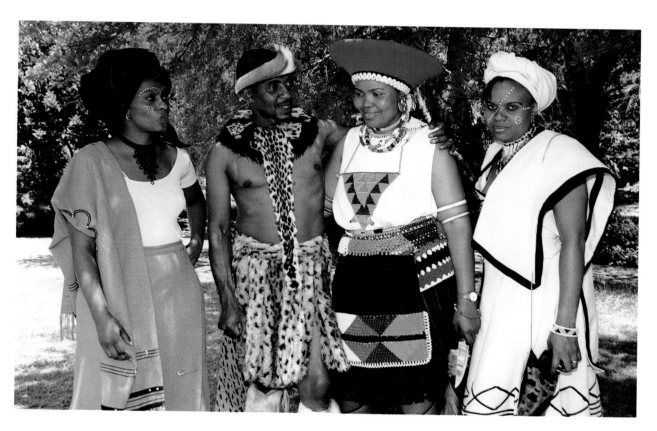

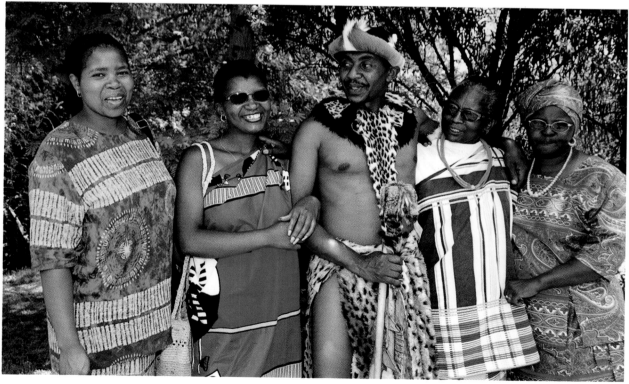

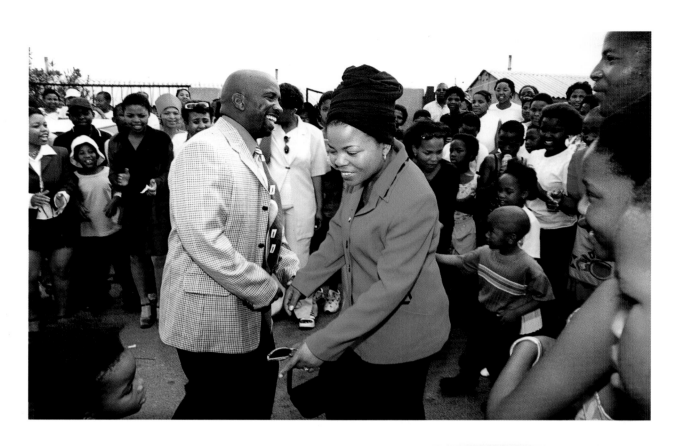

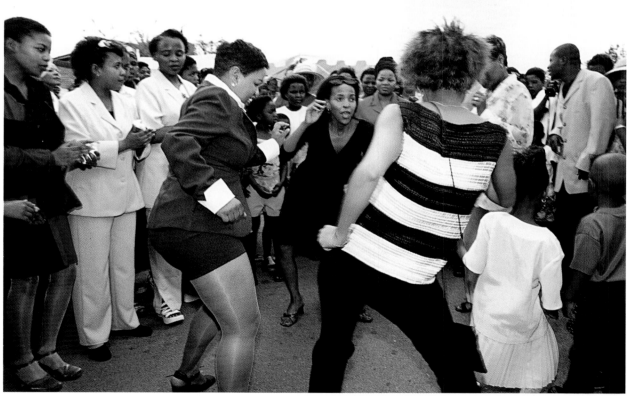

SOWETO
PETER MAGUBANE

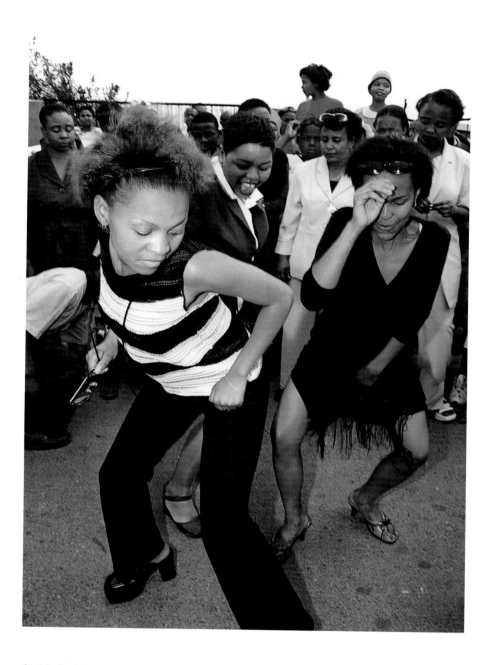

At this fashionable wedding in Diepkloof, Soweto, music gets the guests (*above* and *opposite bottom*) and the bride and groom (*opposite top*) doing the spirited dance that keeps the township moving over the weekends. The 'Soweto jive' is almost as famous as the 'Madiba jive' – the rather stiff dance that former president Mandela is prone to execute when music moves him.

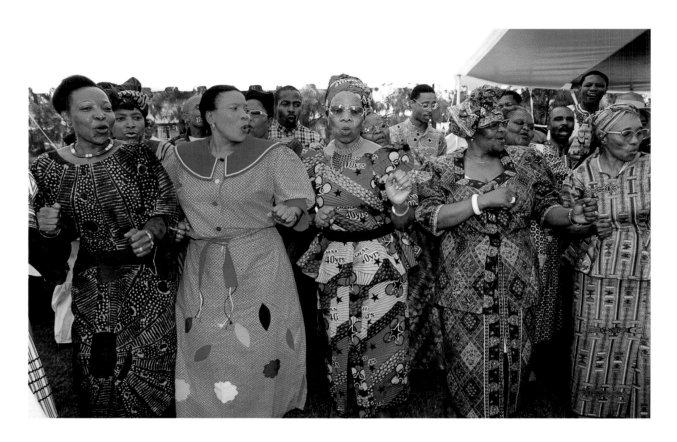

Andrew Mlangeni (*below, third from left*), who was incarcerated on Robben Island in 1963 along with Nelson Mandela and the other Rivonia trialists, was released with Walter Sisulu in 1989. He and his wife June celebrated their 50th wedding anniversary at Ubuntu Kraal in Soweto. Among the guests were Walter Sisulu (*below, second from left*) and Education Minister Kadar Asmal (*below, second from right*). The Soweto Teachers' Choir (*above*) and a trumpeter (*opposite, bottom*) provided some of the entertainment.

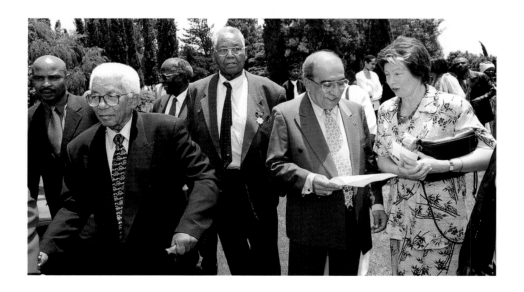

Wearing traditional Pondo dress and surrounded by her 'adoptive' family, the Boqo family of Soweto, is exchange student Maria Walter from Berlin, Germany (*below, second from right*), who attended St Matthew's High School in Soweto for a year. The name bestowed on her by the Boqo family is Nomsa, an Nguni name that means 'kindness is found'.

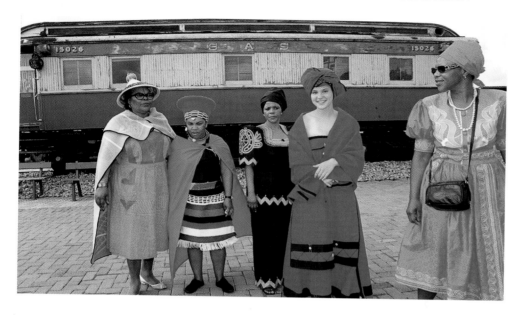

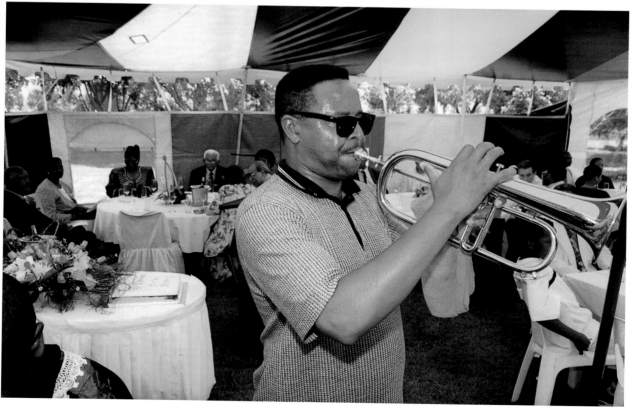

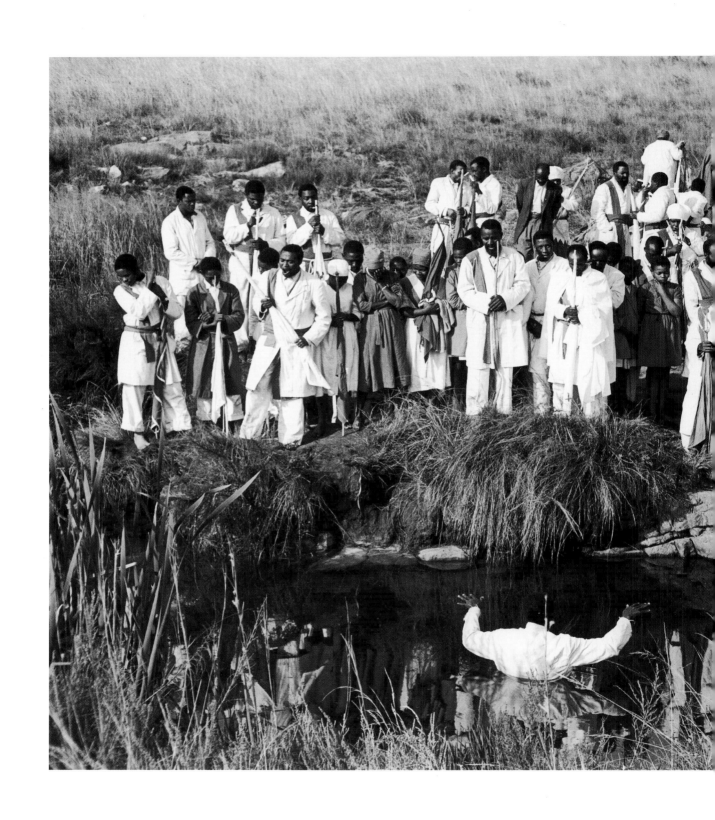

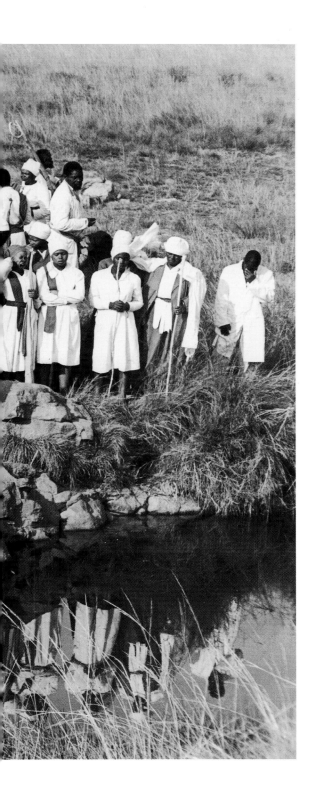

There was an easy path from traditional beliefs to Christianity in many cultures. Among some ethnic groups (for example the Xhosa and Venda) it was believed there was a powerful god in the rivers who, if offerings were made to it, could ensure good crops and peace. Baptism (*left* and page 152) is a short step from such beliefs in terms of symbolism.

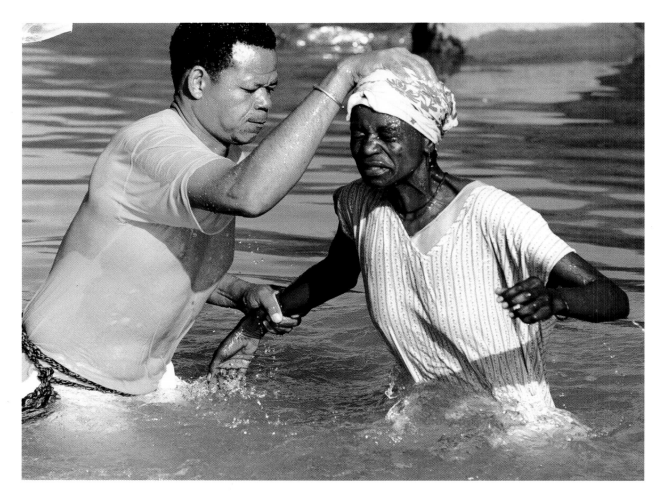

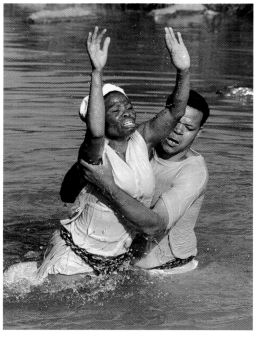

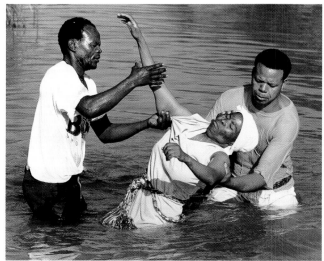

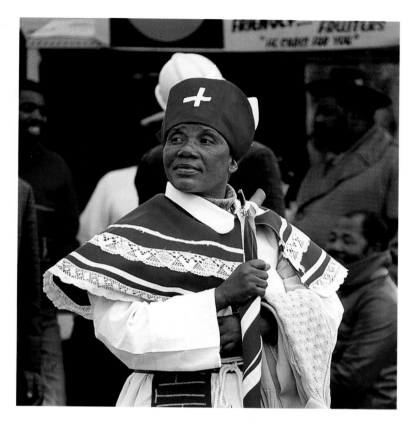

During the apartheid era black people frequently held religious services under trees and around sacred rocks. Elaborate uniforms, in a sense, became the church structure – you could tell the church that a person belonged to from the colours and designs of a stiffly starched, neatly pressed uniform (*left* and *below*).

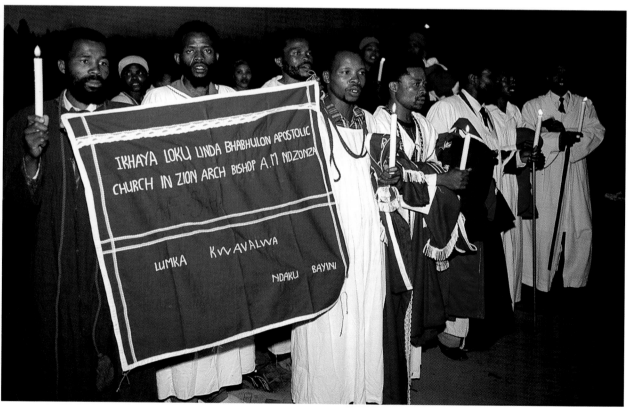

The ritual slaughter of animals at weddings, baptisms and funerals, and to commemorate other important events is an important aspect of African tradition. The animal is, however, not always willing to co-operate.

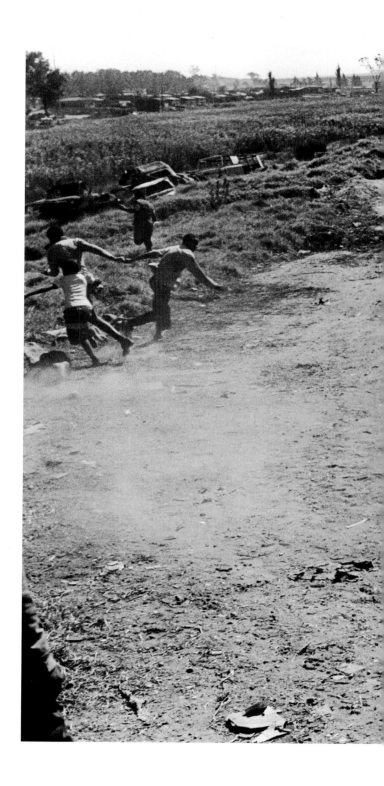

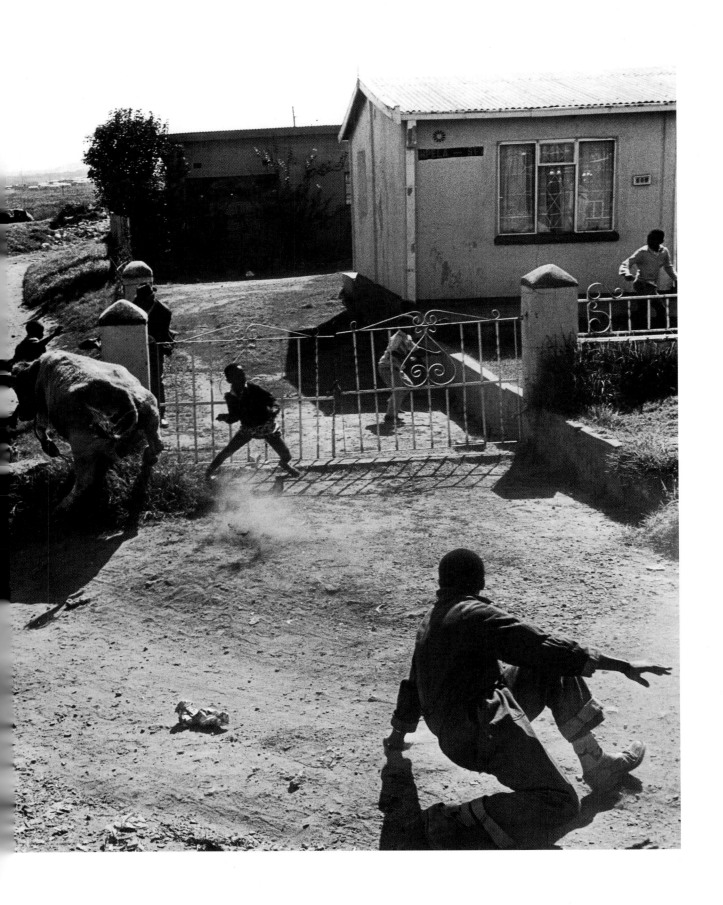

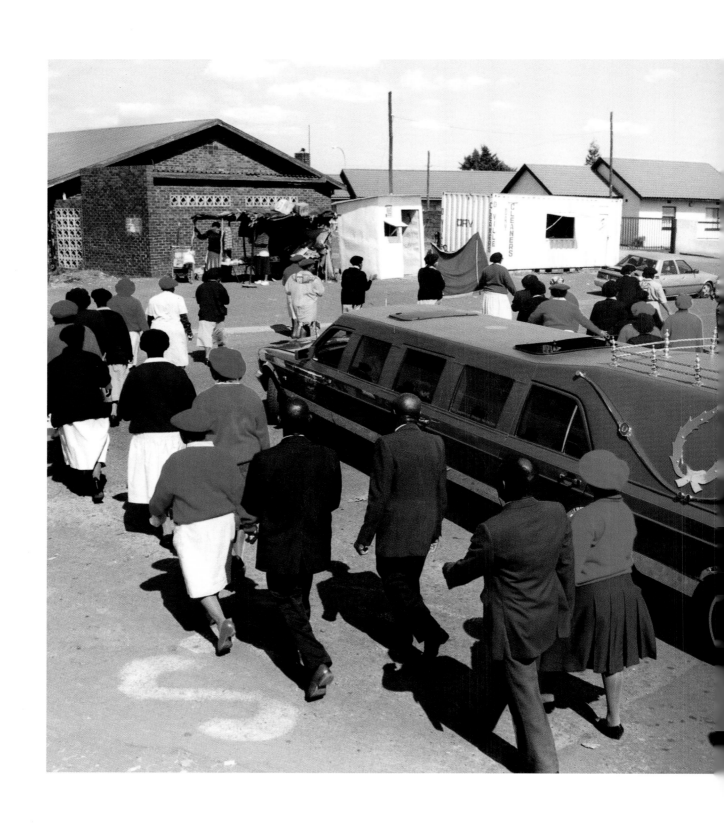

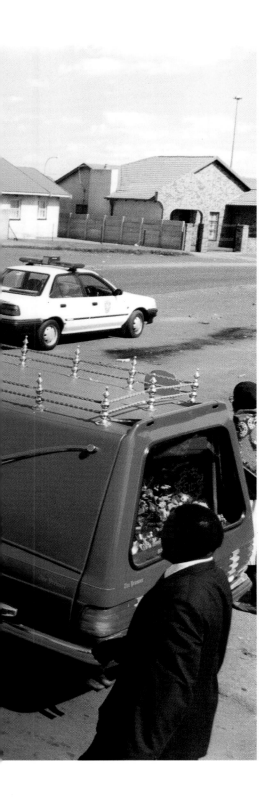

Because of poverty and the high cost of funerals (*left*), people have for decades banded together in burial societies. Each person contributes a monthly tithe, and meetings are held. These societies are an important way of binding communities: when a person dies, the entire burial society attends the funeral, helps with preparations (*below*) and relieves the family of the financial burden. A fine funeral is considered an important signal of a person's status in the community and his or her wealth. In recent times some burial societies were so wealthy that they became major investors in companies such as funeral parlours and coffin manufacturers.

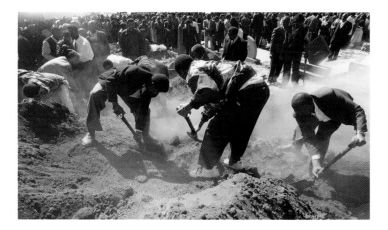

The ascent of the spirit into the world of the ancestors is a time when great respect is shown to the deceased and his or her family. After a death, women sit wrapped in blankets, with a lit candle at their feet, mourning the death. In traditional practice, which a few people still observe in Soweto, the period of mourning lasts a year, during which time people do not sing or call out loudly, nor do they make repairs to their home.

BIBLIOGRAPHY

Bonner, Philip and Segal, Lauren. *Soweto: A History*. Maskew Miller Longman, 1998.

Hammond-Tooke, David. *The Roots of Black South Africa*. Jonathan Ball, Johannesburg, 1993.

Lukhele, Andrew Khehla. *Stokvels in South Africa*. Amagi Books, 1990.

Millard, Arnold (editor). *Steve Biko: Black Consciousness in South Africa*. Vintage Books, 1979.

Mutwa, Vusamazulu Credo. *Indaba, my Children: African tribal history, legends, customs and religious beliefs*.
    Kahn & Averill, London, 1966.

Nakasa, Nathaniel (editor), with submissions from Can Themba, Richard Rive, Ezekiel Mphahlele, Casey Motsisi
    and others. *The Classic, Johannesburg Quarterly*, Volume One, Number 1, 1963.

Smith, Charlene. *Robben Island*. Struik Publishers, 1997.

Tyrrel, Barbara and Jurgens, Pete. *African Heritage*. Macmillan South Africa, 1983.

Younge, Gavin. *Art of the South African Townships*. Rizzoli, 1988.

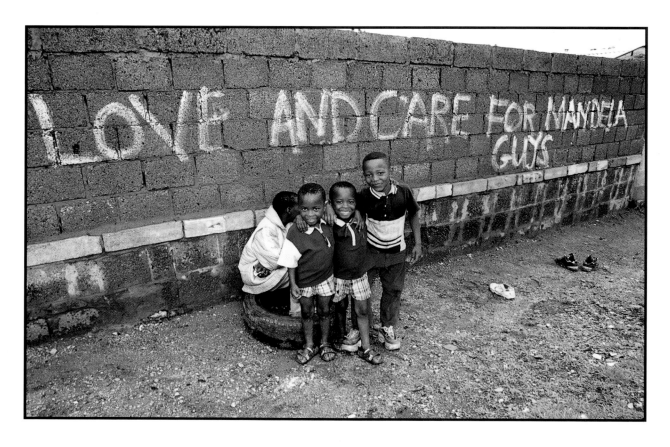

'Love and care for Mandela guys'
... and the children of Soweto so beloved by him.

INDEX